Ocular Trauma

A Comprehensive Text

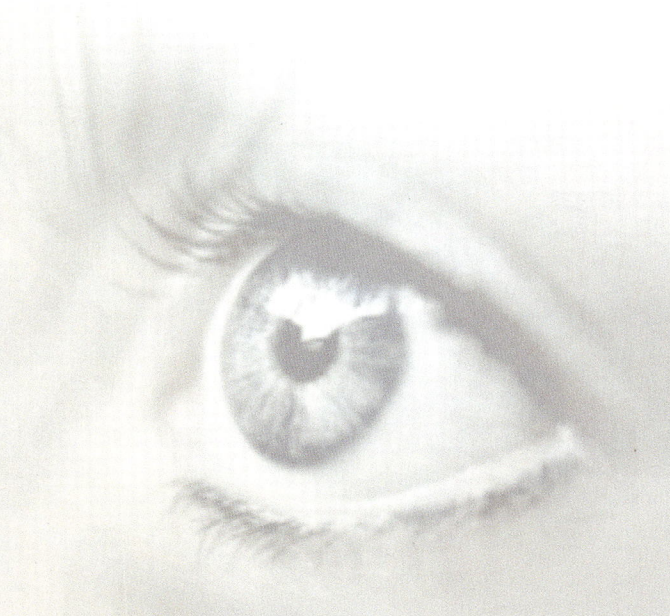

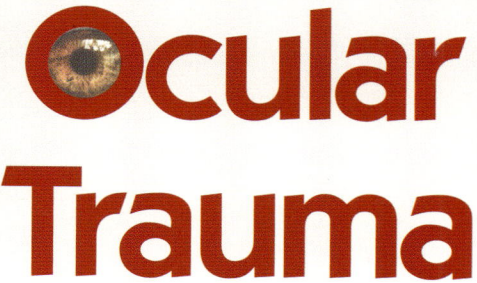

Ocular Trauma

A Comprehensive Text

DK Mehta MS, MNAMS, FIMSA
Professor and Head
Department of Ophthalmology
School of Medical Sciences and Research, Sharda Hospital
Greater Noida, Uttar Pradesh, India

Formerly
Director and Professor
Maulana Azad Medical College and
Guru Nanak Eye Center, Delhi, India

Ex-President Ocular Trauma Society of India

Foreword

MS Boparai

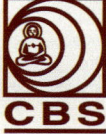

CBS

CBS Publishers & Distributors Pvt Ltd

New Delhi • Bengaluru • Chennai • Kochi • Mumbai • Pune
Hyderabad • Kolkata • Nagpur • Patna • Vijayawada

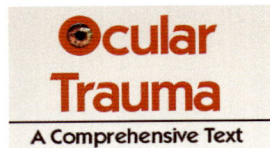

ISBN: 978-81-239-2478-6

Published by Satish Kumar Jain and produced by Varun Jain for

CBS Publishers & Distributors Pvt Ltd

4819/XI Prahlad Street, 24 Ansari Road, Daryaganj, New Delhi 110 002, India.
Ph: 23289259, 23266861, 23266867   Fax: 011-23243014   Website: www.cbspd.com
e-mail: delhi@cbspd.com; cbspubs@airtelmail.in.

Corporate Office: 204 FIE, Industrial Area, Patparganj, Delhi 110 092
Ph: 4934 4934   Fax: 4934 4935   e-mail: publishing@cbspd.com; publicity@cbspd.com

Branches

- **Bengaluru:** Seema House 2975, 17th Cross, K.R. Road,
  Banasankari 2nd Stage, Bengaluru 560 070, Karnataka
  Ph: +91-80-26771678/79   Fax: +91-80-26771680   e-mail: bangalore@cbspd.com
- **Chennai:** No. 7, Subbaraya Street, Shenoy Nagar, Chennai 600 030, Tamil Nadu
  Ph: +91-44-42032115, M: 09500090969   Fax: +91-44-42032115   e-mail: chennai@cbspd.com
- **Kochi:** 36/14 Kalluvilakam, Lissie Hospital Road, Kochi 682 018, Kerala
  Ph: +91-484-4059061-65   Fax: +91-484-4059065   e-mail: kochi@cbspd.com
- **Mumbai:** 83-C, Dr E Moses Road, Worli, Mumbai-400018, Maharashtra
  Ph: +91-22-24902340/41   Fax: +91-22-24902342   e-mail: mumbai@cbspd.com
- **Pune:** Bhuruk Prestige, Sr. No. 52/12/2+1+3/2 Narhe, Haveli
  (Near Katraj-Dehu Road Bypass), Pune 411 041, Maharashtra
  Ph: +91-20-64704058, 64704059, 32392277 Fax: +91-20-24300160   e-mail: pune@cbspd.com

Representatives

- **Hyderabad**   0-9885175004
- **Nagpur**   0-9021734563
- **Kolkata**   0-9831437309, 0-9051152362
- **Patna**   0-9334159340
- **Vijayawada**   0-9000660880

Printed at R. P. Printers, G-68, Sector-6, Noida 201 301(U.P.)

to

Ocular Trauma Society of India (OTSI)
in persuit of
better awareness, prevention, protection and
near zero morbidity management
of ocular injuries

Foreword

Trauma is as old as the human civilization and ocular trauma is no exception. Over the years, the management of ocular trauma has not been satisfactory, as life and limb saving measures took priority over ocular trauma which was considered minor. However, as time progressed, knowledge of ophthalmology improved and so did the understanding of ocular trauma. Development of specialties in ophthalmology gave further impetus to the understanding and management of ocular trauma. This book is yet another step in this direction.

One of the reasons for poor management of ocular trauma has been the non-availability of a standard and uniform system of classifying ocular injuries. This has been amply emphasized in the book. With Kuhn's classification having more or less been uniformly accepted, ocular trauma will be better understood, managed and researched. Incidence of ocular injuries will also be better and more correctly projected. Presently available statistics do not point to correct figures and appear biased. There is, however, still scope for further improving the classification.

The chapters on Epidemiology of Ocular Trauma and Classifications of Ocular Trauma bring a systematic approach towards the problems of ocular injury, its registration and worldwide pattern for better prophylaxis understanding. Separate chapters on Chemical Injuries, War and in Insurgency, Injury by Physical Agents have been dealt in details to cover the less covered hazards. Like lasers and laser based equipment of the modern era.

New modalities of investigations such as ultrasonography (USG), computer tomography (CT), magnetic resonance imaging (MRI) and so on have contributed immensely to the understanding and management of ocular trauma. A sound clinical judgement has to be exercised in selecting the modalities judiciously in appropriate cases. USG has a great potential but has limitations in penetrating injuries. It is important that while ordering investigations, the possibility of causing iatrogenic damage or enhancement of existing damage be kept in mind.

Revolution in industry and agriculture has brought about improvements in the well-being and raised the socioeconomic standards of countries and societies. This has resulted in further adding to the rising levels of ocular trauma. The incidence of visual morbidity and young age blindness has gone up. Better and timely management of eye injuries can bring down this incidence and hence the need for evolving better and ideal strategies by ophthalmic surgeons. Anterior segment injuries need prompt attention and decisions may have to be taken on the operating table for better long term rehabilitation of the patients. Ocular injuries are very often a part of polytrauma rather than being in isolation and therefore likely to be neglected to a "later stage management". This aspect has been well emphasized by the authors. Long term results of posterior segment injuries may not be encouraging and may requires repeated surgeries. A positive and optimistic attitude should therefore be taken by the operating surgeon. Better surgical outcomes are to be expected in the future with improvements in vitreo-retinal procedures. Adnexal injuries are important, both from functional and cosmetic point of view. They may require both immediate and delayed management. The removal of eye after trauma has drastically reduced with advance surgical techniques.

Rehabilitation of individuals going blind needs special attention both at professional and social levels. A new dimension has been added to this need, by the involvement of public at large and deployment of armed forces and police personnel in tackling insurgency. The use of improvized explosive devices by insurgents has markedly increased the incidence of eye injuries. Early evacuation and management of these injuries is highly desirable to reduce incidence of ocular morbidity.

Prevention is the best way of reducing, the incidence of any disease and it is much more important in ocular injuries because of impending possibility of blindness. The book has given a special chapters on Fireworks Injuries and Sports Injuries with epidemiological and preventive priorities. The role of governmental regulatory agencies, socioreligious organizations, media and nongovernmental organizations has been well-emphasized. There is a great scope in further improving the preventive devices. Standardization of protective gears, making effective regulations and implementation of the law can save many eyes from blindness.

This book adds holistically to the knowledge of understanding and management of ocular trauma from the point of view of general ophthalmologists, postgraduate students and ophthalmologists practising ocular trauma as a specialty. The contributors have done justice to their topics.

MS Boparai Air Marshal (Retd)
Director
Armed Forces Medical College
Pune, Maharashtra, India
Founder President Ocular Trauma Society of India

Emeritus Professor
National Academy of Medical Sciences (India)
Member Board of Management
Baba Farid University of Health Sciences, Punjab, India

Preface

Ocular trauma is one of the foremost causes of monocular blindness. Lack of awareness, deficient management facilities and disregard to final outcome prompted us to add useful literature to otherwise scanty integrated knowledge available on ocular trauma. The book is conceptualized to give a comprehensive account of eye injuries, their prevalence, epidemiology, cause and effect, management at primary and higher levels and preventive aspects. I am thankful to all the contributors who have put their expertise and experience in this book with a view to reduce the incidence of ocular trauma and lowering ocular morbidity to near zero level with better diagnosis, timely management, careful and rational medical and surgical treatment and also its prevention.

This book, entitled *Ocular Trauma*, is a very sincere effort to consolidate the data, diagnosis and management, prevention and medicolegal aspects involved in ocular injuries. This book belongs to all the contributors who have integrated their contributions at one place to make it comprehensive. I thank them all for their efforts, time and commitment to reduce the ocular morbidity due to trauma.

I am thankful to Dr Shailley Jain, Dr Neha Goel, Dr Manish Tandon and Dr Vinod Agrawal who have spared time to go through the proofs.

I must thank the publishers and their team for their meaningful, pleasant and esthetic layout of the book.

My special thanks go to Dr Ashma, my wife, for supporting and reminding me about the job I was committed to, and also helping me in proofreading.

DK Mehta

Contributors

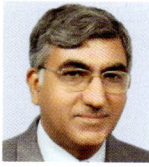

AK Grover (Padma Shri) MD (AIIMS), MNAMS, FRCS (Glasgow) FIMSA, FICO, FAICO
Chairman, Department of Ophthalmology
Sir Ganga Ram Hospital and
Chairman, Vision Eye Centres
New Delhi, India

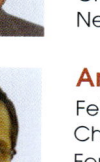

Anand Verma MBBS, MS
Fellow Sadaguru Netra Chikitsalaya
Chitrakoot, Madhya Pradesh, India
Formerly Assistant Professor
School of Medical Sciences and Research
Greater Noida
Director, Anand Eye Centre, Greater Noida
Consultant Max Hospital, Greater Noida
Uttar Pradesh, India

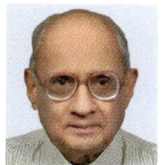

B Shukla MS, MAMS, FAMS, FACS, PhD, DSc, FAICO
Director, Research and Training
Ratan Jyoti Netralaya
Ophthalmic Institute and Research Centre
Gwalior, Madhya Pradesh, India
Formerly Head, Department of
Ophthalmology, Gwalior Medical College
Gwalior, Madhya Pradesh, India

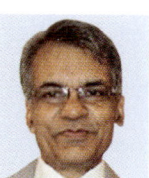

Barun Kumar Nayak MS (AIIMS), DO (London), Fellow Lion's Eye Institute, Australia
Head, Department of Ophthalmology
PD Hinduja Hospital and Medical Research
Centre, Mumbai, Maharashtra, India

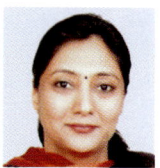

Deepali Garg Mathur MS, DNB, MNAMS
Consultant
Max Eye Care, Panchsheel Park
Consultant Max Superspeciality Hospital, Saket
Netrayatan Eye Hospital
Delhi, India

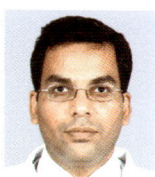

Deepender Chouhan MS, DNB, FRCS, Fellow LVPEI
Consultant, Shroff Eye Centre and
Pushpanjali Crosslay Hospital
Delhi, India

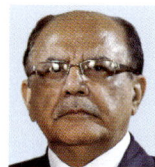

DK Mehta MS, MNAMS, FIMSA
Professor and Head
Department of Ophthalmology, School of
Medical Sciences and Research, Sharda
Hospital, Greater Noida, Uttar Pradesh, India

Formerly Director and Professor
Maulana Azad Medical College and
Guru Nanak Eye Centre, Delhi, India
Ex-President, Ocular Trauma Society of India

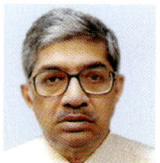

G Mukherjee MD
Vice President
Ocular Trauma Society of India
Formerly Associate Professor, Ophthalmology
RP Centre for Ophthalmic Sciences
All India Institute of Medical Sciences, Delhi
Mukherjee Eye Clinic, CR Park, Delhi, India

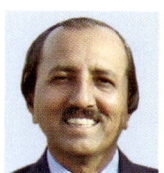

Jagat Ram MD
Professor, Department of Ophthalmology
at the Advanced Eye Centre
Postgraduate Institute of Medical
Education and Research (PGIMER)
Chandigarh, India

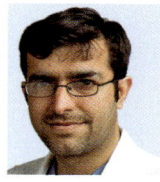

Jay Chhablani MD, Fellow LVPEI
Consultant LV Prasad Eye Institute
Hyderabad, Telangana, India

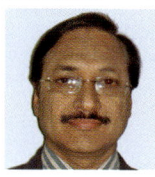

JL Goyal MD, DNB
Director Professor
Department of Ophthalmology
Maulana Azad Medical College
Guru Nanak Eye Centre, New Delhi, India

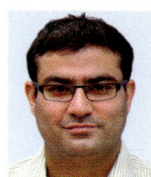

Manish Tandon DNB, MNAMS, Fellow Aravind Eye Hospital
Assistant Professor of Ophthalmology
Postgraduate Institute of Ophthalmology
Aravind Eye Hospital, Madurai
Tamil Nadu, India

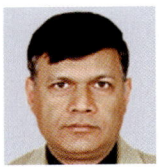

Mukesh Yadav BSc, MBBS, MD, MBA (HCA), LLB, PGDHR
Professor and Head
Department of Forensic Medicine and Toxicology
School of Medical Sciences and Research
Sharda University
Greater Noida, Uttar Pradesh, India

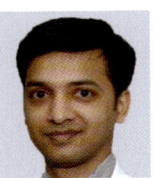

Narayanan Raja MS, Fellow LVPEI
Head, Clinical Research and
Consultant Retina
LV Prasad Eye Institute
Hyderabad, Telangana, India

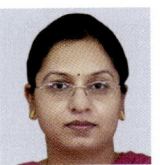

Neelam Verma MS (PGIMER)
Institute of Eye Advance
Postgraduate Institute of Medical Education
and Research, Chandigarh, India

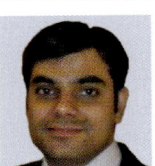

Piyush Mishra DNB
Fellow Pediatric Ophthalmology
Aravind Eye Hospital
Madurai, Tamil Nadu, India

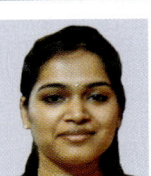

Pragati Gupta MBBS, MS
Assistant Professor
Department of Ophthalmology
Manipal Medical College
Manipal, Karnataka, India

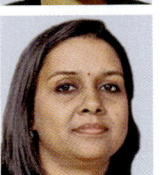

Prerna Agrawal MS, Fellow Venu Eye Institute
Senior Medical Officer
Venu Eye Institute, Delhi, India

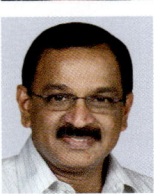

R Kim DO, DNB
Chief Consultant of Vitreo Retinal Services
Aravind Eye Hospital and Postgraduate
Institute of Ophthalmology, Madurai
Tamil Nadu, India

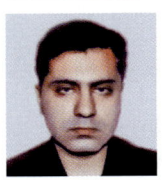

Rajat Chaudhary (Major) MS, DNB, FICO
Graded Specialist, Ophthalmologist
Army Medical Core
Roorkee, Uttrakhand
India

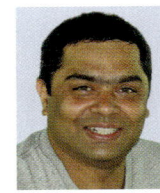

Rajib Mukherjee DNB
Muhkerjee Eye Clinic
Delhi, India

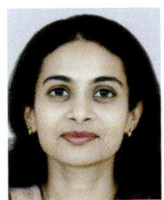

Reema Bansal MS
Assistant Professor
Advance Institute of Eye
Postgraduate Institute of Medical Education
and Research, Chandigarh, India

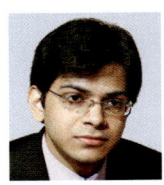

Rigved Gupta MBBS, MS
Lady Hardinge Medical college
New Delhi, India

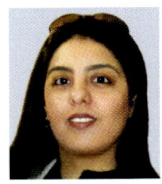

Ritika Sachdev MBBS, MS
Consultant Ophthalmologist
Additional Director, Medical Services
Centre for Sight Group of Eye Hospital,
Delhi, India

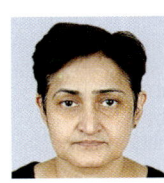

Ritu Arora MD, Dip. Nat. Board
Director Professor, Ophthalmology

Head, Department of Cornea
Maulana Azad Medical College
Guru Nanak Eye Centre, New Delhi, India

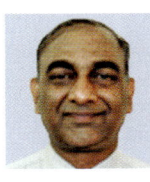

RP Gupta (Colonel), MS
Fellow Sankara Nethralaya
Chennai, Tamil Nadu, India
Professor, Department of Ophthalmology
Dr VV Patil Medical College
Ahmednagar Maharashtra, India
Formerly, Professor and Head
Department of Ophthalmology
Armed Force Medical College
Pune, Maharashtra, India

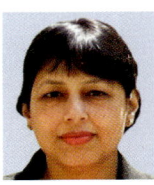

Ruchi Goel MS, DNB, FICS
Professor
Department of Ophthalmology
Maulana Azad Medical College
New Delhi, India

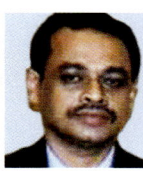

Sanjoy Chowdhury MBBS, DO, DNB
Joint Director
Medical and Health Services SAIL/BHG
Bokaro Steel City, Bokaro, Jharkhand, India

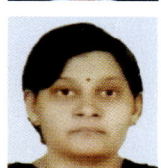

Shailley Jain MS
Specialist, Department of Ophthalmology
Jag Pravesh Chandra Hospital, Delhi
Formerly
Consultant, Max Hospital, Pitampura
New Delhi, India
Consultant, Tirupati Eye Centre, Noida
Uttar Pradesh, India

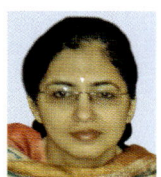

Shaloo Bageja DNB
Consultant
Sir Ganga Ram Hospital, Delhi

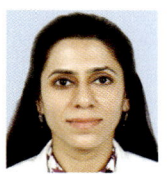

Sonika Gupta MBBS, MS, ICO
Senior Consultant Ophthalmology
Max Health Care, New Delhi
Former Assistant Professor
In-charge Eye Bank Services
Government Medical College
Chandigarh, India

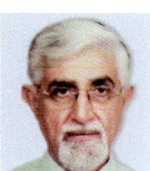

SM Bhatia BE, MBA (Marketing + sales)
Former Deputy Director, General Bureau of
Indian Standard Bahadur Shah Zafar Marg
New Delhi, India
Lead Auditor Medical Devices ISO 138150
Lead Auditor ISO 9000 and ISO14000

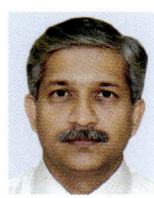

Sunil Kumar Jain MS, Fellow LVPEI
Consultant
Mumbai, Maharashtra, India

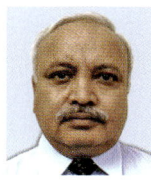

Sushil Kumar MBBS, MD
Director Professor, Ophthalmology

Head, Oculoplasty and Ultrasonography
Maulana Azad Medical College
Guru Nanak Eye Centre, New Delhi, India

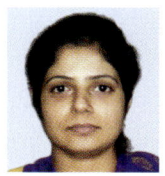

Tarana Sarwat DO
Department of Ophthalmology
School of Medical Sciences and Research
Sharda Hospital, Greater Noida
Uttar Pradesh, India

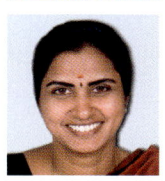

Usha Kim DO, DNB
Professor, Department of Ophthalmology
Head, Department of
Oculoplasty and Ocular Oncology
Director, Mid Level Ophthalmic Personnel
Training, Aravind Eye Care System, Madurai
Tamil Nadu, India

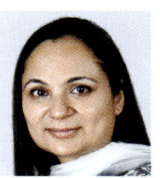

Vishali Gupta MD
Additional Professor
Advance Eye Care
Postgraduate Institute of Medical Education
and Research, Chandigarh, India

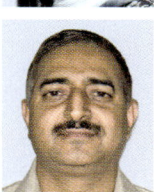

VK Baranwal MBBS, MS
Graded Specialist, Ophthalmologist
Army Medical Core
Lucknow, Uttar Pradesh, India

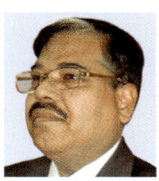

VP Gupta MD (AIIMS), DNB
Professor and Head
Department of Ophthalmology
University College of Medical Sciences and
Guru Teg Bahadur Hospital, Delhi, India

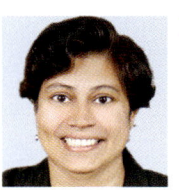

Zia Chaudhuri MS, DNB, MNAMS, FRCS (Glasg)
Professor, Department of Ophthalmology
Lady Hardinge Medical College
New Delhi, India

Jasneet Kang MS
Maulana Azad Medical College and
Associated Guru Nanak Eye Centre, Delhi, India

Shilpa Taneja DNB, MNAMS, FICC, Fellow Arvind Eye Institute, Madurai
ESIC Hospital and Postgraduate Institute
Basaidarapur, Delhi, India

Contents

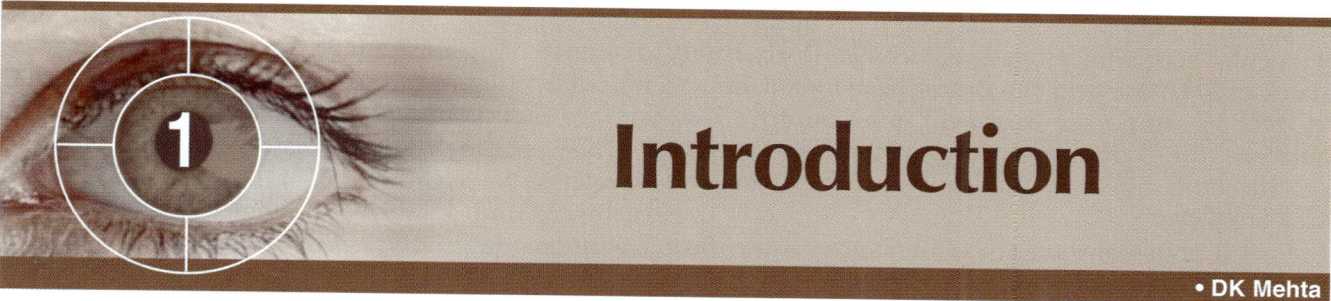

Introduction

• DK Mehta

Visual deprivation is one of the most significant deficit recorded by a human being. Ocular deformity is also very evident in all facial injuries. Ocular trauma assumes an important place in morbidity due to high vulnerability to direct exposure and delicate tissue configuration. Trauma is the leading cause of monocular blindness in people younger than 45 years. Trauma of the eye and its adnexa represents approximately 20% of all eye injuries in children. Incidence of traumatic cataract in children is reported as high as 29% of all pediatric cataracts. Majority of children suffer unilateral eye injury leading to amblyopia and boys are more often affected (over 2/3) than girls. Posterior segment involvement is recorded in nearly 52% of all injuries and out of this 8–11% have pure posterior segment involvement.

It is reported that 37% of total sports injury in United States of America (USA) are in under 16 years of age. In India and Pakistan, most sports injuries are under 25 years. Similar figures are available from Portugal.

Global incidence of corneal trauma reported is widely variable. Corneal injury reported from India also varies from 1 to 5%.

Reporting of the injuries is very patchy and a definite prevalence and incidence has been very inadequate and misleading due to different parameters and data collection. There is no standardized method for medical records and data collection. Definitions used in literature and unification of classification are necessary to be put together for its understanding and usage in data collection. Newer classification of chemical injuries has given a good insight for management and expected outcome.

Ophthalmic injuries presenting as oculo-orbital trauma may be the result of traffic accident, industrial mishaps, sports injury, etc. Ocular involvement may occur alone or as a part of polytrauma with faciomaxillary and head injuries. Initial emergency management should be aimed at stabilization of the general condition of the patient. Preventing inadvertent collateral ocular damage in these critical cases is also very important.

An estimated 16% of fireworks-related injuries affect eyes. Bottle rocket firecrackers and sparklers are the main source of injuries. All types of legally available fireworks need special consideration in manufacture, transportation and consumption.

Apart from corneal blindness, cataract and retino-choroidal injuries are also responsible for blindness. Trauma is responsible for 12–18.8% of all cases of vitreous hemorrhage only after diabetes and Eales' disease.

Lid and adnexal injuries have not been treated well in the past. Proper lid repair its timing and management of drainage system also needs special mention for these eye injuries.

Vehicular accidents often lead to facial injuries apart from chest and limb fractures. Use of airbags and seat belts have reduced the mortality but have lead to more ocular damage due to broken glass and ocular chemical injuries due to gas-filled air bags and broken spectacles with restricted body movement head hitting on the dashboard.

Ocular trauma accounts for substantial proportion of work-related injuries and around 50% of all eye injuries are considered to be industry related. Automation has changed the nature and profile of ocular trauma sustained by the people working there. Still the prevalence of work-related eye injuries among United States (US) workers is 4.4.

World over, 50% of the severe sports eye injuries are below 25 years of age. Younger population is greatly affected leading to substantial loss of man hours and economic loss in the long run. Only 47% of the ocular sports injury patients achieve final visual acuity of 20/200 or better according to an Indian report in 1989 contemporary treatment must improve the outcome. Protective gears, rules of the game, arena specifications can make the sports much safer than they are today.

United States of America ignites more fireworks than any other country on celebration to mark "Thanks Giving Day". This may account for more than two-thirds of annual fireworks-related ocular injuries that occur between June 16 and July 16. Fireworks are most commonly used during festival of Deepawali, Gurupurva, during wedding and other happy occasions also in India. There is increasing trend of using firecrackers in Malaysia, China and Sri Lanka.

Nonconventional combat is present all around the world. In recent years, there has been an increase in insurgents using improvized explosive devices (IED), hand mines, rocket-propelled grenades (RPG) and explosive formed projectiles. Explosive devices tend to accelerate metallic fragments and also propel soil and organic matter.

Posterior segment needs to be investigated properly and managed carefully in all cases of closed globe trauma and also even in presence of simple looking open globe injury. A separate section deals with such injuries.

Relevant investigations in an ocular injury to choose from the list may make the outcome better and treatment more cost-effective. Clinical judgment is critical in deciding the imaging of choice. Frequently, traumatic tissue damage or ocular media opacities such as traumatic cataracts or intraocular hemorrhage prevent adequate direct ophthalmologic evaluation, and the ophthalmologist must rely on available imaging techniques for the detection of intraocular foreign bodies like optical coherence tomography (OCT) is also turning into a potent imaging modality for wide variety of corneal and anterior segment studies. It is a good modality for follow-up and diagnosis of post-traumatic macular pathologies like macular edema, commotioretinae, vitreoretinal surface alterations and macular hole.

Therapeutics of trauma may not be very different in relation to cause and effect to specifics and mode of injury and extent of damage. Initial care and treatment definitely affect the outcome. Efficient antibiotic umbrella is needed in management of ocular injuries nearly 25% of endophthalmitis is seen in trauma cases and 2.4–7.4% eyes with penetrating ocular trauma develop endophthalmitis.

Eighty percent of ocular injuries are preventable yet ocular trauma is one of the most common causes of uniocular blindness. According to different studies, patients with open globe injuries only 22–42% obtain a final visual acuity of 20 of 40 or better. Loss of man-hours, compensation and need for notification in many cases as per factory rules and in cases of road side accidents may be required by the ophthalmologist. Safety factors in different situations awareness and there enforcement also have been incorporated in different sections.

Casualty management of an injury often leaves a lacuna for early eye injury management. Pole to pole surgery or superspecialist intervention may have to be decided and managed in different situations from primary care to tertiary intervention. Casuality officer if they are not ophthalmologist should be trained so that they can examine and inspect above mentioned ocular injuries in cases of polytrauma. This book in different sections has given a good support to all stakeholders in management and prevention of ocular injuries.

This book covers the different aspects of ocular injuries including classification, epidemiology, diagnostic modalities, injury in different situations, management and preventive aspect. The contributors have made serious efforts to deal with the different aspects of ocular injuries comprehensively.

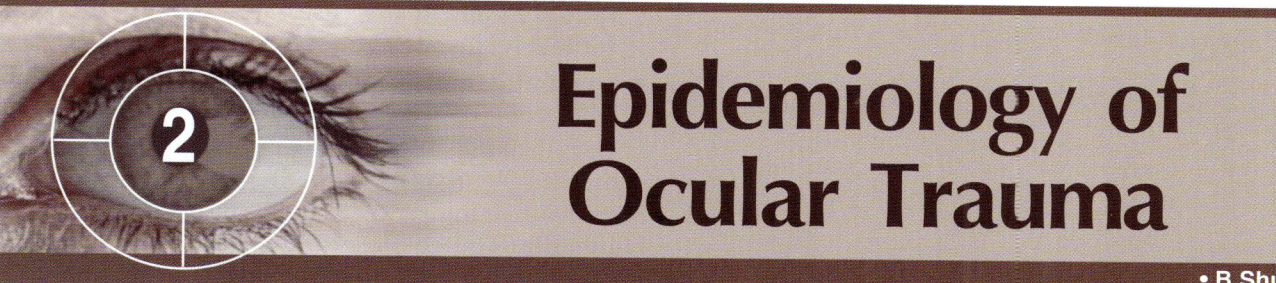

Epidemiology of Ocular Trauma

• B Shukla

INTRODUCTION

Epidemiology is a study of disease frequency, distribution, determinants and methods of control. It could be descriptive, analytical or inerventional (experimental).[1] Epidemiology of ocular trauma is usually of descriptive type.

The incidence and prevalence of ocular trauma in a defined population is the basic requirement. Prevalence is the number of cases (old and new) existing at a given point or period in time (usually a year) in a given population. It is known by a cross-sectional study. Incidence is the number of new cases occurring in a defined population during a specific period of time and is usually known by a longitudinal study. In most studies on epidemiology of ocular trauma incidence has been studied and in some studies this point is not very clear. The results are expressed differently for hospital or population based studies. Though population based study is ideal, for a relatively uncommon condition like ocular trauma it is difficult, time taking and expensive and extrapolation from large hospital based studies are justifiable.

Thus, we express the result in a ratio in which the numerator is actual number of cases seen and is constant whereas the denominator may be all eye, all hospital cases or the whole-defined population. When denominator is all eyes cases the result are usually expressed in percentage. Depending on the rarity of the condition population based studies are expressed as per 1,000, per 10,000 or even per 100,000 as in ocular trauma cases. With the above considerations an effort is made to compare some of the similar type of studies.

Ocular trauma includes many clinical entities. For a long-time the terminology was not clear and different authors used the same term for different condition or the same condition was defined by many different terms. The terminology has been now standardized by Kuhn et al.[2]

Malik and Gupta[3] reported only 349 major cases in 1968. The line of demarcation between major and minor is not clear. Similarly, Glynn et al[4] have studied only adult eyes and reported an incidence of 0.97%. Parver[5] has stated that 2–4 million eye injuries occur in USA every year (Tables 2.1 and 2.2).

Shukla[6] analyzed 1,600 cases of ocular trauma for 8 years (1981–88) in the only major eye center in the region of a population of about 1 million. Year-wise distribution is given in Fig. 2.1 and structure-wise distribution in Fig. 2.2.

Table 2.1: Incidence of ocular trauma in all eye cases

Author	Year	Place	Number	%
Malik and Gupta[3]	1968	Delhi	349	2.7
Shukla and Verma[7]	1969	Raipur	400	2.27
Canavan et al[8]	1980	N. Ireland	-	8.7
Parver[5]	1986	Maryland	-	5.0
Koval and Teller[9]	1988	Israel	-	4.4
Mukherjee[10]	1984	Jabalpur	166	1.34
Shukla[11]	2002	Gwalior	1600	1.0

Note. Delhi, Raipur, Jabalpur, and Gwalior are in India.

Table 2.2: Incidence of hospital based ocular trauma

Author	Year	Place	Number/100,000
Karlson and Klein[12]	1979	Madison	423 acute hospitalized cases
Tielsch et al[13]	1986	Maryland	13.2 from hospital discharge cases
Desai et al[14]	1966	Scotland	0.41 incidence of blindness
Fong L[15]	1955	Australia	15.2 cases requiring hospitalization
Byhr E[16]	1944	Sweden	3.3 cases of perforation injuries

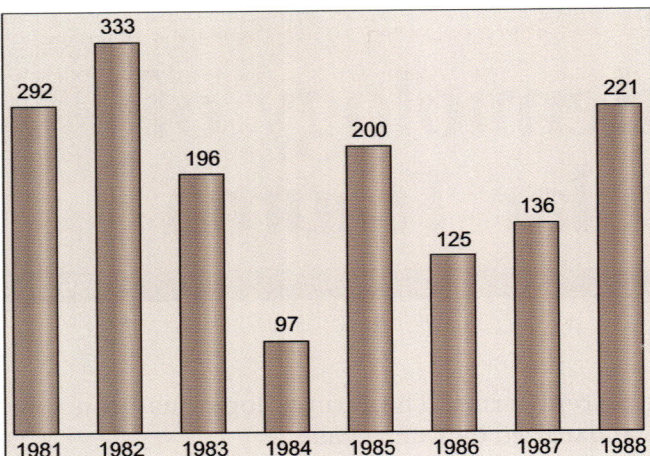

Fig. 2.1: Incidence of ocular injuries

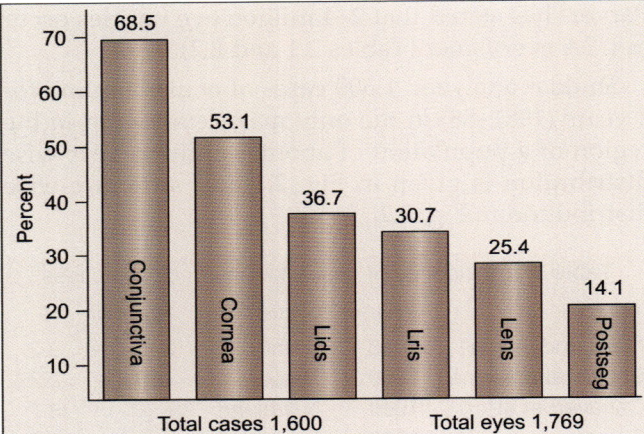

Fig. 2.2: Structures in ocular trauma

It would be appreciated that most of the data presented cannot be compared properly for the following reasons:

- Number of cases studied and their duration is very variable.
- Some studies are based on all eye cases whereas some on all hospital cases or even larger population based.
- Many studies have restricted their focus on serious/major/hospital admitted cases admission to hospital depends on many factors apart from seriousness of a case. The criteria for major/minor cases may vary. From the last two decades admission to hospital and stay in hospital is rapidly

declining and many cases are discharged on the same day despite their seriousness.

- Type and nature of injury have been defined differently by different authors.

Inspite of the above problems many trends emerge out quite clearly from the above data. Currently, National Eye Injury Registries have been formed like Hungarian, United States and even World Eye Injury Registry. Recently, Indian Eye Injury Registry has also been formed. They are broad based and collect a more representative data from large areas of population. However, they are limited to "injuries resulting in permanent and significant structural and functional loss to the eye".[17] We need to have a dividing line between significant and non-significant and between temporary and permanent. A system of Trauma Index (TI) was proposed for this purpose based on the degree of structural and functional loss.[18] When TI was 10 or less the injury was minor, between 11 and 50 it was moderate and above 50 it was severe. We shall consider the epidemiology with regard to major factors, like age, sex, occupation and residence. There are other factors also for consideration but the discussion of all factors will be beyond the scope of a chapter on the subject.

SEX INCIDENCE

Males are more employed in all types of factories and manual jobs. They also indulge more in sports and games, rash driving and crimes and hence they have outnumbered the females as shown in Table 2.3.

Lambah[19] had studied the industrial population at Wolverhampton. Moreira[20] studied Brazilian children in whom sex ratio is not marked. It can be said that

Table 2.3: Sex ratio in ocular trauma		
Author	*Year*	*Male: famale ratio*
Lambah[19]	1968	4.00:1
Malik	1968	3.00:1
Olurin[21]	1971	5.00:1
Mehrotra[22]	1978	5.62:1
Shukla[7]	1979	5.10:1
Canavan[8]	1980	5.25:1
Moreira[20]	1988	1.73:1
Glynn[4]	1988	5.50:1
MacEwan[23]	1999	6.50:1
Shukla[11]	2002	4.16:1
Kuhn[24]	2002	4.16:1

Table 2.4: Maximum age group incidence in ocular trauma			
Author	*Year*	*Maximum age group*	*Percentage*
Malik[3]	1968	0–10	29.1
Olurin[21]	1971	20–30	33.0
Canavan[8]	1980	15–29	36.9
Koval[9]	1988	06–12	23.6
Moreira[20]	1988	0–15	36.8
Shukla[11]	2002	21–30	27.3

Table 2.5: Incidence of occupational injuries		
Author	*Year*	*Occupational injuries (%)*
Malik[3]	1968	19.7
Glynn[21]	1988	48.0
Koval[9]	1988	28.2
Kuhn[24]	2002	21.0
Shukla[11]	2002	29.2

the number of males are 4 to 6 times higher than females.

AGE INCIDENCE

Here also there is considerable variation in the maximum age group incidence in different studies perhaps due to selection of cases or some regional or geographical factors. However, it is clear that ocular trauma is a problem of young or very young. Sudden drop in number was seen after 30 years. However, Klopfer[25] found a second peak after the age of 75 years though only a few cases were observed (Table 2.4).

OCCUPATION IN OCULAR TRAUMA

There is a considerable ambiguity about the terminology. Excluding very young and very old most people have some occupation and as such these injuries could be called occupational. However, it usually implies specific type of work and does not include students or house wives. Now, the word "Work related" is widely used for occupational injuries. Classification of occupation has also been done in different ways. Inspite of these problems, Table 2.5 shows distribution of such injuries.

In general, it may be said that the incidence of occupational injuries is higher in Western countries but the incidence is declining due to more awareness and application of safety measures.

RESIDENCE IN OCULAR TRAUMA

Although Saari[26] has pointed out that agricultural settings are also important in ocular trauma but a division into rural and urban areas is not well demarcated in Western countries as in India and some other Asian countries. In India, this is very important as about 70% of population lives in rural areas where the lifestyle is very different from urban areas. In rural areas, agriculture is the main occupation and ocular injuries are also related to that. Usually, they are caused by wooden or metal articles used for work, branches or twigs or animal injuries like bull horn or a buffalow's tail. Dust injuries are seen and fungal infections are also common. However, only 39.75% cases are reported from rural area as opposed to 61.25% from urban area (Shukla).[11] This appears due to lack of education, awareness, finances, transport and medical facilities.

OTHER CONSIDERATIONS

Epidemiology of ocular trauma is a big subject. There are many other aspects which can be considered as socioeconomic status, type of sports and games, pattern of crimes and road traffic accidents. Non-mechanical injuries by chemicals and burns are also important. A detailed consideration of all of them is beyond the scope of a chapter on epidemiology.

REFERENCES

1. Park K. Park's Text Book of Preventive and Social Medicine, 14th ed. M/s Banarsidas Bhanot Publishers, Jabalpur, 1995. p. 54.
2. Kuhn F, Morris R, et al. A standardised classification of ocular trauma terminology, Ophthalmology, 1996;103:240–3.
3. Malik SRK, Gupta AK. J All Ind Oph Soc. 1968;16:178.
4. Glynn RJ, Seddon J, Berlin B. The incidence of eye injuries in New Negland adults. Arch Ophthal. 1988;106:785.
5. Parver LM. Arch Ophthal. 1986;104:1452.
6. Shukla B. Epidemiology of ocular trauma, 1st Ed. Jaypee Brothers Medical Publishers, New Delhi, 2002 p.21.
7. Shukla IM, Verma RN. Ind J Oph. 1979;1:33.
8. Canavan YM, et al. Brit J Ophth. 1980;64:618.
9. Koval R, Teller J, et al. Arch Ophthal 1988; 106:771.
10. Mukherjee AK, et al. Ind J Ophthal 1984;32:269.
11. Shukla B. Epidemiology of Ocular Trauma, 1st Ed. Jaypee Brothers Medical Publishers, New Delhi 2002. p.20.
12. Karlson T, Klein B. The incidence of acute hospital treated eye injuries. Arch Ophthal. 1986;104:1473–6.
13. Tielsch J, Parver L, Shankar B. Time trends in the incidence of hospitalised ocular trauma. Arch Ophthal. 1989;107:519–23.

14. Desai P, MacEwen C, Bains P, et al. Incidence of cases of ocular trauma admited to hospital. Brit J. Ophthal. 1966; 80:592–6.

15. Fong L. Eye injuries in Victoria, Australia, Med J Aust, 1995;162:64–8.

16. Byhr E. Perforating eye injuries in the western part of Sweden. Acta Ophthal. 1994;72:91–7.

17. Kuhn F, Pieramici DJ. Ocular Trauma, Priciples and Practice, 1st Ed. Thieme Publication, New York, 2002 p.15.

18. Shukla B, Khanna B. Trauma Index. Ind J Ophthal. 1983;31:439.

19. Lambah P. Adult eye injuries at Wolverhampton. Trans Oph Soc UK, 1968;88:661–73.

20. Moreira CA, Debert-Rebeiro M, Belfort R. Epidemio-logical study of eye injuries in Brazilian children. Arch Ophthal. 1988;106:781–4.

21. Olurin MB. Ameri J Ophthal. 1971;72:72.

22. Mehrotra AS, Ignatius NK. Ind J Ophthal. 1978;26:17.

23. MacEwen CJ, Bains PS, Desai P. Eye injuries in children: the current picture. Brit J Ophthal. 1999;83:933–6.

24. Kuhn F, Pieramicic DJ. Ocular Trauma, Principles and Practice, 1st Ed. Thiems Publication, New York, 2002, 15–16.

25. Klopfer J, Tielsch J, et al. Ocular Trauma in the United States, Eye injuries resulting the hospitalisation, 1984–87, Arch Ophthal. 1992;110:838–42.

26. Saari M, Parvi V. Occupational eye injuries in Finland. Acta Ophthal. 1984;161 (Suppl.):17–28.

Classification of Ocular Trauma

3.1 CLASSIFICATION OF MECHANICAL OCULAR TRAUMA

• Tarana Sarwat • DK Mehta

INTRODUCTION

Advancement in lifestyle and working techniques parallels the incidence of trauma including the ocular ones. As this incidence of ocular trauma has increased, it has also led to more of its understanding as well as building up of newer techniques for its management.

Why Need a Classification System for Ocular Trauma?

Best management of ocular trauma can be done only if its reporting is standardized. This is because it permits authentic statistical assessment of outcomes among the treating institutions. A classification system has immediate clinical and research application. It also helps retrospectively as well as prospectively, to evaluate the efficacy of treatment modalities, thereby establishing the best possible guidelines for the first contact person be it a physician or an ophthalmologist.

BASIS OF CLASSIFYING OCULAR TRAUMA

1. According to the mode of injury, for example:
   • Intrauterine
   • Birth
   • Domestic
   • Sports
   • Occupational.
2. According to the nature of injury, for example:
   • Mechanical
   • Non-mechanical, e.g. chemical, thermal, electrical, radiation.
3. According to the ocular tissue involved
   • Globe and its contents
   • Ocular adenexa.
4. According to the type of injury inflicted
   • Blunt
   • Penetrating
   • Perforating.

The classification in this manner has little to serve the purpose of proper recording and giving proper treatment. It was in 1996 that Kuhn came with the classification to cover the clinical aspects to relate to treatment modalities.

KUHN'S CLASSIFICATION

This classification was given by Dr Ferenc Kuhn. In this classification, trauma has been categorized into two major types: (1) closed globe, and (2) open globe. These have further been subcategorized as follows:

Closed Globe

• Contusion
• Lamellar laceration
• Superficial foreign body.

Open Globe

• Laceration
  – Penetrating
  – Perforating
  – Intraocular foreign body
• Rupture.

Definition of Ocular Trauma Terms

- *Closed globe injury*—in this type of injury, there is no full thickness wound on the eyeball.
- *Open globe injury*—eyeball suffers a full thickness wound in this type.
- *Contusion*—is a closed globe injury caused by a blunt object.
- *Lamellar laceration*—closed globe injury caused by a sharp object not reaching full thickness.
- *Superficial foreign body*—foreign body lying either on the cornea or on the conjunctiva.
- *Laceration*—it is an open globe injury caused by a sharp object with irregular margins.
- *Penetrating injury*—it is a single full thickness wound caused by a sharp object.
- *Perforating injury*—in this injury, there are two full thickness wounds (entry wound and exit wound)
- *Intraocular foreign body*—in this, the foreign body gets retained inside the eyeball leaving only a single entry wound.
- *Rupture*—full thickness wound caused by a blunt object.

This classification was endorsed initially by:

- Board of directors of the international society of ocular trauma
- The US eye injury registry
- The Hungarian eye injury society
- The American academy of ophthalmology.

BIRMINGHAM EYE TRAUMA TERMINOLOGY SYSTEM (BETTS) CLASSIFICATION

This classification was given in 1996, by Dr Kuhn, et al. The US eye injury registry was setup with the University of Alabama at Birmingham as the nodal centre. The professional association headed by Dr Ferenc Kuhn, tried to standardize the terminology related to ocular trauma. Henceforth specific terminology to define subcategories of trauma emerged which were predictive of the visual prognosis. Following is the BETTS classification:

Injury

1. Closed globe
   - Contusion
   - Lamellar laceration
2. Open globe
   - Laceration

- – Penetrating
- – IOFB
- – Perforating
- Rupture.

Glossary of Terms

- *Eyewall*—sclera and cornea (though technically the eyewall has three coats post to limbus, for clinical and practical purposes violation of only the most external structure is taken into consideration.
- *Closed globe injury*—no full thickness wound of eyeball.
- *Open globe injury*—full thickness wound of eyeball.
- *Contusion*—there is no full thickness wound (the injury is either due to direct energy delivered by the object, e.g. choroidal rupture or to the changes in the shape of the globe, e.g. angle resection.
- *Rupture*—full thickness wound of the eyewall caused by a blunt object.
- *Laceration*—full thickness wound of the eyewall, caused by a sharp object.
- *Penetrating injury*—is a full thickness injury cause by sharp top high speed object.
- *Entrance wound*—if more than one wound is present each must have been caused by a different agent .
- *Retained foreign objects*—technically a penetrating injury, but grouped separately because of different clinical implications.
- *Perforating injury*—entrance and exit wounds (both wounds caused by the same agent).

BETTS satisfies all criteria to standardize ocular classification by:

1. Providing a clear definition for all injuries.
2. Placing each injury type with in the framework of a comprehensive system.

The key to BETTS logic is to understand that all terms relate to the whole eyeball as the tissue of reference while in BETTS "a penetrating corneal injury" is unambiguously an open globe injury with a corneal wound, the same term had two potential meanings before:

1. An injury penetrating into the cornea (i.e. a partial thickness corneal wound: closed globe injury)
2. An injury penetrating into the globe (i.e. full thickness corneal wound: an open globe injury)

This classification was endorsed by:

- World Eye Injury Registry

- American Academy of Ophthalmology
- International Society of Ocular Trauma
- Retina Society
- United States Eye Injury Registry
- Vitreous Society
- World Eye Injury Registry
- American Society of Ocular Trauma.

THE OCULAR TRAUMA SCORE

The US Eye Injury Registry (USEIR) developed the ocular trauma score (OTS) with support from the centers for disease control and prevention. Modeled on the APGAR (activity, pulse, grimace, appearance and respiration) test, the OTS uses initial visual acuity (VA) and injury type to predict on outcome at the time of presentation. It provides a single probability estimate of an eye trauma patient will obtain a specific visual range by 6 months after injury. The OTS can be used as an aid in the counseling and treatment of eye injury patients, and is able to direct attention toward resource needs and rehabilitation the treatment process. The OTS is meant to be a continually evolving scoring system to be used by the clinician to facilitate patient counseling, treatment, rehabilitation and research.

OCULAR TRAUMA SCORE EVALUATION

Upon presentation, the physician evaluates the patient's eyes as well as his or her general condition. The patient's VA upon presentation is assigned a numerical score between 60 and 100 (Table 3.1.1), with 100 being the best. The doctor then assesses the

Table 3.1.2: Estimated probability of follow-up VA category by the OTS score

Raw score sum	OTS score	NLP (%)	LP/HM (%)	1/200–19/200 (%)	20/200–20/50 (%)	>=20/40 (%)
0–44	1	73	17	7	2	1
45–65	2	28	26	18	13	15
66–80	3	2	11	15	28	44
81–91	4	1	2	2	21	74
92–100	5	0	1	2	5	92

patient's vision-threatening injuries (injuries that are not sight-threatening, e.g. dislocated lenses, hyphema, or traumatic cataract, are not factored in because, if there's modern equipment in the trauma center, these injuries can be easily repaired by a skilled surgeon. Sight-threatening injuries are assigned a number, which was determined and weighted by a computerized assessment of hundreds of past eye records weighing their outcome. These are then deducted from the visual acuity point score (Table 3.1.1) for a patient with more than one tissue diagnosis [i.e. globe rupture and retinal detachment (RD)] patients should be deducted for both diagnosis values from the VA point score.

After all calculations are made, the physician is left with a raw score up to 100. The raw score is then factored into a scale that roughly divides 100 into five parts. Each part is then assigned a number between 1 and 5 (Table 3.1.2). An injury with an OTS score of 1 is considered the most sight-threatening, leaving a patient with the least chances of good visual recovery. Injuries with OTS score of 5 indicate that a patient has a 96% chance of achieving vision of 20/40 or better.

THE OCULAR TRAUMA CLASSIFICATION SYSTEM

The ocular trauma classification system was developed as the next step in ocular trauma standardization by establishing a system to classify mechanical injuries of the eye. The classification group comprised of a committee of 13 ophthalmologists from seven premier institutions. Among these are the Emort University, Atlanta; University of Southern California, LA; John Hopkins University, Baltimore; University of Alabama, Birmingham; St Louis University, Missouri; Medical College of Wincounsin, Milwaukee and University of Miami, US. The group reviewed trauma classification systems in ophthalmology and general

Table 3.1.1: Computerized method for driving OTS score

Initial visual factor	Raw points
A. Initial visual acuity category	NLP = 60
	LP to HM = 70
	1/200 to 19/200 = 80
	20/200 to 20/50 = 90
	> = 20/40 = 100
B. Globe rupture	– 23
C. Endophthalmitis	– 17
D. Perforating injury	– 14
E. Retinal detachment	– 11
F. Afferent pupillary defect (MGP)	– 10
Raw score sum = Sum of raw points	

Abbreviations: OTS, ocular trauma score; NLP, no light perception; LP, light perception; HM, hand motion; MGP, Marcus Gunn pupil

medicine and reported on the characteristics and outcomes of eye trauma, then established a classification system based on standard terminology and features of eye injuries at initial examination. The classification is based upon anatomic and physiologic variables that have been shown to be prognostic of visual outcome in ocular injuries. These variables can be assessed clinically on initial examination or surgical procedure.

The four specific variables chosen are:
1. *Type of injury:* Open globe, closed globe
2. *Grade of injury:* It is based on VA at initial examination
3. *Pupil status relative afferent pupillary (RAPD):* Present or absent
4. *Zone of injury:* Location of opening in open globe injuries and posterior most structure in closed globe injuries.

How these variables help in categorizing the ocular injuries, is clear from the following discussion:

Types of Injury

The circumstances and nature of injury reported by the patient or witness to the incident are to be noted. If the patient is unconscious or no witness is available, typing is based on overall findings from examination of patient. If intraocular foreign body is suspected, ancillary testing is used to define the injury.

Closed Globe Injury

This injury is further divided into four types:
1. Contusion—which is labelled as "A"
2. Lamellar laceration—labelled as "B"
3. Superficial foreign body—as "C"
4. Mixed (if it has all the above characteristics present)—labelled as "D".

Similarly *open globe injury* is divided into five types which are labelled as A to E.
1. Rupture—A
2. Penetrating—B
3. Intraocular foreign body—C
4. Perforating—D
5. Mixed—E.

Grade of Injury

As mentioned earlier, it is based on the VA at initial examination. Inspite of VA being a physiological

variable and its subjective nature, it is considered the strongest predictor of future visual outcome. Distance acuity is assessed using Snellen's acuity and near vision is recorded with Rosenbaum's card.

Acuity of no perception of light (PL) is confirmed by a bright source such as an indirect ophthalmoscope at its high intensity.

Based on the recorded VA, following five grades are defined:

Grade	Visual acuity
I	>20/40
II	20/50–20/100
III	19/100–5/200
IV	4/200–PL
V	No PL

Relative Afferent Pupillary Defect

This grossly measures optic nerve and retinal function. Swinging flash light test is used to elicit this. If one pupil is mechanically or pharmacologically non-reactive or not visualized, relative afferent pupillary defect (RAPD) is assessed by consensual response in the other eye.

RAPD cannot be assessed in monocular patients or in eyes with bilaterally fixed, non-reacting pupils. It is reported as positive or negative thereby labelling as "P" or "N" subsequently.
- Positive—P
- Negative—N.

Zone of Injury

Both closed and open globe injuries have been divided into three zones depending upon their location on the eyeball.

Closed Globe Injury

- *Zone 1:* Superficial or external injuries limited to bulbar conjunctiva, sclera or cornea are grouped in zone 1 injuries.
- *Zone 2:* Anterior segment injuries, internal to cornea up to posterior lens capsule or pars plicata are grouped in zone 2 injuries.
- *Zone 3:* Injuries involving all other internal structures fall in zone 3.

Open Globe Injury

Location of the most posterior full thickness aspect of globe opening is considered as follows:

- *Zone 1:* Globe opening isolated to cornea or limbus.
- *Zone 2:* Globe opening involving anterior 5 mm of sclera.
- *Zone 3:* Globe opening posterior to anterior 5 mm of sclera.

In case of multiple openings, zone is defined as that of most posterior opening.

In intraocular foreign body, entry site defines the zone.

In case of perforating injuries, zone is defined as the most posterior defect (mostly the exit site).

On the basis of above classification, an ocular injury at the first examination site, can be categorized completely and prognosis explained, e.g. a closed globe contusional injury lying between limbus and anterior 5 mm of sclera with vision between 20/50 and 50/100 and RAPD present, can be written as A2PII (Fig. 3.1.1). Similarly, a corneal perforation with vision between 4/200 to PL and no RAPD can be labelled as B4N1 (Fig. 3.1.2).

This classification, thus gives the complete description of an ocular injury when examined initially and can be used to explain the visual prognosis but there are certain things which this classification does not reflect or talk about.

It does not comment on the status of lens while examining the injury, which can dramatically alter the visual prognosis, e.g. dislocation, subluxation or rupture of lens can alter the visual prognosis.

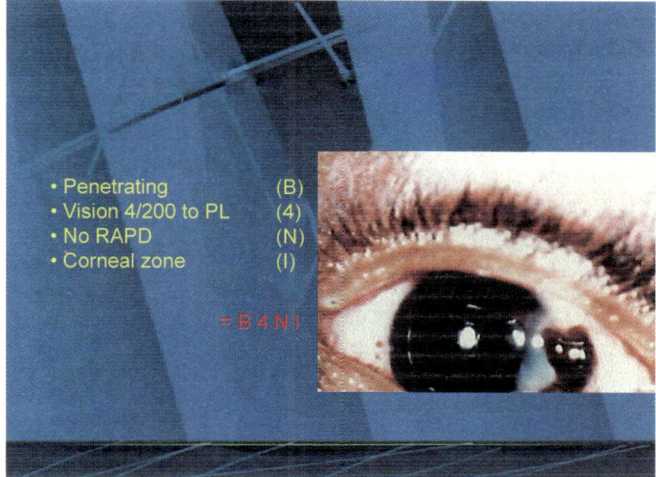

Fig. 3.1.2: Representing parameters in a open globe injury

It does not mention the angle damage or recession which again can alter the visual prognosis.

Retinal or choroidal insult, like detachment, tear or edema which can result in poor prognosis have again, not been talked about.

No adenexal deficits have been discussed, e.g. traumatic ptosis, muscular injuries or orbital wall injuries which play an important role in determining the visual prognosis.

FUTURE

If the above mentioned structural injuries are taken into consideration, a better diagnostic and prognostic criteria can be established, e.g. if lens and angle injuries are considered, the visual prognosis can be explained in a better way, as the later on deterioration of VA by a delayed formation of traumatic cataract or a late rise of IOP by angle recession or hyphema can be kept in mind. Similarly, retinal or choroidal tears leading to detachment later on, can again alter the visual prognosis; just like a retained IOFB leading to siderosis can. Squint and ptosis are other delayed sequelae of trauma which can markedly deteriorate the vision later on but can very efficiently dealt with surgically to improve the visual outcome.

These injuries, therefore deserve a special terminology and place in the nomenclature.

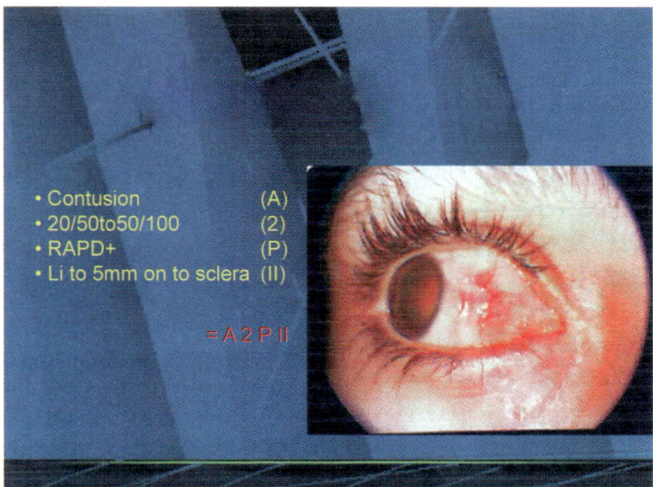

Fig. 3.1.1: Representing parameters in a closed global injury

An example will make the description very clear and same may be applied for a detailed recording:

Adnexal damage	y	n
Open globe	O	o
Penetrating injury	P	(D)double perforation
Vision grade	4	4
No RAPD	N	P
Zone	I	I
Lens intact	LI	LI

The observations marked green can be incorporated to give a complete description with details for documentation and follow-up. The inspiration is taken from the floral formula applied to describe the details of structural details of any flower. A case of trauma can be represented as:

YOD4NILi = adnexal damage, open globe, vision 6/200, no RAPD, corneal injury, lens intact.

BIBLIOGRAPHY

1. Ference Kuhn, Richard Maisink, Lo Rette Mann, Morris Robert M, Witherspoon C. Douglas: OTS: predicting the final vision of the injured eye. Ocular Trauma Principles and Practice, Theime Medical Publishers inc 2002;7–9.

2. Kuhn F, Morris R. A standardized classification of Ocular Trauma, Ophthalmology 1996:103:240–243.

3. Kuhn F, Morris R, Witherspoon C. Douglas: Bett: The terminology of Ocular Trauma P3.5 Ocular Trauma Principles and practice, Theime Medical Publishers inc 2002.

4. Mehta DK, T Deven. New classification system for ocular trauma. Management of Ocular trauma, 1st edition. CBS publishers, India 2002;8–11.

5. Pieramici DJ. The classification of eye injuries p 2–11, Modern management of Ocular trauma. Jaypee Highlights Medical Publishers.inc.

6. Sharanth C Raja, Pieramici Dante J. Classification of ocular Trauma. Ocular Trauma Principles and practice. Theime Medical Publishers inc 2002;6–8.

7. Sternberg P, A system for classifying Mechanical injuries of the Eye. American J Opthalmology 1997:123,820–31.

3.2 CLASSIFICATION OF CHEMICAL OCULAR TRAUMA

• Ritu Arora • Shailley Jain

Ocular chemical burns can be devastating and its sequelae can result in permanent blindness.

Clinical findings present immediately after injury are related to the area of involvement (extent of fluorescein staining), depth of penetration (loss of stromal clarity, limbal ischemia and/or necrosis of limbal and bulbar conjunctiva, hypotony and cataract) and toxicity of the substance.[1]

Historically it has been recognized that the extent of tissue damage is an indicator of prognosis of recovery following ocular surface injury, hence, a classification of these injuries has been attempted by various authors. There is however, no ideal grading or classification because of the many variables associated with these injuries.

Hughes[2] first proposed a classification of alkali burns in 1946 taking into account the epithelial defect and stromal opacity (Table 3.2.1). This classification provides a base to estimate prognosis and plan treatment. However, this classification does not evaluate injuries to other ocular surfaces and deeper tissues; hence prognosis of the injury may be estimated wrongly.

Table 3.2.1: Hughes classification

Grade	Clinical findings	Prognosis
Mild	Erosion of corneal epithelium Faint haziness of the cornea No ischemic necrosis of conjunctiva or sclera	Good
Moderately severe	Corneal opacity blurs iris details Minimal ischemic necrosis of conjunctiva and sclera	Guarded
Very severe	Blurred pupillary outline Blanching of conjunctiva and sclera	Poor

In 1965, Roper Hall[3] emphasized the relation between limbal ischemia and prognosis thus attempting to rectify the inadequacies of Hughes classification. This new classification included quantification of conjunctival and episcleral ischemia (area of whitening) and also emphasized that total loss of corneal epithelium is significant in determining the ultimate prognosis. This is presently the most commonly used classification (Table 3.2.2).

Table 3.2.2: Roper Hall classification

Grade	Clinical findings	Prognosis
I	Corneal epithelial damage No limbal ischemia	Excellent
II	Cornea hazy but iris details seen Ischemia affects <1/3 of the limbus	Good
III	Total loss of corneal epithelium Stromal haze obscures iris details Ischemia affects 1/2–1/3 of the limbus	Guarded
IV	Cornea opaque, no view of iris or pupil Ischemia affects >1/2 of the limbus	Poor

However, in the following years, the knowledge and understanding of ocular surface healing and approach to surgical management has changed dramatically. The concept of limbal and forniceal stem cells and its application in management of severe burns has significantly improved the outcome of treatment in these patients. Using a limbal stem cell injury based model, Thoft[4] classified chemical injuries as:

- *Grade I:* Little or no loss of stem cells (Hughes grade I) (Fig. 3.2.1)
- *Grade II:* Subtotal stem cell loss (Hughes grade II/III)
- *Grade III:* Complete stem cell loss with retention of some proximal conjunctival epithelium and vascularity (Hughes grade IV) (Fig. 3.2.2)

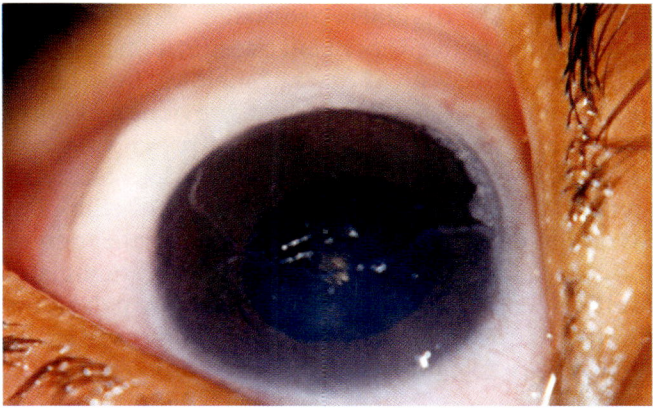

Fig. 3.2.1: Grade I injury (Roper Hall and Dua's classification): corneal epithelial defect with no limbal ischemia

Table 3.2.3: Dua's classification

Grade	Prognosis	Limbal involvement	Conjunctival involvement	Analog scale
I	Very good	0 O'clock hours	0	0/0
II	Good	≥ 3 O'clock hours	≥ 30	0.1–3/1–29
III	Good	> 3–6 O'clock hours	> 30–50	3.1–6/31–50
IV	Good-guarded	> 6–9 O'clock hours	> 50–75	6.1–9/51–75
V	Guarded-poor	> 9–< 12 O'clock hours	> 75–100	9.1–11.9/75–99.9
VI	Very poor	Total limbus	Total conjunctival involvement	12/100

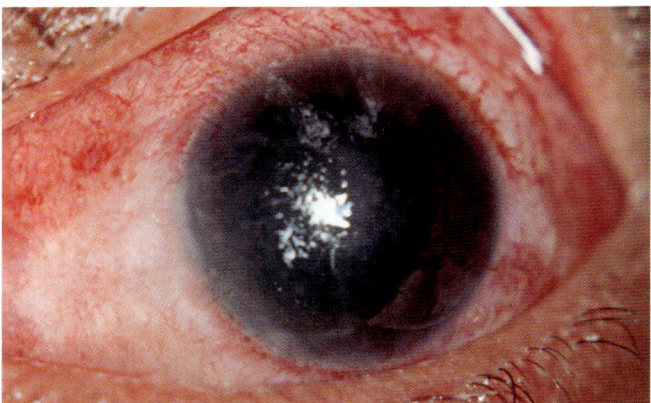

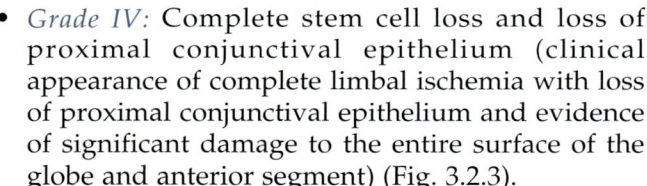

Fig. 3.2.2: Grade III injury (Roper Hall classification): corneal epithelial defect with stromal haze with limbal ischemia affecting < ½ of the limbus with guarded prognosis. Same injury is classified as grade III injury as per Dua's classification with good prognosis

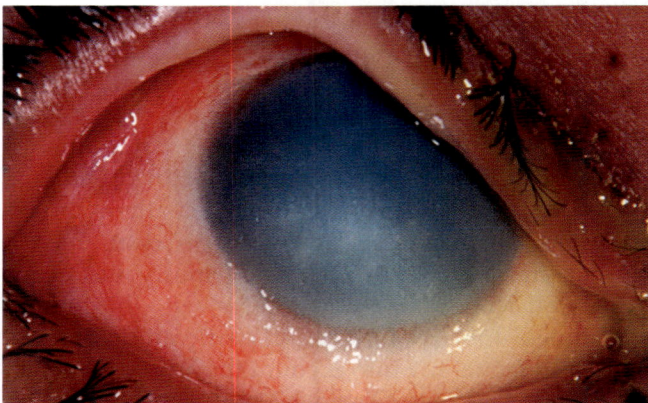

Fig. 3.2.3: Grade IV injury (Roper Hall classification): cornea opaque with ischemia affecting > ½ of the limbus with poor prognosis. Same injury is classified as grade IV injury as per Dua's classification with good-guarded prognosis

- *Grade IV:* Complete stem cell loss and loss of proximal conjunctival epithelium (clinical appearance of complete limbal ischemia with loss of proximal conjunctival epithelium and evidence of significant damage to the entire surface of the globe and anterior segment) (Fig. 3.2.3).

Dua et al[5] in 2001 proposed a significant modification to the Roper Hall classification based on their experience with 67 cases of chemical burns of all grades of injury. They felt that the previous classifications were inadequate especially in prognostication of grade IV burns. In cases with 100% loss of limbal stem cells, any surviving conjunctival epithelium is a favorable prognostic factor as conjunctivalization of the cornea prevents progressive corneal thinning and melting. The ensuing vascularization promotes healing and facilitates repair and provides an opportunity to carry out restorative procedures at a later date. However, in eyes with 100% limbal as well as 100% conjunctival involvement, a very poor outcome would be expected even with a maximum

intervention. As per the Roper Hall classification both these injuries would be classified as grade IV injury with the same prognosis but it is not so as has been noted by Dua et al. Therefore, the Roper Hall classification is inadequate in planning management and prognosis (Table 3.2.3).

Dua et al took into account the extent of limbal involvement in o'clock hours and the percentage of conjunctival involvement was estimated by dividing the bulbar and forniceal conjunctiva into quadrants and determining the area involved. They preferred the term limbal involvement over limbal ischemia as it included areas where a complete or full thickness loss of limbal epithelium occurred without significant ischemia and vice versa. They proposed that the extent of limbal involvement be based on the o'clock hours of limbal staining observed which can be reviewed frequently and reclassified. When attributing a grade to a given clinical situation, the extent of limbal involvement takes precedence over the extent of conjunctival involvement (Fig. 3.2.4).

Grade	Epithelial defect/opacity	Stromal edema	Stromal opacity	Conjunctival involvement	Limbal ischemia
Minimal	Mild haze, punctate epithelial erosions	None	None	Erythema, chemosis	None
Mild	White, opacified	None to minimal	None	Erythema, opacification, chemosis	None
Moderate	White, opacified, common at 24–36 hours	Mild to moderate	None	Opacification, chemosis, petechia/subconjunctival hemorrhage	None to minimal
Severe	Entire epithelium opacified white, usually large after 24–36 hours	Moderate to severe	Mild	Opacification, hemorrhage, necrosis	≥ 1/3
Very severe	Opacified white if present, sloughs rapidly	Marked	Severe	Necrosis may be extensive	> 1/3

Table 3.2.4: Classification of acid burns

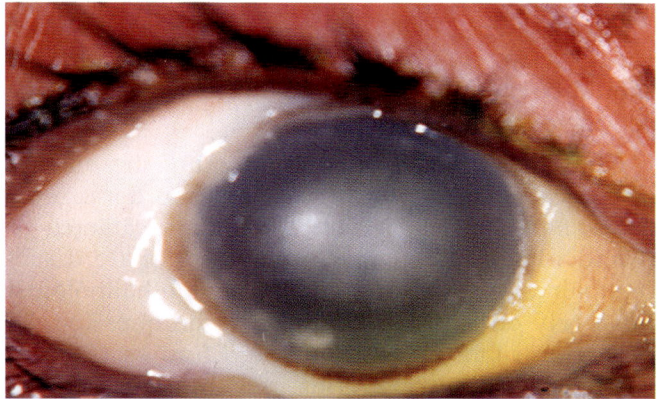

Fig. 3.2.4: Grade IV injury (Roper Hall classification) cornea opaque with a cataractous lens. Ischemia affects 360° of the limbus. Same injury is grade VI injury (Dua's classification) with total limbal and conjunctival involvement. Prognosis is very poor in both classifications

Thus, the classification proposed by them allows flexibility in documenting the changes in the post-injury period. It has the added advantage that it can be presented in an analog manner rather than the stepped progression of other classifications allowing a crossover between grades. The scores can be recorded on a daily basis and reclassified as the patient improves or worsens. While being simple and easy to use, this classification defines the extent of injury and helps in planning management and predicts the prognosis with greater precision.

ACID BURNS

No specific classification system has been proposed for acid burns. However, a modification of Hughes classification of alkali burns has been proposed by Pfister and Pfister[6] to classify acid burns (Table 3.2.4). In using the classification, a delay of 24–48 hours may be needed as the initial clinical impression may be better or worse than the actual injury.

For any acid, the degree of tissue damage correlates with the quantity and concentration of the acid to which the eye is exposed and with the duration of exposure. Generally, the fumes containing hydrogen ions and droplets of acidic solutions cause only minor injury; more severe injuries result from a direct splash. If the epithelium is intact, acids tend to cause severe tissue damage only if their pH is less than 2.5. If the epithelium is absent prior to exposure, acids at a higher pH can cause severe damage. Clinical signs suggesting a poor prognosis after acid injury reflect the degree of acid penetration of the tissue. They include complete corneal anesthesia, conjunctival and episcleral ischemia, severe iritis and lens opacity.

REFERENCES

1. Smolin, Thoft's. The cornea, Scientific foundations and Clinical Practice, 4th ed. In: Foster CS, Azar DT, Dohlman CH (eds). Lippincott Williams and Wilkins Pfister RR Chemical trauma 2005;781–796.
2. Ralph RA. Chemical burns of the eye. In: Duane TD, Jaeger EA, eds. *Clinical Ophthalmology*. Philadelphia, Pa: Harper and Row; 1987:4.
3. Roper Hall MJ. Thermal and chemical burns: Trans Ophthalmol Soc UK 1965;85:631–53.
4. Wagoner MD. Chemical injuries of the eye: Current Concepts in Pathophysiology and Therapy. Surv Ophthalmol 1997;41(4):275–313.
5. Dua HS, King AJ, Joseph A. A new classification of ocular surface burns. Br J Ophthalmol 2001;85:1379–83.
6. Pfister DR, Pfister RR. Acid Injuries of the Eye. In: Krachmer JH, Mannis MJ, Holland EJ. Cornea 2nd edn Elsevier; Mosby 2005;1277–84.

Investigational Tools in Ocular Trauma

4

• Reema Bansal • Vishali Gupta

4.1 RADIOLOGICAL INVESTIGATIONS IN OCULAR INJURIES

INTRODUCTION

Accidental injury to the eye is a major public health issue accounting for permanent visual loss and monocular blindness. Severe trauma can present significant emotional challenges in adults and developmental concerns in children especially if a cosmetic defect is present. Prompt diagnosis of ocular injuries coupled with timely treatment can limit the sight-threatening sequelae of ocular trauma and it is possible to obtain a good to excellent visual result even with serious injuries.

The injury may involve lids, lacrimal apparatus, bony orbit, the adjacent structures, eyeball and the visual pathway. The visual loss is pronounced in penetrating injuries of the eye. The cornea bears the main brunt and lacerations of this result in iris prolapse, endophthalmitis and even phthisis bulbi. Lens changes, retinal detachment, macular and optic nerve damage are more common with blunt injury. Vitreous hemorrhage can occur in both penetrating and blunt trauma.

Prior to ordering any radiological imaging, a complete history should be taken and ocular examination performed on all patients presenting with ocular injury. Specific information such as occupation, prior eye trauma, the mechanism of the current injury and whether eye protection was worn at the time of the injury should be obtained. Clinical examination is aimed at looking for direct or indirect evidence of blunt trauma or an open-globe injury. If a globe is ruptured, systemic antibiotics and tetanus prophylaxis should be administered, and further examination should be deferred until surgical exploration can be conducted.

Clinical judgment is critical in deciding the imaging of choice. Frequently, traumatic tissue damage or ocular media opacities such as traumatic cataracts or intraocular hemorrhage prevent adequate direct ophthalmologic evaluation, and the ophthalmologist must rely on available imaging techniques for the detection of intraocular foreign bodies (FBs).[1-6] Radiological investigations help in assessing the anatomy of the injured eye and the surrounding adnexa. Imaging is essential for proper diagnosis and treatment of ocular/orbital trauma. Orbital fractures are often associated with facial injuries. A thorough ophthalmic evaluation is mandatory to detect ocular injuries and to preserve vision. Treatment of patients with ocular trauma and suspected intraocular foreign bodies (IOFBs) require an accurate and reliable determination of the number and location of FBs before surgery. Failure to recognize a retained IOFB may lead to a fulminant infection or inflammatory endophthalmitis, with ultimate loss of sight or the eye itself.[7-9] If the ocular media are clear, an ophthalmologist may examine the globe and indirect ophthalmoscopy is certainly a very important examination to visualize the FBs and also post-segment evaluation; however in many cases of ocular trauma, having a compromised media transparency radiologic imaging[10] and ultrasonography (USG) are the only options.

Once a complete ophthalmic examination has been performed, selected studies such as plain film radiography, computed tomography (CT) or magnetic

16

resonance imaging (MRI) can be ordered with defined parameters to provide meaningful results.

PLAIN FILM RADIOGRAPHY (ROENTGENOGRAPHY)

Although they have been largely replaced by the CT scans, plain radiographs are still valuable for orbital fracture and IOFBs, especially in settings where more advanced imaging modalities are not available. Plain films are relatively inexpensive and almost universally available. However, soft-tissue definition is poor. The standard projections for orbital evaluation are anteroposterior (AP) occipitofrontal (Caldwell's view), lateral-occipito-oral (Waters' view) and oblique views. The Caldwell's view provides a view of the size and shape of the orbit, the orbit floor, zygomaticofrontal suture and lamina papyracea. The lateral view demonstrates the sella turcica, anterior and posterior clinoids, anterior and posterior walls of the frontal sinus, sphenoid sinus, and nasopharyngeal soft tissues. The Waters's view provides the best projection of the maxillary antra and inferior orbital rim and is particularly useful for evaluating orbital floor blow-out fractures. Oblique views are used to assess the shape and diameter of the optic canal.[11] Plain radiography is a readily available and inexpensive method for primary evaluations of IOFBs and orbital fractures (Figs 4.1.1a to c). It is, however, inadequate for evaluating internal orbital fractures. If plain films reveal an internal orbital fracture that possibly warrants surgical intervention, then CT scans should be obtained. The fracture can then be fully evaluated for surgical treatment planning.

Localization of FBs is unreliable with plain films alone. Nonmetallic, radiolucent FBs, such as wood, plastic, or glass, are not easily seen on plain X-ray films and may be missed. Suturing a limbal ring to the eye and repeating AP and lateral views is an effective means of localizing the position of an FB within the globe.[12] When there are multiple radiopaque FBs such as in wind-screen injuries, plain films permit a rapid assessment of the number and shape of the objects.

COMPUTED TOMOGRAPHY

CT scans have become the standard of care in evaluating traumatized eye and the orbit.[13] Non-contrasted CT is the primary imaging modality currently used for evaluating blunt or penetrating ocular injuries, as well as for localizing most orbital FBs.[14] Current generation CT machines can detect nonmetallic radiolucent FBs 1 mm in size. CT allows excellent visualization of orbital soft tissues and permits simultaneous assessment of the cranial vault and brain. A CT image is a mathematical reconstruction of data obtained from multiple radiographic projections of an object. The basic principle of the CT scan involves an X-ray source and an array of detectors mounted in a gantry. The CT study ideally includes both axial and coronal sections. For coronal sections, the patient must either be in a prone position with the head resting on the chin or in supine position with the head extended back on the vertex. Coronal scans offer improved resolution. Direct coronal scans are particularly useful to evaluate the orbital roof, orbital floor and superior and inferior rectus muscles[15] (Figs 4.1.2 a to c). Axial images provide good cross-sectional anatomical views of the orbit, globe and the skull (Fig. 4.1.2d). Axial sections of the orbit should be no greater than 1.5 mm apart and in the case of a suspected small FB, overlapping slices may be requested. Modern CT scanners have a

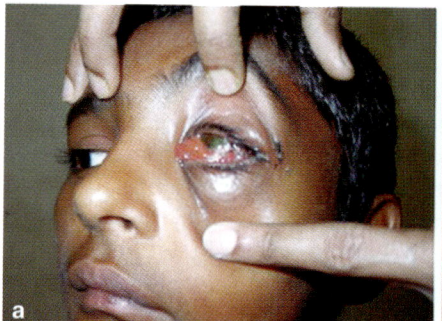
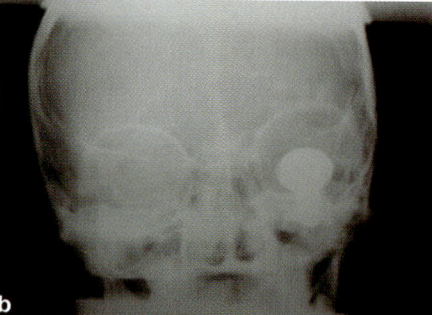
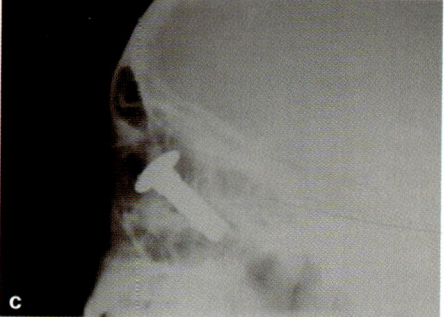

Figs 4.1.1a to c: (a) Severe lid edema and conjunctival chemosis after an iron screw perforated the left eye; (b) The iron nail seen as a radio-opaque shadow in the left orbit in the posteroanterior view of the plain skull radiograph; (c) Lateral view of the plain skull radiograph of the same eye shows anteroposterior extent of the foreign body

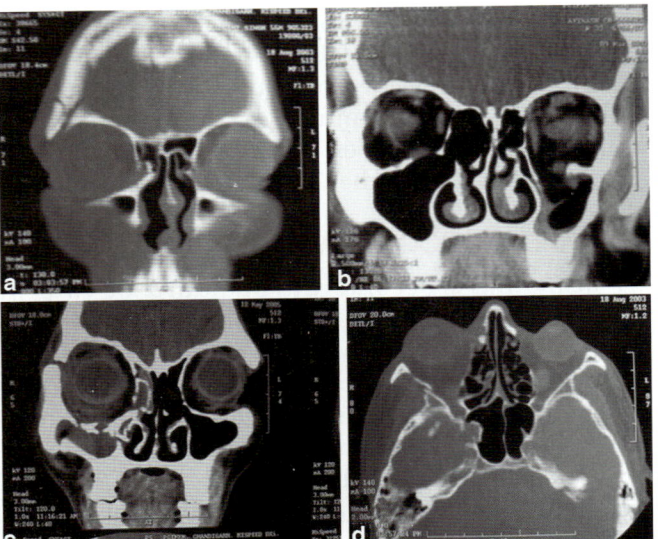

Figs 4.1.2a to d: (a) Coronal view of the CT scan showing right lateral orbital wall fracture after a road-side accident in a patient, (b) Coronal view of the CT scan showing left inferior orbital wall fracture with herniation of orbital fat into the maxillary sinus in another patient after a road-side accident, (c) Coronal view of the CT scan showing multiple fractures of the right orbital walls after a road-side accident in another patient, (d) Axial view of the same patient as shown in Fig. 4.1.2a, showing overriding of the bony fragments of fractured right lateral orbital wall

fixed array of detectors with a rapidly moving source, permitting decreased scan times and higher spatial resolutions. Relatively new scanners move the patient through the gantry continuously at the rate of one slice thickness per revolution of the X-ray source. This is called a helical or spiral CT; scan time is shortened further and patient movement artifact is limited.[16-18] Bone-free projections are used to detect small radiolucent FBs.

CT scans adequately assess lens dislocation, vitreous hemorrhage, ruptured globe, retrobulbar hemorrhage, or avulsion of the optic nerve. CT is the imaging of choice in localizing metallic and most nonmetallic FBs in relation to the globe, muscular cone, and the optic nerve.[19,20] The location and extent of any subperiosteal hematoma formation, with possible mass effects, can also be adequately assessed with CT imaging.

CT is not sensitive enough to be solely relied upon for diagnosis of all open globe injuries.[21,22] The sensitivity and specificity of CT in the detection of open globe injury are 73% and 95%, respectively.[21]

Some typical CT findings suggesting open-globe injuries are intraocular air, loss of eyewall contour, IOFB or intraocular hemorrhage. However, no conclusion regarding the existence of perforating ocular injury should ever be drawn based on CT alone. The ophthalmologists should be warned against considering the CT as a gold standard in the diagnosis of ocular perforation. The other disadvantages of CT scan include artifact formation with metallic foreign material and bone artifact at the skull base, which limits visualization. Patients experience difficulty in positioning themselves comfortably for direct coronal imaging. Thus, CT scan is difficult in cases who are restless and cannot maintain steady posture. Also, CT scan can miss wooden FBs.

CT has been used in the detection and localization of IOFBs since 1977.[23] Overtime, conventional CT technology has evolved from axial to helical CT. Helical CT offers the advantage of continuous imaging in one plane with no time gap in image acquisition, reduced motion artifacts, a decreased radiation dose to the lens, and the ability to obtain multiplanar reconstructions without additional scanning.[1,2] Of the imaging modalities currently available, helical CT is considered the most sensitive method overall for the detection of IOFBs. Computer-generated three-dimensional CT is usually available in most hospitals; it is fast and less expensive than MRI.

MAGNETIC RESONANCE IMAGING

Magnetic resonance imaging (MRI) demonstrates superior visualization of the optic nerve, intracranial injuries and wooden FBs. The principle of MRI is that the nuclei of certain atoms become aligned when placed in a magnetic field.

MRI can be useful in the setting of orbital trauma to assess soft tissue injury or entrapment of extraocular muscles. Standard radiographs or CT scans should be obtained before MRI is performed on patients with suspected intraocular or intraorbital ferromagnetic bodies because of the potential for displacement of the metallic fragments, resulting in further significant ocular or brain injury.[24,25] The most common of these images are the T1-weighted, T2-weighted, and proton density-weighted. The parameters used to produce a T1-weighted image result in a characteristic appearance of ocular structures. The views produced with an MRI scan are similar to those produced by CT. There are axial and coronal images, and sagittal images are also produced. Unlike CT, though, the coronal and sagittal images are always reconstructions.

MRI can detect a wide variety of vegetable, plastic, glass, and radiolucent FBs in the eye. If the history or clinical examination indicates that fragments of wood may have penetrated the orbit or globe, then an MRI should be ordered. It has certain advantages, such as the ability to generate axial, coronal, and sagittal views simultaneously (eliminating the need for patient repositioning), an image quality superior to that provided by CT for soft tissues and nonmagnetic IOFBs (wood, glass), and its availability for pregnant patients. However, MRI is not useful, and is potentially harmful, in identifying magnetic FBs and may not be readily available preoperatively. MRI does not provide good visualization of bone detail, and thus is not helpful in the setting of fractures. It is expensive and requires longer scanning times. Also, MRI may be difficult to perform emergently.

ULTRASONOGRAPHY

Ultrasound is defined as sound frequency greater than 20 kHz. When an electrical potential is applied across the crystal, the crystal is mechanically deformed, and an ultrasonic pulse is emitted. The echoes can be displayed in two formats: amplitude (A) or brightness (B) modulation. Amplitude modulation, or A-scan, displays a series of spikes along a baseline. The height of the spikes correlates with the density of the structure displayed, whereas the distance between spikes corresponds to the distance between structures. This modality is useful in the measurements of intraocular length for intraocular lens calculations and in diagnosis of intraocular and intraorbital tumors. The usefulness of the A-scan in the evaluation of ocular injuries is, therefore, limited. Brightness modulation or B-scan, is a two dimensional representation of the eye and orbit.[26] This permits a rapid assessment of location, size, and configuration of any abnormal structures within the globe or orbit by changing the orientation of the ultrasound probe, thus providing the maximum amount of information. B-scan can be an invaluable tool in the diagnosis and evaluation of ocular injuries. It is the only imaging modality in which the ophthalmologist controls the access to and quality of the study.

In ocular injuries, USG is useful to assess the posterior segment when visualization is limited by anterior segment pathology such as hyphema, traumatic cataract, and corneal edema. It is reliable in detecting retinal detachment, radio-opaque as well as radiolucent IOFB (Figs 4.1.3a to e), posterior perforation, vitreous incarceration, choroidal detachment (serous or hemorrhagic), vitreous hemorrhage, posterior vitreous separation, retinal tears and areas of vitreoretinal adhesion and scleral ruptures. This imaging should be done only if an open globe injury is ruled out or has been repaired primarily. It is less expensive than CT scan and allows outstanding resolution with real-time images of the eye and to a lesser extent, the orbit.

Ultrasound has several advantages over CT scan and MRI. Multiple cross-sectional and radial cuts of the eye can be rapidly obtained at the bedside or in an operating room because of its transportable equipment. It is less expensive than CT and MRI. It is the preferred modality for following the clinical course of conditions like choroidal detachment resolution, membrane or retinal detachment development. However, certain disadvantages are associated with its use in ocular injuries. Ruptured globe is a relative contraindication. Ocular ultrasound may be difficult to do immediately in cases with lid injuries and cases with severe pain in eyes. It is not useful in diagnosing orbital fractures, and requires training and skill. The site and size on an IOFB may pose a challenge sometimes. Nevertheless, it is a useful diagnostic tool when media opacities preclude using standard means to view the ocular structures and is especially helpful when used in conjunction with other imaging modalities. USG is discussed in subsequent pages (Ch 4.2).

ULTRASOUND BIOMICROSCOPY

Posterior segment FBs are detected by clinical examination and imaging techniques such as CT scan and low-frequency (5–10 MHz) USG.[27-29] However, accurate localization of anterior segment IOFBs is difficult when conventional imaging techniques are employed.[30] Ultrasound biomicroscopy (UBM) is a high-frequency (50 MHz), high-resolution imaging technique that offers cross-sectional images of the anterior segment to a depth of 5 mm.[31-33] Frequencies of 35 MHz and above provide over a threefold improvement in resolution compared with conventional ophthalmic ultrasound systems. UBM allows imaging of anatomy and pathology involving the anterior segment, including regions obscured by

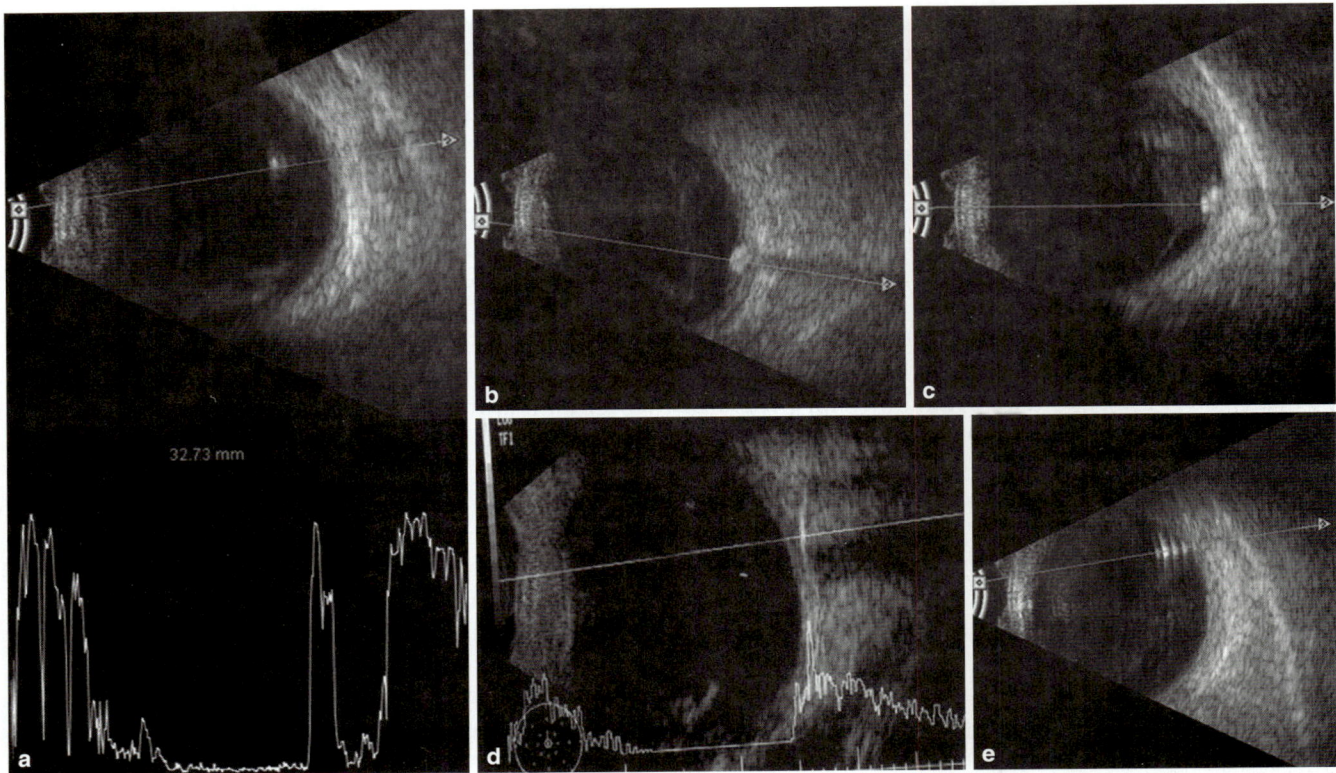

Figs 4.1.3a to e: (a) Ultrasound of the left eye showing an intraocular foreign body in the posterior vitreous with mild vitreous hemorrhage inferiorly, (b) Ultrasound of the right eye showing an intraocular foreign body lying on the retina, (c) Ultrasound of the left eye showing an intraocular foreign body lying on the retina with dense vitreous hemorrhage, (d) Ultrasound of the eye showing an intraocular foreign body within the optic nerve, (e) Ultrasound of the right eye showing a glass foreign body in the posterior vitreous. The ultrasound waves must strike the glass foreign body perpendicular to the long flat surface to produce dense echogenic shadow. If the waves strike obliquely, most sound reflects away resulting in a weak echo. A glass foreign body may easily be missed on the ultrasound

overlying optically opaque anatomic or pathologic structures. Besides providing useful information in conditions such as glaucoma, cysts and neoplasms, UBM provides diagnostically significant information in trauma and FBs (UBM is discussed in details in subsequent pages). The role of UBM in biometric information regarding anterior segment structures, including the cornea and its constituent layers and the anterior and posterior chambers is well known.[34]

Conventional USG is a valuable imaging modality in evaluating injured eyes in that it not only detects and localizes IOFBs of the posterior segment, but is also useful in demonstrating associated posterior ocular damage as highlighted above.[29] However, B-scan ultrasound cannot be used to assess anterior segment structures as its resolution is not sufficiently high.[30] CT can detect IOFBs about 1 mm in size but its

use is constrained by eye movements and the poor quality of reconstructed computer images.[35] Clinical detection of ocular FBs after trauma can be hindered by small size, haziness of the optical media, poor patient cooperation, or hidden location. UBM is a valuable adjunct in the evaluation of suspected ocular FBs, especially in cases involving small, nonmetallic objects[36,37] (Fig. 4.1.4) especially in the angle.

Recently, UBM has been used to identify and localize a cyclodialysis cleft when direct visualization is difficult.[38,39] The sequelae of cyclodialysis include shallow anterior chamber, cataract, retinal and choroidal folds, hypotonous maculopathy, and loss of vision in cases of prolonged hypotony. UBM has been used for cleft identification, localization, and measurement. While gonioscopy allows evaluation from the anterior face of the ciliary cleft only, UBM

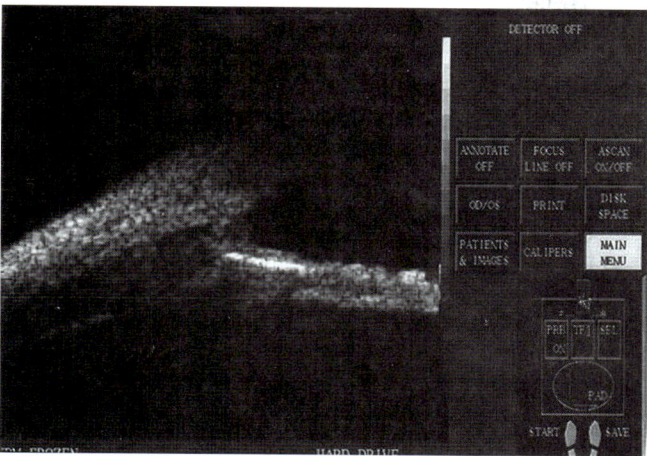

Fig. 4.1.4: Ultrasound biomicroscope of the right eye of a patient after trauma showing a metallic foreign body in the iris stroma

provides cross-sectional information on the iridocorneal angle. In addition, it can easily picture a cyclodialysis when direct communication between the anterior chamber and the supraciliary space is present owing to the contrasting reflectivity of the aqueous and the adjacent tissue. UBM is also particularly useful during follow-up.

Although UBM has now been in use for over 15 years, new technologies, including transducer arrays, pulse encoding and combination of ultrasound with light, offer the potential for significant advances in high-resolution diagnostic imaging of the eye.

UBM is discussed more in subsequent pages (Ch 4.5).

SUMMARY

Preoperative information is vital to critical decision-making. Though X-ray is still a mandatory investigation for medicolegal purposes but it does not give details of ocular and orbital injuries. Whereas ultrasound proves to be a handy bedside imaging tool for providing accurate information about ocular injury, CT scan is a must for orbital wall and orbital injuries. It provides accurate information about injury, delineates extent and severity of associated bony injuries and precisely localizes FBs like splinters and bullets. CT scan assumes greater role in evaluation of these injuries as MRI is contraindicated in localizing metallic IOFB because the magnetic field produced during scanning can cause the FBs to become high velocity intraocular projectiles with catastrophic ocular effects.

CT is a useful imaging option that can aid in the thorough clinical ocular examination. When available, spiral CT scanning utilizing 3 mm axial and coronal cuts through the orbit should be obtained as a first-line study; conventional CT scanning with 3 mm cuts is an acceptable alternative. Plain film X-rays and B-scan USG are convenient to obtain and may be used as adjuncts to CT scanning, but are generally less sensitive and so "negative" results should be interpreted with caution. Software is now available for reconstruction of three-dimensional images of the entire skull. Although not useful in every case, these images can be useful in the reconstruction of severe orbital trauma.

The effects of injuries to eye are much more serious than in any other part of the body, partly because of delicacy of ocular tissues and partly because a trauma which elsewhere would cause little temporary inconvenience, can rapidly result in permanent blindness. Successful management of ocular injuries depends on teamwork of ophthalmologist as well as the radiologist at the primary level. Penetrating ocular injuries are serious and pose a threat to permanent loss of sight. B-scan USG and CT scan are additive to each other for knowing the site, extent and nature of trauma.

REFERENCES

1. Latkis A, Prokesch R, Scholda C, et al. Orbital computed tomography in the diagnosis and management of eye trauma. Ophthalmology 1999;106:2330–5.
2. Latkis A, Steiner E, Scholda C, et al. Evaluation of intraocular foreign bodies by spiral computed tomography and multiplanar reconstruction. Ophthalmology 1998;105:307–12.
3. Gaster RN, Duda EE. Localization of intraocular foreign bodies by computed tomography. Ophthalmic Surg 1980;11:25–9.
4. Kollarits CR, Chiro DG, Christiansen J, et al. Detection of orbital and intraocular foreign bodies by computed tomography. Ophthalmic Surg 1977;8:45–53.
5. Chacko JG, Figueroa RE, Johnson MH, et al. Detection and localization of steel intraocular foreign bodies using computed tomography. Ophthalmology 1997;104:319–23.
6. Tate E, Cupples H. Detection of orbital foreign bodies with computed tomography: current limits. AJNR 1981;2:363–5.
7. Deramo VA, Shah GK, Baumal CR, et al. Ultrasound biomicroscopy as a tool for detecting and localizing occult foreign bodies after ocular trauma. Ophthalmology 1999;106:301–5.
8. Jonas JB, Knorr HL, Budde WM. Prognostic factors in ocular injuries caused by intraocular or retrobulbar foreign bodies. Ophthalmology 2000;107:823–8.

9. Thompson JT, Parver LM, Enger CL, et al. Infectious endophthalmitis after penetrating injuries with retained intraocular foreign bodies: National Eye Trauma System. Ophthalmology 1993;100:1468–74.

10. Lindahl S. Computed tomography of intraorbital foreign bodies. Acta Radiol 1987;28:235–40.

11. Weber AL. Imaging techniques and normal radiographic anatomy. In: Albert DM, ed. Principles and Practice of Ophthalmology. Philadelphia, Pa: WB Saunders Company; 1994:5:3505–10.

12. Moseley L. The orbit and eye. In: Sutton D, ed. A Textbook of Radiology and Imaging. London, England: Churchill Livingstone; 1993;2:1287–1309.

13. Coleman DJ, Rondeau MJ. Diagnostic imaging of ocular and orbital trauma. In: Shingleton BJ, Hersh PS, Kenyon KR, eds. Eye Trauma. St Louis: Mosby-Year Book, 1991;25–40.

14. Kelly JK, Lazo A, Metes JJ. Radiology of orbital trauma. In: Spoor TC, Nesi FA, eds. Management of ocular, orbital and adnexal trauma. New York: Raven Press; 1988;247–68.

15. Koornneef L, Zonneveld F. The role of direct multiplanar high resolution CT in the assessment and management of orbital trauma. Radiol Clin North Am 1987;25:753–66.

16. Wiesen EJ, Miraldi F. Imaging principles in computed tomography. In: Haaga JR, ed. Computed Tomography and Magnetic Resonance Imaging of the Whole Body. St Louis, Mo: Mosby; 1994;1:3–25.

17. Chacko JG, Figueroa RE, Johnson MH, Marcus DM, Brooks SE. Detection and localization of steel intraocular foreign bodies using computed tomography: A comparison of helical and conventional axial scanning. Ophthalmology 1997;104:319–23.

18. Lakits A, Prokesch R, Scholda C, Bankier A, Weninger F, Imhof H. Multiplanar imaging in the preoperative assessment of metallic intraocular foreign bodies: Helical computed tomography versus conventional computed tomography. Ophthalmology 1998;105:1679–85.

19. Kelly JK, Lazo A, Metes JJ. Radiology of orbital trauma. In: Spoor TC, Nesi FA, eds. Management of ocular, orbital and adnexal trauma. New York: Raven Press; 1988;247–68.

20. Lindahl S. Computed tomography of intraorbital foreign bodies. Acta Radiol 1987; 28:235–40.

21. Joseph DP, Pieramici DJ, Beauchamp NJ. Computed tomography (CT) in the diagnosis and prognosis of open-globe injuries. Ophthalmology 2000;107:1899–1906.

22. Pikkel J, Beiran I, Ophir A, Miller B. Computed tomography: Not an ophthalmic polygraph. IMAJ 2004;6:63.

23. Topilow HW, Ackerman AL, Zimmerman RD. Limitations of computed tomography in the localization of intra-ocular foreign bodies. Ophthalmology 1984;91:1086–91.

24. Kelly WM, Paglen PG, Pearson JA, et al. Ferromagnetism of intraocular foreign body causes unilateral blindness after MR study. Am J Neuroradiol 1986;7:243–5.

25. Otto PM, Otto RA, Virapongse C, et al. Screening test for detection of metallic foreign objects in the orbit before magnetic resonance imaging. Invest Radiol 1992;27:308–11.

26. Puodziuviene E, Paunksnis A, Kurapkiene S, Imbrasiene D. Ultrasound value in diagnosis, management and prognosis of severe eye injuries. ISSN 2005;3(56):1392–2114.

27. Coleman DJ, Rondeau MJ. Diagnostic imaging of ocular and orbital trauma. In: Shingleton BJ, Herssh PS, Kenyon KR, eds. Eye Trauma. St Louis: Mosby-Year Book, 1991;25–40.

28. Coleman DJ. Reliability of ocular and orbital diagnosis with B-scan ultrasound. 2. Orbital diagnosis. Am J Ophthalmol 1972;74:704–18.

29. Das T, Namperumalsamy P. Ultrasound in ocular trauma. Indian J Ophthalmol 1987;35:121–5.

30. Nouby-Mahmoud G, Silverman RH, Coleman DJ. Using high-frequency ultrasound to characterize intraocular foreign bodies. Ophthalmic Surg 1993;24:94–9.

31. Pavlin CJ, Harasiewicz K, Sherar MD, Foster FS. Clinical use of ultrasound biomicroscopy. Ophthalmology 1991;98:287–95.

32. Deramo VA, Shah GK, Baumal CR, Fineman MS, Correa ZM, Benson WE, et al. Ultrasound biomicroscopy as a tool for detecting and localizing occult foreign bodies after ocular trauma. Ophthalmology 1999;106:301–5.

33. Looi ALG, Gazzard G, Tan DTH. Surgical exploration minimised by ultrasound biomicroscopy localization of intraocular foreign body. Eye 2001;2:234–5.

34. Silverman RH. High-resolution imaging of the eye- a review. Clin Experiment Ophthalmol 2009;37:54–67.

35. Topilow HW, Ackerman AL, Zimmerman RD. Limitations of computerised tomography in the localisation of intraocular foreign bodies. Ophthalmology 1984;91:1086–91.

36. Guha S, Bhende M, Baskaran M, Sharma T. Role of ultrasound biomicroscopy in the detection and localization of anterior segment foreign bodies. Ann Acad Med Singapore 2006;35:536–40.

37. Deramo VA, Shah GK, Baumal CR, fineman MS, Correa ZM, Benson WE, Rapuano CJ, Cohen EJ, Augsburger JJ. Ultrasound biomicroscopy as a tool for detecting and localizing occult foreign bodies after ocular trauma. Ophthalmology 1999;106:301–5.

38. Bhende M, Lekha T, Vijaya L, Gopal L, Sharma T, Parikh S. Ultrasound biomicroscopy in the diagnosis and management of cyclodialysis clefts. Indian J Ophthalmol 1999;47:19–23.

39. Malandrini A, Balestrazzi A, Martone G, Tosi GM, Caporossi A. Diagnosis and management of cyclodialysis cleft. J Cataract Refract Surg 2008;34:1213–6.

4.2 ULTRASONOGRAPHY IN OPHTHALMIC TRAUMA

• Sushil Kumar • Ruchi Goel

INTRODUCTION

Ophthalmic injuries presenting as oculo-orbital trauma may be the result of traffic accident, industrial mishaps, sports injury, etc. Ocular involvement may occur alone or as a part of polytrauma with faciomaxillary and head injury. Initial emergency management aims at stabilization of the general condition of the patient. A complete radiological work-up comprising of plain X-rays, CT scan and even MRI is then carried out to assess the orbital and globe injuries. Bony injuries and radio-opaque foreign bodies are best evaluated on CT scan. For assessment of structural damage to the eyeball, echography has a significant role. It is of particular value when the light conducting media are opacified and direct visualization by ophthalmoscopy is difficult or impossible.[1] Initially, echography may be difficult to perform due to an open globe injury, massive lid edema and pain. An open globe needs to be repaired before an echographic examination is performed to avoid fallacious results and the risk of introduction of infection. Different types of trauma result in different pathological changes in the globe as well as the orbital cavity.

CLOSED GLOBE INJURY

Even a trivial trauma can result in severe structural damage therefore, a thorough evaluation of both the anterior and posterior segment is mandatory. Zone I and some of the zone II injuries are better evaluated by slit lamp examination.

In the anterior segment, one needs to look for hyphema, iridodialysis or lens status that is whether displaced or cataractous following capsular rupture. For anterior segment evaluation, *immersion scan* (B-scan with scleral cup) or ultrasound biomicroscopy (UBM) is required. Sometimes, an experienced echographer may be able to opine with high frequency B-scan probe applied over the closed lids.

Hyphema is seen as a blood clot in the anterior chamber. The anterior chamber becomes abnormally deep in cases with posterior displacement of lens or may be obliterated due to anteriorly displaced lens. A clear lens, normally is seen with anterior and posterior borders with minimal or low reflectivity. A dense cataractous lens shows high reflectivity internal echospikes.[2]

In the posterior segment, one must look for the following:
- Vitreous hemorrhage
- Retinal tears/dialysis/detachment
- Retinochoroidal layer edema/hemorrhage
- Posteriorly displaced crystalline lens/intraocular lens.

Vitreous hemorrhage may be mild, moderate or severe quantitatively and localized to the core of the vitreous body with or without posterior vitreous detachment (PVD). PVD may be stained with hemorrhage especially if there is pre-retinal hemorrhage or subhyaloid hemorrhage (Figs 4.2.1 to 4.2.3). Mild trickle of hemorrhage into the vitreous cavity, if traced may lead the examiner to the site of either retinal break. When the retinal break is big (dialysis), one usually encounters retinal detachment of the peripheral retina (Fig. 4.2.4).

Retinal detachment (RD) on B-scan is seen as lifted retina from the choroidoscleral complex but shows attachment at the optic nerve head (Figs 4.2.5 and 4.2.6). RD may co-exist with total PVD with blood staining and organized vitreous hemorrhage.

In old cases of vitreous hemorrhage, there may be vitreous membrane formation after the hemorrhage organizes and it may exert traction on the retina to produce tractional retinal detachment. Sometimes, following absorption of vitreous hemorrhage, a few debri dots along with a thickened retinochoroidal layer is the only tell tale sign.

OPEN GLOBE INJURIES

These injuries are associated with marked disruption and/or distortion of normal eye structures.

The spectra of findings in the *anterior segment* include:
- Hyphema
- Traumatic cataract
- Foreign body like a glass piece embedded in the lens (Fig. 4.2.7)

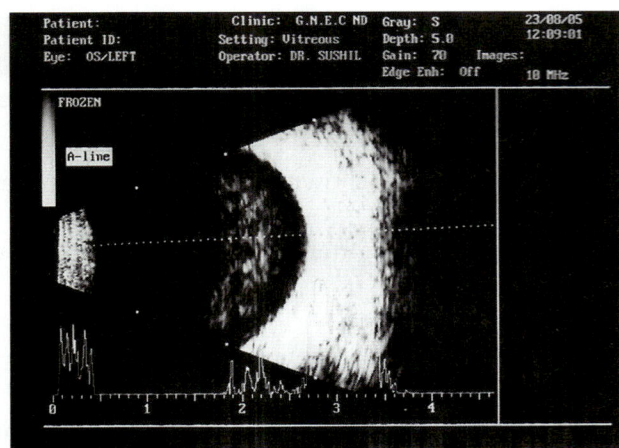

Fig. 4.2.1: Vitreous hemorrhage in posterior one-thirds of vitreous cavity with clear retrovitreal space

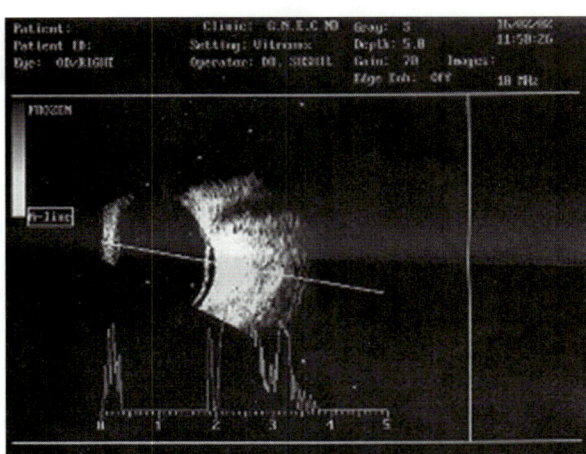

Fig. 4.2.4: Shallow retinal detachment

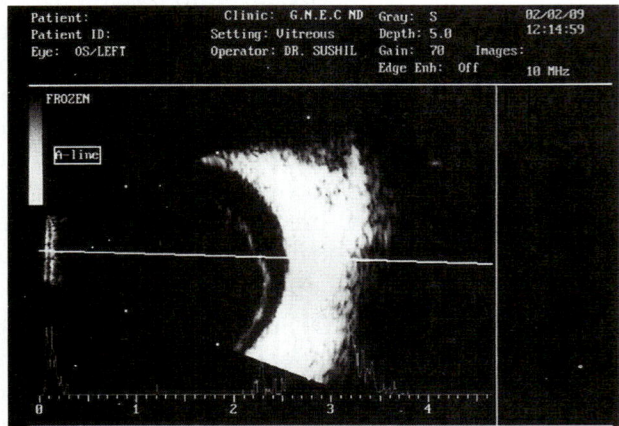

Fig. 4.2.2: Vitreous hemorrhage with blood staining of posterior vitreous detachment

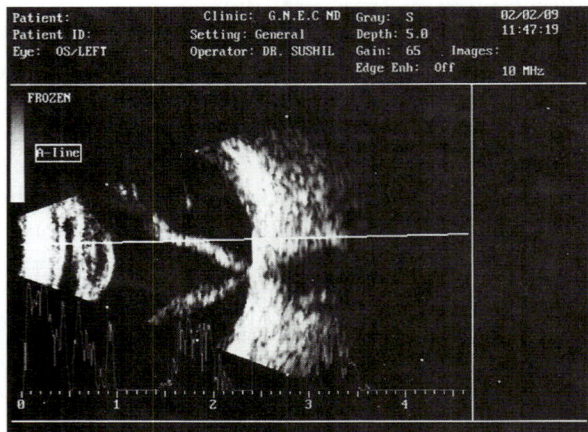

Fig. 4.2.5: Old retinal detachment with attachment at optic nerve head

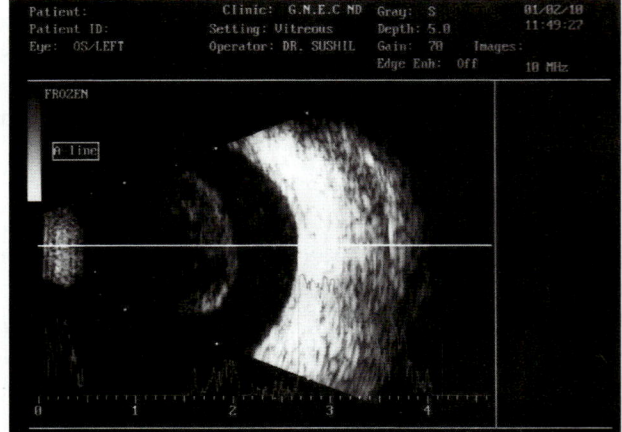

Fig. 4.2.3: Vitreous hemorrhage with blood stained posterior vitreous detachment with blood in preretinal area

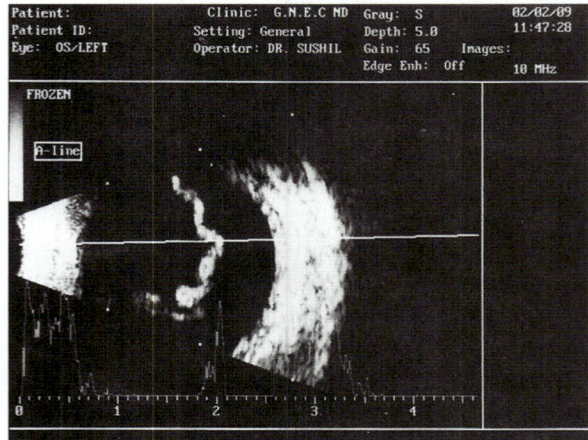

Fig. 4.2.6: Old retinal detachment with convolutions

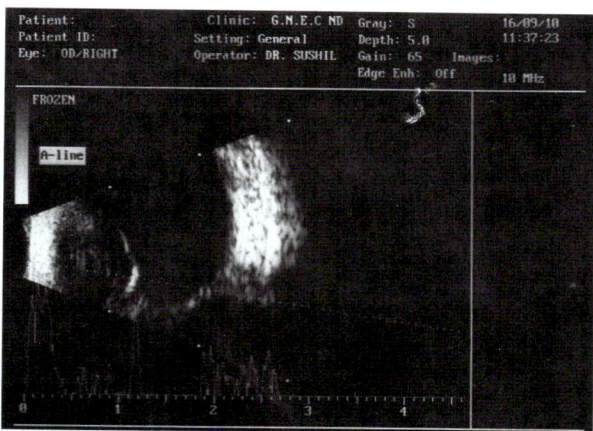

Fig. 4.2.7: Intralenticular foreign body

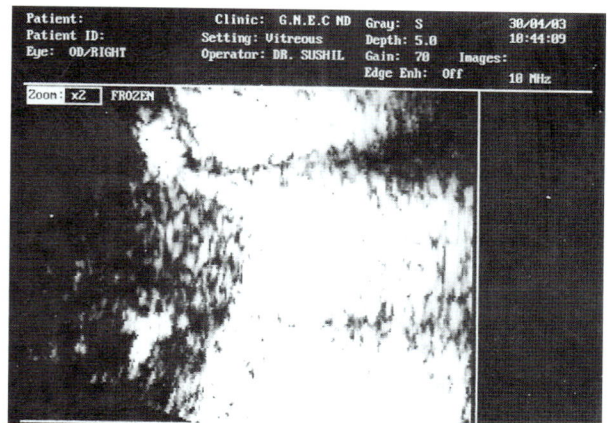

Fig. 4.2.8: Track leading to site of scleral rupture

- Ciliochoroidal effusion/hemorrhage
- Posterior capsular rupture (better picked up on UBM).

Posterior segment may demonstrate
- Vitreous hemorrhage with or without posterior vitreous detachment
- Posterior scleral rupture
- Retinal detachment
- Hemorrhagic choroidal detachment
- Scleral folds
- Intraocular FBs of different types.

Posterior scleral rupture varies in size widely. If the rupture is large, then the globe shall be soft on digital palpation and the vitreous cavity will be full of hemorrhage. There may be a co-existing RD or a posteriorly displaced crystalline lens. Diagnosis of smaller ruptures is difficult both clinically as well as on echography. Indirect indicators that can be picked up on B-scan are as follows:
- Trickle of hemorrhage from the outer coat into the vitreous cavity (Fig. 4.2.8)
- Organized hemorrhage over the retina or a localized thickening of the retina
- Incarcerated vitreous band into the rupture site producing traction
- Hemorrhage in the immediate episcleral space.

Vitreous hemorrhage seen in penetrating trauma is seen as a hemorrhagic track through the vitreous cavity if the injury is with a sharp object like needle, nail, pointed pencil or pen nib. This track may end in the vitreous body or extend further to the site of scleral rupture or IOFB. A proper alignment of probe is critical to demonstrate this (Fig. 4.2.9).

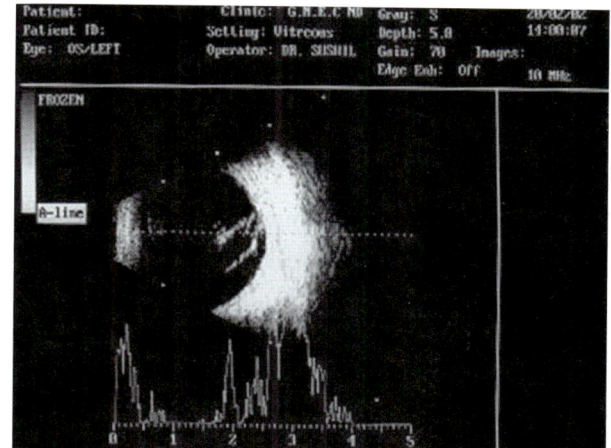

Fig. 4.2.9: Scleral dehiscence with "T" sign with vitreous hemorrhage following perforating injury of the globe

Traumatic retinal detachment may occur immediately following injury or develop later on. Late RD is usually the result of vitreous traction on the retina. There may also be incarceration of retina in the scleral rupture site. Subretinal hemorrhage is usually seen in very severe injuries.

Choroidal hemorrhage with or without detachment is seen with bigger scleral lacerations/dehiscence as discontinuity in the outer coat. Hemorrhagic choroidal detachment may be dome shaped or flat surfaced and these may extend posterior to the equator up to the optic nerve head. If the eye is aphakic, the hemorrhagic choroidal detachment may be highly elevated and appear to "kiss" centrally (Fig. 4.2.10). The presence of choroidal detachments can alter the timing of

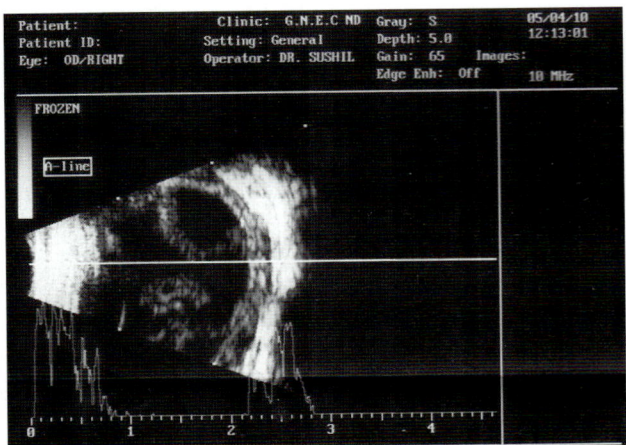

Fig. 4.2.10: Choroidal detachment

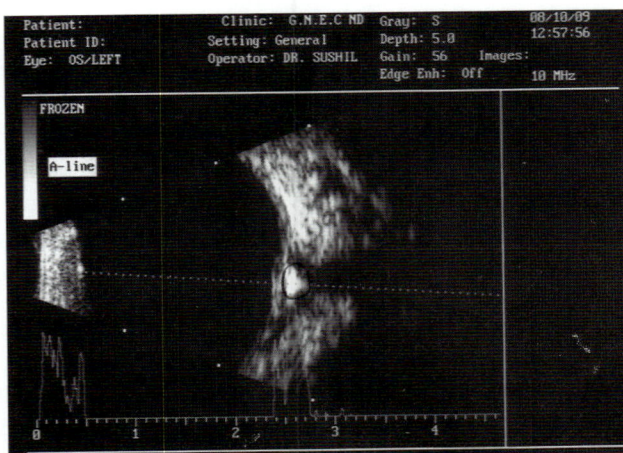

Fig. 4.2.11: Intraretinal foreign body with acoustic shadowing

surgical intervention as well as the surgical approach used in ruptured globes.[3]

Scleral folds if present indicate low intraocular pressure and have to be differentiated from FBs and scleral explants.

Intraocular foreign bodies may be of different nature that is metallic/nonmetallic, glass pieces and organic/vegetable materials. These foreign bodies may be of various shapes and sizes. Radio-opaque FBs can be picked up and localized by X-rays and CT scan but collateral damage is better assessed by echography. USG can pick up even non-radio-opaque FBs. Another merit is the ability to differentiate between intraocular and extraocular FBs when they are located in the vicinity of sclera. In addition, the mobility, magnetic properties and shift in position of the FBs between the time of initial study and the time of surgery can be accurately evaluated. However, this modality does have some limitations. Softer materials, which are only intermediately reflective (wood and vegetative material) are more difficult to detect.[4] Echography also helps in confirming and localizing FBs as small as 0.2 mm.

In general, all FBs are seen as echodense spots with shadowing effect (Fig. 4.2.11) behind them and have 100% reflectivity even on decreasing the overall gain. These echodense spots may be surrounded with organized hemorrhage in fresh cases or fibrosis in old cases. An old forgotten iron FB may be suspected in a patient with signs of siderosis bulbi. The presence of corneal opacity, localized scleral ectasia, iris hole with corresponding area of lens showing cataractous

changes or signs of siderosis should always alert an echographer to look for a FB.

Spherical FBs (e.g. ballistic balls or gun shot pellets) produce very unique and specific multiple signals.[5] It is because of the reverberation occurring due to the return of some sound waves to the probe after striking the foreign body so that reduplication of signals occurs.

In detection of glass FBs, the alignment of sound beam plays an important role. If the sound beam is directed along the long axis of the FB, it may sometimes be missed or may appear very small in size. However, if the beam falls perpendicular to the long axis or flat surface of it, a highly reflective signal is obtained. Similar situation occurs with a dropped intraocular lens (Fig. 4.2.12).

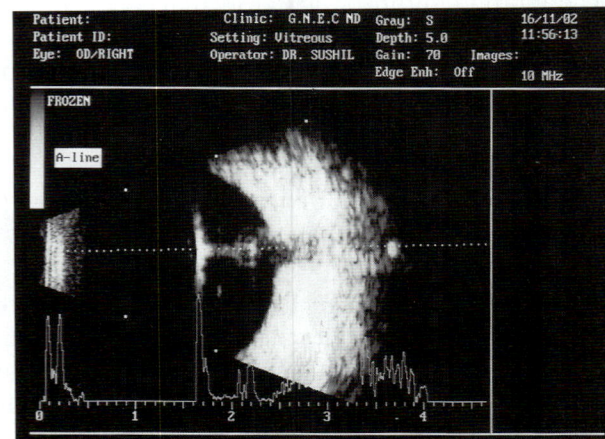

Fig. 4.2.12: Posteriorly dislocated intraocular lens showing 100% reflectivity

Organic/vegetable material as FB can produce variable echoreflectivities, i.e. high reflectivity initially and low reflectivity over passage of time due to its decay. Thus, at times diagnosis of FB becomes difficult and one has to resort to the history and clinical findings.

SURGICAL TRAUMA

B-scan is of immense help in diagnosis and follow-up of surgical complications. *Endophthalmitis* is picked up by seeing multiple vitreous debris or exudation with low reflectivity in the vitreous cavity while the patient presents with severe inflammation clinically. Additional findings seen on B-scan may be posterior vitreous detachment, thickened retinochoroidal layer or sometimes RD.

Vitreous hemorrhage may appear as endophthalmitis on echography but clinically there will be absence of inflammation. Posterior vitreous detachment is more extensive in hemorrhage as compared to endophthalmitis. Organizing hemorrhage with membrane formation is commonly seen in the lower part of vitreous cavity (effect of gravity) whereas organized exudation with membrane formation

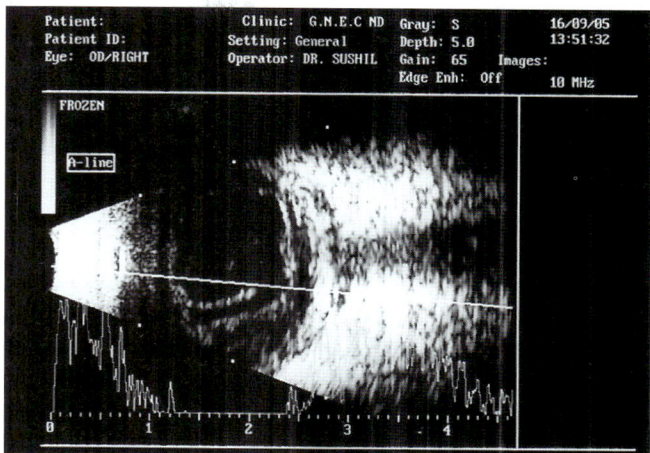

Fig. 4.2.14: Vitreous exudates, membrane formation and "T" sign in endophthalmitis

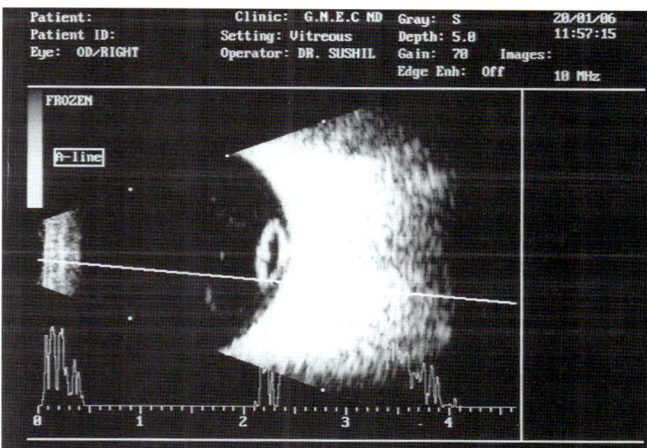

Fig. 4.2.15: Nucleus drop seen on the retinal surface with vitritis

occurs throughout the vitreous cavity in endophthalmitis (Figs 4.2.13 and 4.2.14).

A dropped nucleus may be seen in case of posterior capsular rupture (Fig. 4.2.15).

In *expulsive choroidal hemorrhage* vitreous cavity is full of hemorrhage along with massive subchoroidal hemorrhage producing dome-shaped elevation or detachment. It may involve one or two quadrants of the globe whereas in severe cases there may be a 360° choroidal detachment producing "kissing configuration".

If serial echography is performed in expulsive hemorrhage cases, there is flattening of choroidal detachment domes, the clearing of vitreous hemorrhage and appearance of vitreous debris in its place. There may be peripheral RD as well.

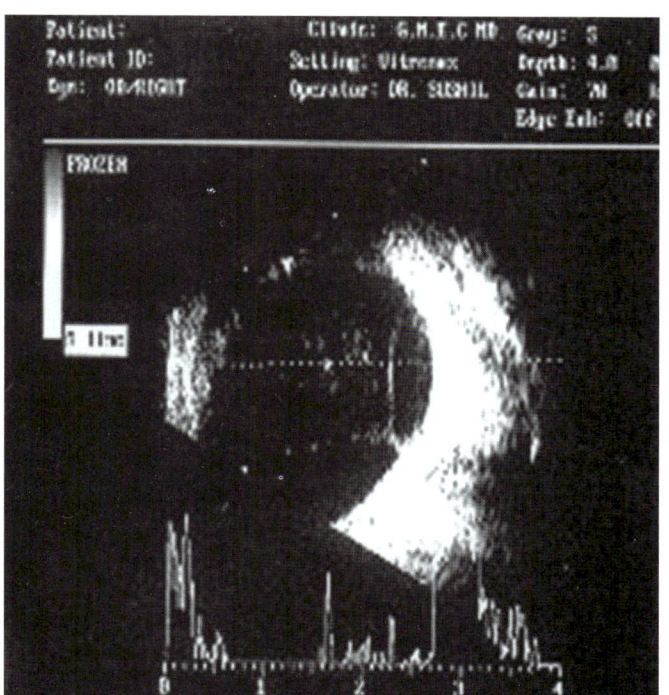

Fig. 4.2.13: Early endophthalmitis with membrane formation and cells in posterior one-third of vitreous cavity

In cases of posterior capsular tear, there can be lens matter/nucleus or even IOL drop into the vitreous cavity. They appear as highly reflective structures, sometimes mobile with surrounding vitritis.

Macular edema if present appears as localized thickening of retino choroidal layer in the region of macula. If the media is clear it is better documented on optical coherence tomography (OCT).

In cases of *sympathetic ophthalmitis*, the injured eye shows echopicture suggestive of vitreous hemorrhage along with RD, PVD and sometimes IOFB; whereas the sympathising eye shows diffuse, low reflective thickening of choroids in the posterior pole region along with shallow RD and vitreous haze.

Phthisis bulbi can occur as an end result of severe damage to the globe and is seen as deshaped globe with low intraocular pressure, thickened retinochoroid with or without calcification and RD (Fig. 4.2.16).

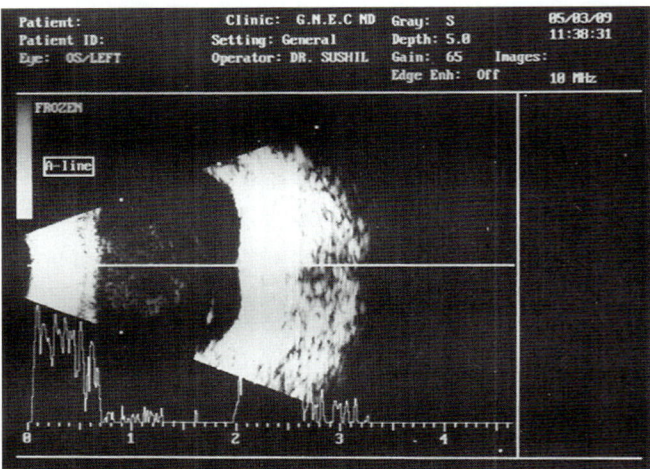

Fig. 4.2.16: Prephthisical eye with small, deshaped globe, thickened retinochoroidal complex and vitreous debri

ORBITAL TRAUMA

The bony orbit is best evaluated radiologically on plain X-ray or CT scan. For soft tissue, MRI scan and B-scan (to a limited extent) are the investigations of choice. Clinical conditions which can be commented upon in the B-scan are as follows:

- Orbital hemorrhage/hematoma
- Orbital cellulitis
- Orbital abcess
- Orbital FB
- Orbital fracture
- Extraocular muscle injury
- Optic nerve trauma.

Orbital hemorrhage/hematoma is seen as diffuse or localized collection. When it is diffuse, there is total obliteration of soft tissue details. When localized, it may be in any surgical space in any of the orbital quadrant. Subperiosteal collections take weeks to months to resolve. It may be difficult to differentiate hematoma from abcess on B-scan however, clinically, in the absence of intervention, hematoma tends to regress whereas an abcess increases with passage of time.

Orbital cellulitis with abscess formation presents as a diffuse swelling of all the soft tissue structures. The normal orbital fat pattern is replaced with widening of spaces and persistent high reflectivity. Any decrease in reflectivity in certain areas of orbit on follow-up may be an early indication of abcess formation.

Orbital abcess may be single or multiloculated. These are seen as echoluscent spots on B-scan and have variable shapes and sizes. Subperiosteal abcesses are very painful and need urgent drainage.

Orbital FBs can be of various types such as glass, metal, stone or vegetative material. These can be detected easily if present in anterior two-thirds of orbital cavity. FBs in the posterior one-third or those near the orbital apex are likely to be missed.

FBs appear as echodense spots with high A-scan reflectivity (Fig. 4.2.17). They may be surrounded with localized hemorrhage or abcess. FBs of vegetative material (wooden splinters) can be picked up easily in

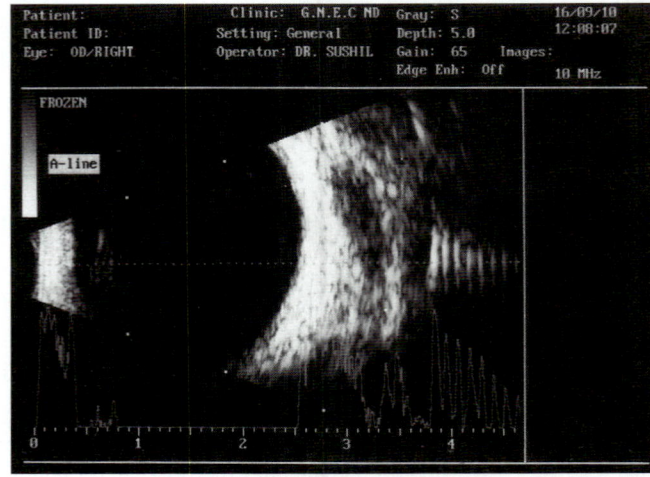

Fig. 4.2.17: Orbital foreign body

the early phase of injury but may go undetected at a later phase due to the process of decay.

Spherical FBs (lead pellets, ballistic balls) are easily picked up because they produce a characteristic chain of multiple signals.

EMPHYSEMA AND ORBITAL FRACTURES

Orbital fractures are best diagnosed on CT scan but with B-scan indirect evidences such as bony fragment appearing as FB surrounded with hematoma, incarceration of orbital soft tissues in the floor of the orbit and subperiosteal hematoma can be picked up. USG is used as intraoperative visualizing tool in all midfacial fractures with displacement of the zygomatic arch.[6] Air can enter the orbit from the paranasal sinuses following fracture of orbital wall and clinically the patient presents with proptosis and crepitus. In closed globe injury, the air bubble in the orbital cavity is seen as echolucent spot with a chain of multiple signals.

Extraocular muscle injuries can occur in the form of muscle sheath hemorrhage, incarceration into the fracture site, avulsion or dislodgement from the globe. The best option for diagnosing such injuries is MRI scan. Only an experienced echographer shall be able to diagnose these in the early phase of trauma.

Optic nerve trauma results in partial or complete avulsion or optic nerve sheath hemorrhage. A complete avulsion is seen as a big hollow echolucent area in the sclera. Partial avulsion or optic nerve sheath hemorrhage is suspected if there is increased optic nerve thickness/widening of optic nerve shadow. MRI and visual-evoked potential (VEP) are valuable in both diagnosis and prognosis of such patients.

To conclude, B-scan with cross vector examination is an extremely useful investigation in all varities of trauma for management, follow-up and prediction of visual prognosis. It also provides quick documentary evidence in medicolegal cases. Road traffic accident is the most common cause of traumatic ocular injury affecting the globe. RD and vitreous hemorrhage are the most frequent injuries to the globe diagnosed by ultrasound scan.[7]

Recently, emergency bedside ultrasound is being used for ruling out and diagnosing ocular pathology in patients presenting to the emergency department.[8] Furthermore, it accurately differentiates between pathology that needs immediate ophthalmologic consultation and that which can be followed up on an outpatient basis.

REFERENCES

1. Fielding J. The assessment of ocular injury by ultrasound. Clinical Radiology 2009;59:301–2.

2. Byrne SF, Green RL. Trauma. Ultrasound of the eye and orbit. Mosby Year book 1992;95–131.

3. Ligget PE, Mani N, Green RL, et al. Management of traumatic rupture of the globe in aphakic patients. Retina 1990;10(suppl 1):59.

4. Chugh JP, Susheel, Verma M. Role of ultrasonography in ocular trauma. Indian J Radiol Imaging 2001;11:75–9.

5. Ossoinig KC, Bigar F, Kaefring SL, et al. Echographic detection and localization of BB shots in the eye and orbit. Bibl Ophthalmol 1975;83:109.

6. Gülicher D, Krimmel M, Reinert S. The role of intra-operative ultrasonography in zygomatic complex fracture repair. International Journal of Oral and Maxillofacial Surgery 2006;35(3):224–30.

7. Eze KC, Enock ME, Eluehike SU. Ultrasonic evaluation of orbito-ocular trauma in Benin-City, Nigeria. Niger Postgrad Med J 2009;16(3):198–202.

8. Blaivas M, Theodoro D, Sierzenski PR. A Study of Bedside Ocular Ultrasonography in the Emergency Department. Academic Emergency Medicine 2002; 9:791–799.

4.3 OPTICAL COHERENCE TOMOGRAPHY IN POSTERIOR SEGMENT TRAUMA

• DK Mehta • Deepender Chouhan

INTRODUCTION

Visual prognosis in trauma cases is strongly related to the posterior segment status. Documenting such clinical findings helps not only in surgical planning and patient counseling regarding the possible outcomes of such an event, but is also important from medicolegal aspect. There is no better alternative to an astute clinical examination but if direct visualization of the vitreous and retina with the ophthalmoscope or at the slit lamp is not possible because of media opacity, several diagnostic tests like USG, CT, MRI and UBM can provide important indirect information.[1,2]

Also, electrophysiological tests like pattern-evoked (VER) and electroretinography (ERG) provide important clues regarding visual prognosis.

Optical coherence tomography (OCT) is a noninvasive, noncontact technique which is essentially analogous to ultrasound B-mode imaging, However, OCT employs optical reflectivity rather than acoustic reflectivity as measured with B-scan. OCT uses near infra-red, low coherent light passing through a Michaelson interferometer.[3] Cross-sectional scanning of the tissue obtained by OCT is an "anatomic" tomographic representation of the retinal layers highlighting the retinal pathologies with an exceptionally high resolution (approximately 10 pm) and reproducibility.

OCT provides detailed diagnostic information which is an adjunct to conventional diagnostic modalities such as fundus photography and fluorescein angiography, thus making it extremely useful in the diagnosis and monitoring of retinal disorders especially the posterior pole, optic nerve and retinal nerve fiber layer analysis. The limitations of OCT are media haze and need for fixation.

In addition, OCT is also turning in to a potent imaging modality for wide variety of corneal and anterior segment studies.

It is a good modality for follow-up and diagnosis of post-traumatic macular pathologies like macular edema, commotio retinae, vitreoretinal surface alterations and macular hole. It has also been used to study ultrastructural changes in choroidal rupture, subhyaloid hemorrhages and subsequent underlying photoreceptor level damage. OCT has also enhanced the understanding of photic retinopathy and laser induced retinal injuries. However, there is a lack of large, systematic studies on OCT findings in ocular trauma and the present knowledge is largely contributed by isolated case reports. In this chapter, we shall be discussing role of OCT in patients with ocular trauma.

OCT is an increasingly utilized test, although it requires clear media and its usefulness is mostly restricted for the chronic cases. OCT plays an important role when evaluating small retinal changes like a traumatic macular hole or unexplained suboptimal vision, that are difficult to observe by biomicroscopy. OCT is also effective when the direct or indirect view of the retina is obscured (e.g. small pupil or a media opacity obscuring a large section of papillary aperture), because only part of the pupil aperture is necessary for OCT imaging (puliafito).

POSTERIOR VITREOUS DETACHMENT

Significant ocular injury is often associated with posterior vitreous detachment (PVD). PVD is often reported to occur in eyes with post-traumatic vitreous hemorrhage.[1,4] However, recent evidence has shown that the vitreous is much less commonly detached after trauma than generally presumed. Only 19% of eyes undergoing vitrectomy for posterior segment IOFB had PVD, however, the duration of trauma was short, a median 9 days (range 5–18 days) after the injury.

PVD is a clear cut diagnosis however, a shallow PVD can be missed clinically and OCT helps in confirming the diagnosis especially when planning a VR surgery. Some authors contest that many cases reported as PVD are actually vitreoschisis. However, it is very difficult to differentiate this condition from PVD even with binocular biomicroscopic, ultra-sonographic, or even OCT examination. Clinically, even a Weiss ring may be present in a case of vitreoschisis. Such a finding has important therapeutic implications, e.g. PVD either spontaneous or surgically induced holds key to successful outcome in macular surgeries. Staining the remaining posterior cortical vitreous with triamcinolone may help to differentiate the two conditions.

OCT provides important information in regards to the vitreomacular interface as in post-traumatic proliferative vitreoretinopathy and vitreomacular traction.[5,6]

CONTUSION RETINOPATHY

Contusion injury of retina produces a white/opaque edematous retina, most pronounced at the posterior pole.[2,4,7,8] This condition, often referred as Berlin edema or commotion retinae usually produces transient/reversible vision loss. However, a severely contused retina may develop persistent edema and traumatic macular hole. It may be associated with few scattered hemorrhages and at times choroidal rupture.

The severity and extent of involvement vary in accord with the severity of trauma. If only the outer segments of the photoreceptors are involved, these regenerate and the retina regains its normal appearance and function.[1,2,5] Subsequently, minor to major RPE disturbance is seen. The vision may improve or remain unchanged.

There are reports of a full thickness macular hole with extensive disruption of the photoreceptor outer segment and RPE on OCT.[8,9]

Ismail et al. reported a spontaneous closure of the macular hole; however, the photoreceptor disruption was extensive and persisted on OCT. Another individual case report documented the separation of the neurosensory retina and the RPE on OCT.[7]

This condition is not caused by edema, as previously presumed, but by photoreceptor death,[4,7] a finding recently confirmed on OCT.[3,5] Optical coherence tomography shows loss of definition of alternate layers of hyper-reflectivity and increased reflectivity in the area of the photoreceptor outer segment probably representing photoreceptor disruption. And marginal increased in retinal thickness in the involved area.

OCT scan at 2 months showing well-defined alternate layers of hyper-reflectivity, with normal appearing zone of outer photoreceptor segment with altered and increased reflectivity with retinal thinning (white arrowheads) limited to the nasal area. Follow-up OCT showed thinning along with hyper-reflectivity segment, suggesting scarring (Fig. 4.3.9).[1-3]

The major site of retinal trauma appeared on OCT to be at the level of the photoreceptor outer segment/RPE interface. The OCT images are consistent with fragmentation of photoreceptor outer segments and damaged cell bodies, as suggested by Sipperley et al[1] in their study of the histological changes in commotio retinae in primates.

Histopathology studies done by Mansour et al have shown disruption of the photoreceptor outer segment and retinal pigment epithelium (RPE) damage which corresponds to the area of whitening in commotion retinae.[1-3] Mild commotio retinae presents with transient visual loss which settles down spontaneously with minimal sequelae. However, more severe cases may be associated with permanent visual loss due to varying degrees of photoreceptor layer atrophy.[1-7]

The final visual prognosis is severely limited by the extent of initial photoreceptor damage, and the excessive pigment atrophy and clumping that follows.

MACULAR EDEMA, MACULAR PUCKER

Collagen production by metaplastic RPE cells and proliferative cells like fibrous astrocytes, fibrocytes, myofibroblasts, macrophages and glial cells on the retinal surface in the macula leads to focal traction with partial- or full-thickness wrinkling of the ILM and (cystoid) macular edema. Because of some similarity in etiopathogenesis, some call epimacular pucker as a "mini-PVR". It usually occurs after contusion, especially after vitreous hemorrhage, retinal detachment, or incomplete vitrectomy (i.e. if PVD was not achieved) and postoperative inflammation. Symptoms include decreased visual acuity,[9] metamorphopsia, micropsia or macropsia due to foveal dragging. The most important diagnostic tools are slit lamp biomicroscopy and OCT (Fig. 4.3.2).

TRAUMATIC MACULAR HOLE

Usually a late sequel, macular hole can occur within a matter of few days after severe trauma. Though the mechanism by which a traumatic macular hole forms is not well understood it is a relatively common posterior segment complication of severe contusion injury.

In cases, the hole is not present initially but develops weeks to months following the incident, the most accepted theory of macular hole formation is tangential vitreoretinal traction epiretinal proliferation (Fig. 4.3.1).

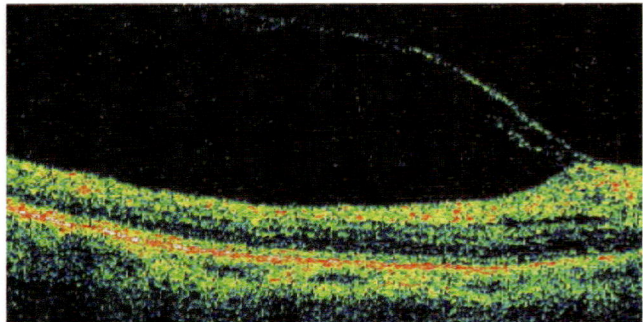

Fig. 4.3.1: Partial PVD and retinal edema at the edge where vitreous band is causing traction at one end

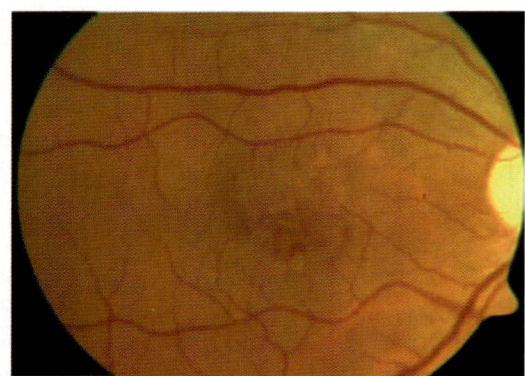

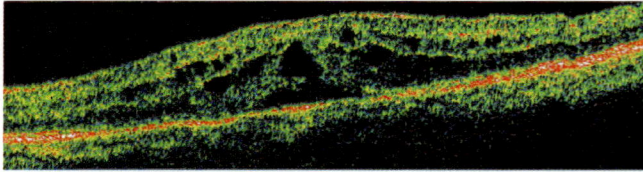

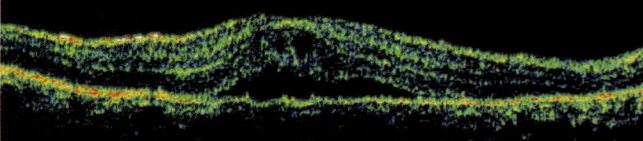

Fig. 4.3.2: Diagnosis of macular edema is straight forward. Cystic spaces suggestive of cystoid changes in a ling standing edema can be easily made out. As these spaces coalesce, they may lead to formation of lamellar or at times a full thickness macular hole. Lower OCT scan shows an underlying serous retinal detachment with early cystic changes and loss of foveal contour with macular edema

However, in cases which develop a macular hole immediately following contusion injury, rapid changes in the anteroposterior dimension with equatorial elongation and rebound may result in rapid creation of anteroposterior vitreoretinal traction in the area of the fovea (Fig. 4.3.2). This acute event in a

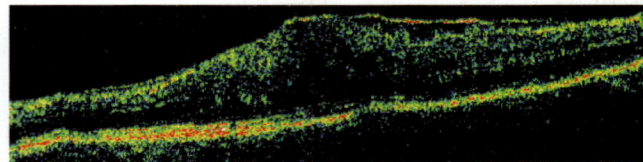

Fig. 4.3.3: OCT showing epiretinal membrane and diffuse macular edema. There is loss of alternating reflectivity pattern in long-standing edema

young patient with an attached posterior hyaloid and rigid internal limiting membrane (ILM) may lead to a small dehiscence of the fovea after trauma.[10]

The success of surgical treatment in terms of anatomical closure of the hole and improvement of vision varies by study, but overall appears to be similar to idiopathic macular holes. Final visual acuity in many of these patients may be limited because of associated intraocular injuries, and the surgeon anticipating traumatic macular hole repair must anticipate this in the preoperative evaluation (Figs 4.3.3 and 4.3.4). It is particularly important to regard the possibility of concomitant optic nerve injury. We generally recommend obtaining preoperative visual field tests in these patients to rule out pre-existing nerve injury, which without baseline tests for comparison may be later incorrectly ascribed to the macular hole repair.[11-13]

The OCT allows following the patient with a post-traumatic macular hole in more detail than what biomicroscopy can provide. Giant macular holes have

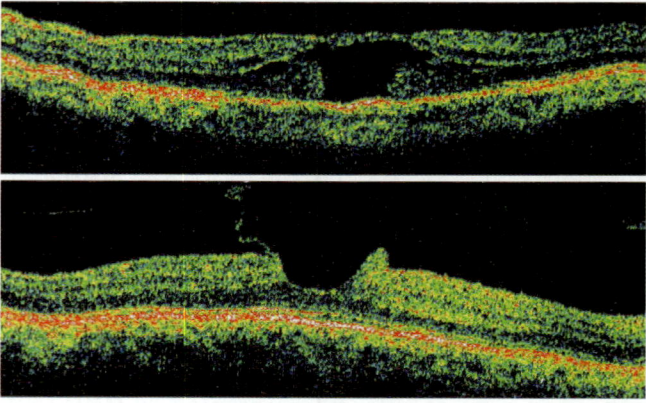

Fig. 4.3.4: Lamellar hole as a result of coalescing cystic spaces in long standing case of cystoid macular edema. Lower OCT picture is of a case of acute traumatic macular hole (partial thickness). Note the vitreous detachment and a vitreous band attached to the edge of macular hole

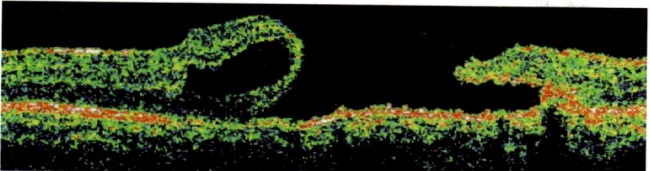

Fig. 4.3.5: OCT provides information regarding vitreomacular interface, epiretinal membranes and secondary changes in the retina in case of macular hole. Calculation of hole forming factor also helps assessing visual prognosis and anatomical success of macular hole

been reported after trauma OCT provides a good measure of prognosis (Fig. 4.3.5).[14-16]

SUBHYALOIDAL HEMORRHAGE

The blood is not dispersed in the vitreous gel but gets trapped in the subhyaloid space. The mechanism of injury to small blood vessels may a direct trauma to the eye or indirectly due to sudden pressure changes in capillary vessels as in valsalva mechanism. When located in front of macula, it causes a dramatic fall in vision, even though the media are clear. Subhyaloid hemorrhage attains a classical boat shape appearance and this may improve the vision to some extent as the red blood cells settle down and later a spontaneous dispersion of the blood occurs over few months (Fig. 4.3.6). OCT is useful in serial monitoring of its resolution and changes at macula. Rare but reported complications like PVR and subsequent retinal detachment have been described vision.

Treatment like yttrium aluminium garnet (YAG) laser hyaloidotomy should be considered if the hemorrhage is large or thick. Vitrectomy is the definite treatment, indicated primarily if additional pathologies are present or the hyaloidotomy attempts have failed.

A sub-ILM hemorrhage, also called as submembranous hemorrhagic macular cyst is a differential diagnosis of this condition. The condition mimics subhyaloid hemorrhage, however, it is dome-shaped and tense. Treatment includes a surgical evacuation usually with YAG laser puncture the ILM and drain the cyst if other pathologies do not interfere.[17,18]

SUBRETINAL HEMORRHAGE

A subretinal hemorrhage is easier to diagnose as retinal blood vessels can be seen over the hemorrhagic retina. It needs early treatment as underlying

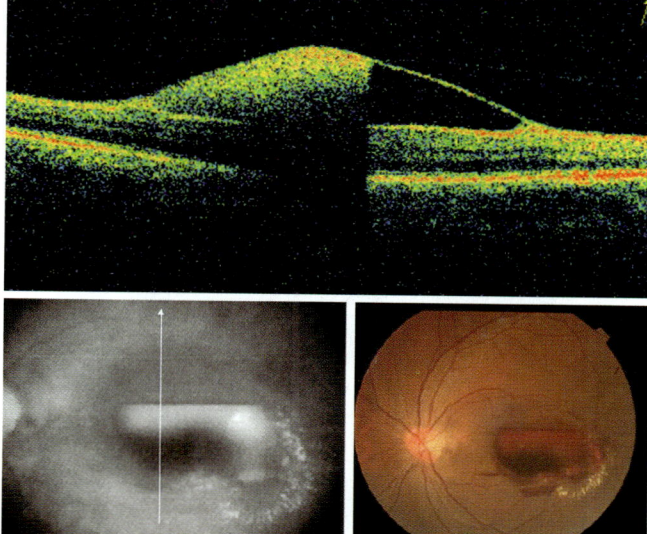

Fig. 4.3.6: Subhyaloid hemorrhage: a vertical tomogram; (white line) shows two well-defined regions. The superior region shows a brightly reflective band just beneath the detached posterior hyaloid that shadowed the retina below while inferior portion of the line scan shows mild backscattering between the retina and the posterior hyaloid

photoreceptors start dying as early as 24 hours if the blood is not evacuated. Late subretinal scarring is another threat that should force the ophthalmologist to consider fairly acute intervention if the blood is thick and submacular (Fig. 4.3.7).

A large subretinal hemorrhage should be considered as hemorrhagic RD. The blood may be located between retinal pigment epithelium (RPE) and neurosensory retina or it may be truly subretinal. If the hemorrhage is very large, a retinotomy has to be performed to allow direct access to the blood. Also, there is an increased risk of PVR (Figs 4.3.8 to 4.3.10).

TRAUMA-RELATED RETINAL DETACHMENT

Trauma cases with RD usually have a poor prognosis. It may be detected late especially in cases with retinal dialysis and vitreous base avulsion. Traumatic RD is the most common type of RD in children.[1,2] In open globe injury, the retinal tears may be due to direct trauma. However, attached vitreous gel over this area may prevent immediate RD. The reason for the slower rate of progression from retinal defect (tear, dialysis) to frank detachment relates to the fact that the vitreous is formed and may be attached in these young patients.

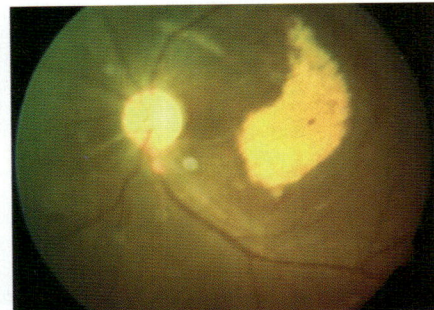

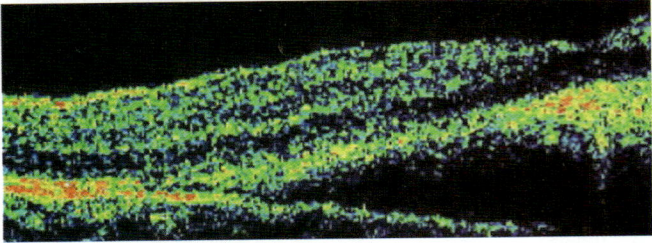

Fig. 4.3.7: Long standing, partly resolved subretinal hemorrhage. OCT showing dome shaped elevation and high optical reflectivity and backscattering under macula. Shadowing in the submacular elevated region is seen as the optical signal gets attenuated by altered blood

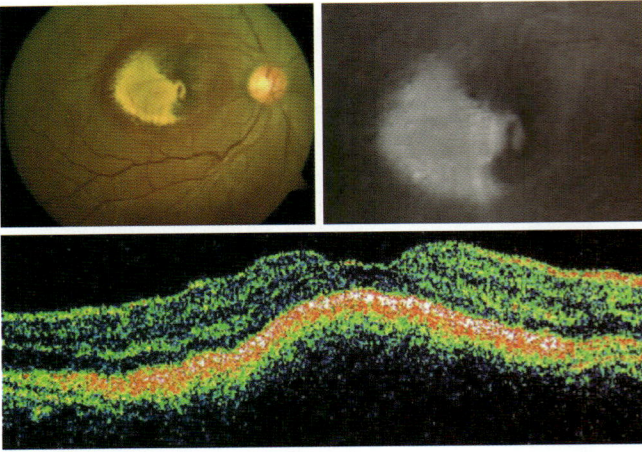

Fig. 4.3.8: Longstanding submacular hemorrhage with cuff of relatively fresh blood. Note the pigmentary alterations in the macular area where the hemorrhage has cleared. OCT shows a subretinal zone of very high optical reflectivity in the area of hemorrhage. The overlying foveal cup is relatively preserved and retina is minimally thickened

For patients developing giant retinal tears following trauma, the progression to detachment is much more rapid, and these types of tears appear to be more common following contusion injury in myopic male patients (Fig. 4.3.11).[19,20]

A more common mechanism of retinal tears and detachment in open globe injuries is due to proliferative vitreoretinopathy as a result of intraocular fibrovascular healing response and formation of vitreous membranes from the wound site. OCT plays an important role in studying the vitreoretinal interface change (Figs 4.3.12a and b).

CHOROIDAL TEARS

Choroidal rupture is a common finding in cases of blunt injury. The Bruch's membrane lacks the relative

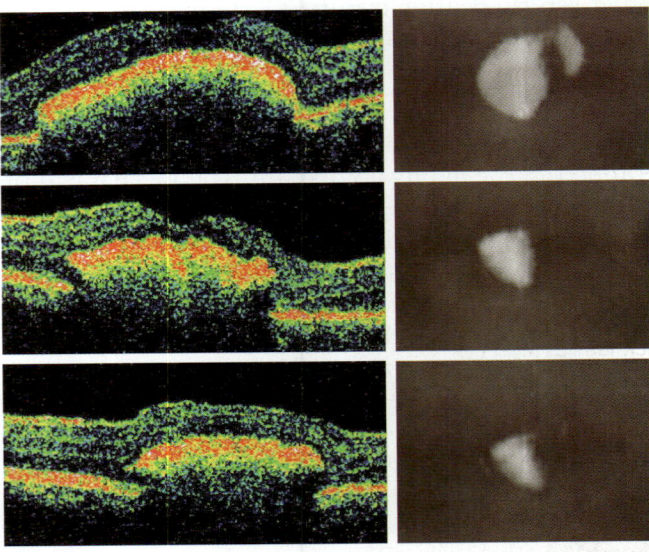

Fig. 4.3.9: Sequential OCT scans over the next few months showing a shrinking zone of optical hyper-reflectivity. Thinning of the overlying retina and loss of alternating reflectivity bands is suggestive of atrophic changes in retina

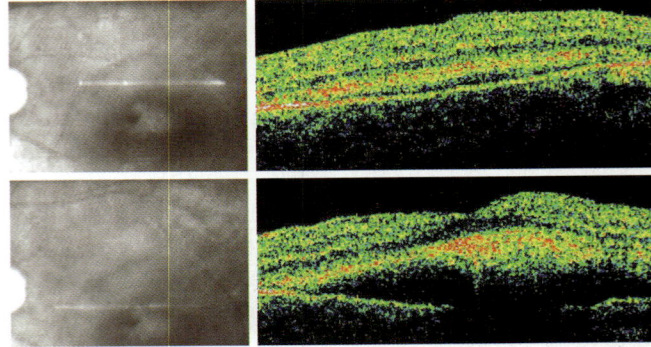

Fig. 4.3.10: Recent subretinal hemorrhage with shallow detached retina at its superior margin and a dome-shaped detachment at fovea. The foveal contour is relatively preserved and OCT shows dome-shaped elevation, high optical reflectivity and backscattering with underlying optical shadowing

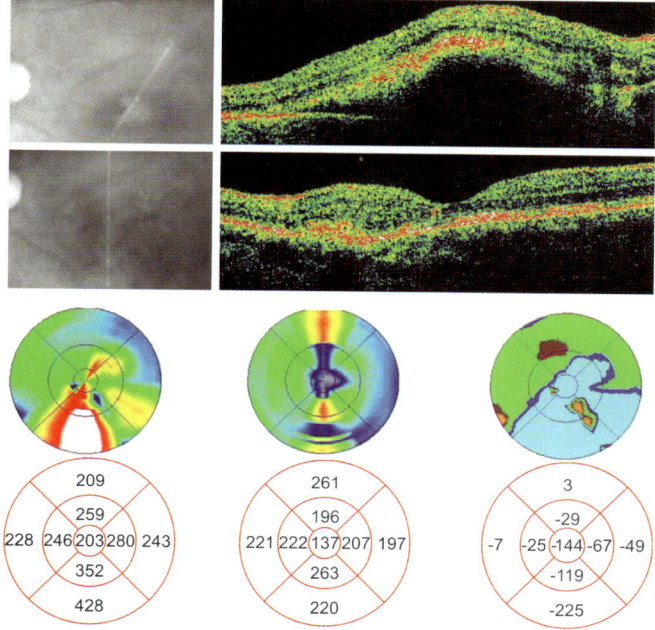

Fig. 4.3.11: Quantitative volumetric data gives an estimate of subretinal fluid collection. It may be better than using retinal thickness analysis for follow-up of subretinal hemorrhages and fluid collection like subretinal detachment. Note the flattening of foveal contour and atrophic changes in the retinal layers. Residual RPE pigment changes are suggested by patchy hyper-reflective changes in these areas

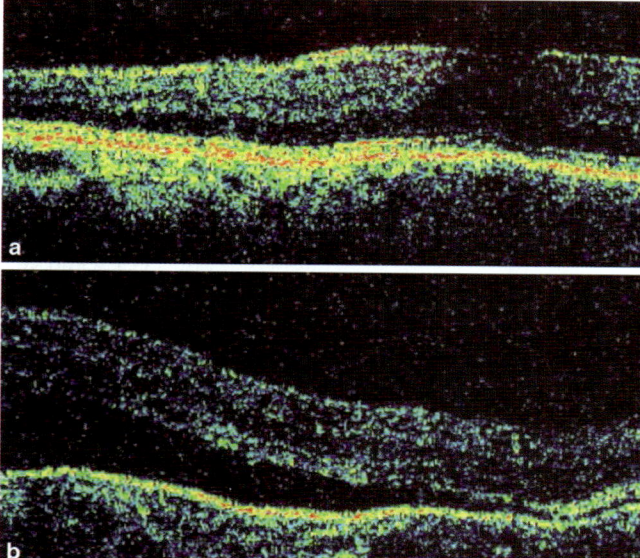

Figs 4.3.12a and b: (a) Shallow retinal detachment inferior to fovea; (b) Missed on indirect ophthalmoscopy and diagnosed as persistent macular edema on biomicroscopy

elasticity of retina and mechanical strength of the sclera. When Bruch's membrane gets ruptured, the choriocapillaris and the RPE also tear. Breaks in the choroid, Bruch's membrane, and the RPE are a relatively common findings than either scleral rupture or even post-equatorial retinal breaks. Associated rupture and retraction of both choroid and retina may accompany severe injuries; as described by the term Chorioretinitis sclopetaria but this condition is rare (Fig. 4.3.13). While peripherally located choroidal

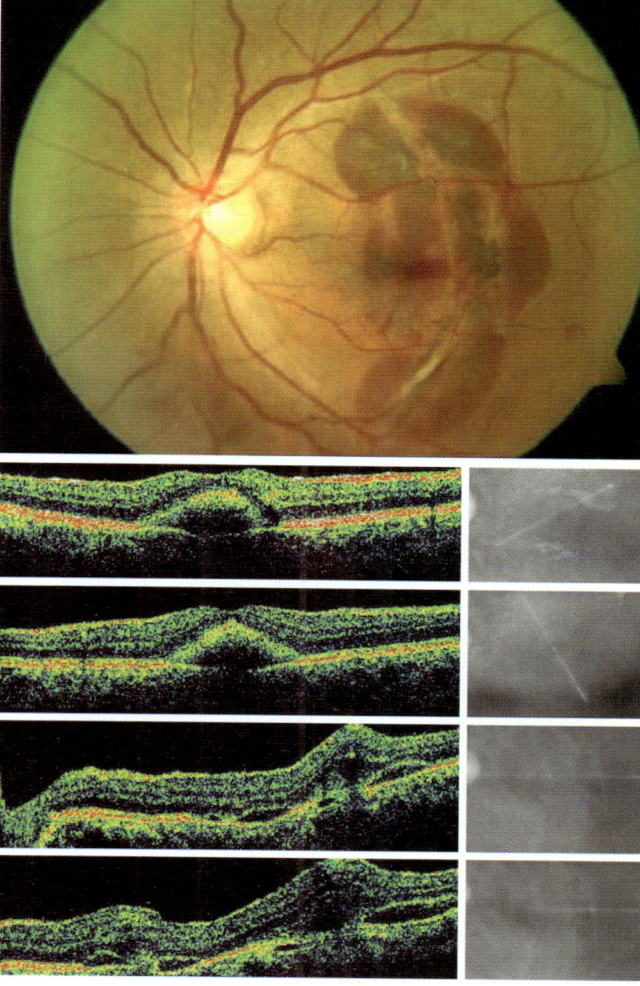

Fig. 4.3.13: Fresh blood, subretinal fluid and retinal edema can obscure an underlying choroidal tear. OCT scans of choroidal rupture show a band of optical hyper-reflectivity at the level of RPE choriocapillaris. There is no break or loss of continuity in the choroidal layer. There is progressive resolution of overlying retinal edema or hemorrhage, leaving behind a narrow band of hyper-reflectivity at the RPE level perhaps as a result of fibrosis

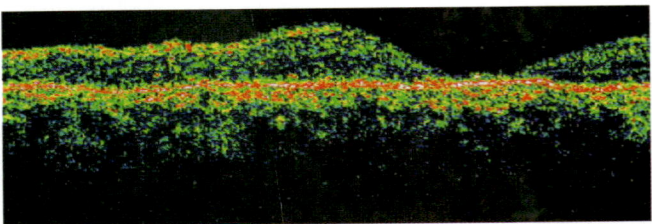

Fig. 4.3.14: Flattened foveal contour, loss of alternate band of hyper-reflectivity and complete atrophy of retinal tissue in the fovea suggestive of macular atrophy. There is enhanced reflectivity from the retinal pigment epithelium beneath consistent with a pigmented scar

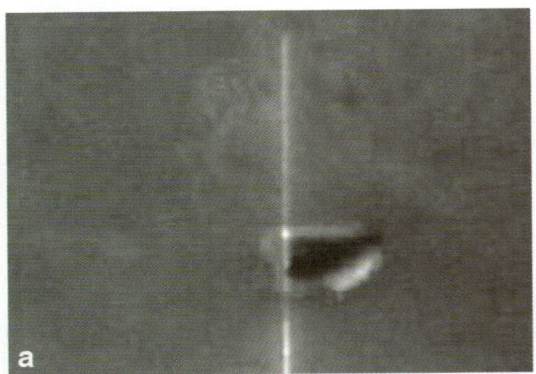

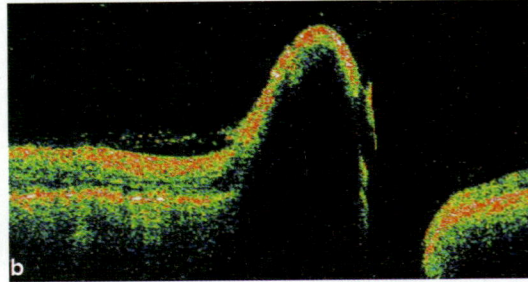

Figs 4.3.15a and b: (a) Vertical OCT image (b) showed an elevation of the retina over the foreign body at the superior margin while the lower margin shows a downward sloping of retina. It implies the direction of entry/impact of foreign body was from below. The elevated retinal layers show reduced thickness, hyper-reflectivity and backscattering suggestive of atrophy. The reflective band corresponding to the retinal pigment epithelium was thickened and highly backs-cattering in this region consistent with pigment aggregation. A few dot like reflectivity in the vitreous near the superior elevated retina

ruptures are caused by adjacent injury forces, a choroidal rupture located at the posterior pole is often when indirect forces are transmitted concentric to the optic nerve.[16] Location, extent of rupture, associated

hemorrhage, and subsequent fibrosis or vascularization dictate the visual prognosis. Often obscured by overlying hemorrhage and edema, choroidal ruptures become evident over few days as the edema and hemorrhage subside.

ATROPHIC MACULOPATHY

Findings like an abnormal foveal contour consistent with the loss of photoreceptors in the foveal pit on OCT. Changes at the RPE level like enhanced backscatter are usually seen with the clinical like a small subretinal hemorrhage or pigment hypertrophy (Fig. 4.3.14).

INTRAOCULAR FOREIGN BODIES

Optical coherence tomography provides images of the ultrastructural changes like RPE hyperpigmentation, retinal photoreceptor atrophy, etc. In localized siderosis, these changes extend beyond the immediate proximity of the FB. OCT also shows vitreous thickening, attachment or PVD in relation to the involved area (Figs 4.3.15a and b).

REFERENCES

1. Blanch RJ, Good PA, Shah P, Bishop JR, Logan A, Scott RA. Visual outcomes after blunt ocular trauma. Ophthalmology. 2013;120(8):1588–91.
2. DJ Pieramici, et al. Vitreoretinal trauma. Ophthalmol Clin N Am 15 226 (2002) 225–234.
3. Hee, Michael R., et al. Optical coherence tomography of ocular diseases. Slack Incorporated, 1996.
4. Yu W, Zheng L, Zhang Z, Dai R, Dong F. Spectral-domain optical coherence tomography characteristics of macular contusion trauma. Ophthalmic Res. 2012;47(4):220–4.
5. Lorusso M, Micelli Ferrari L, Leozappa M, Modoni AP, Micelli Ferrari T. Transient vitreomacular traction syndrome caused by traumatic incomplete posterior vitreous detachment. Eur J Ophthalmol. 2011;21(5):668–70.
6. Shao L, Wei W. Vitreomacular traction syndrome. Chin Med J (Engl). 2014;127(8):1566–71.
7. Kung J, Leung LS, Leng T, Liao YJ. Traumatic airbag maculopathy. JAMA Ophthalmol. 2013;131(5):685–7.
8. Erdurman FC, Sobaci G, Acikel CH, Ceylan MO, Durukan AH, Hurmeric V. Anatomical and functional outcomes in contusion injuries of posterior segment. Eye (Lond). 2011 Aug;25(8):1050–6.
9. Gao Y, Smiddy WE. Morphometric analysis of epiretinal membranes using SD-OCT. Ophthalmic Surg Lasers Imaging. 2012;43(6 Suppl):S7–15.

10. Saleh M, Letsch J, Bourcier T, Munsch C, Speeg-Schatz C, Gaucher D. Long-term outcomes of acute traumatic maculopathy. Retina. 2011;31(10):2037–43.

11. Huang J, Liu X, Wu Z, Sadda S. Comparison of full-thickness traumatic macular holes and idiopathic macular holes by optical coherence tomography. Graefes Arch Clin Exp Ophthalmol. 2010;248(8):1071–5.

12. Arevalo JF, Sanchez JG, Costa RA, Farah ME, Berrocal MH, Graue-Wiechers F, Lizana C, Robledo V, Lopera M. Optical coherence tomography characteristics of full-thickness traumatic macular holes. Eye (Lond). 2008; 22(11):1436–41.

13. Huang J, Liu X, Wu Z, Lin X, Li M, Dustin L, Sadda S. Classification of full-thickness traumatic macular holes by optical coherence tomography. Retina. 2009;29(3):340–8.

14. Kelkar AS, Bhanushali DR, Kelkar JA, Shah RB, Kelkar SB. Spontaneous Closure of a Full-Thickness Stage 2 Idiopathic Macular Hole without Posterior Vitreous Detachment. Case Rep Ophthalmol. 2013;4(3):188–91.

15. Yamashita T, Uemara A, Uchino E, Doi N, Ohba N. Spontaneous closure of traumatic macular hole. Am J Ophthalmol. 2002;133(2):230–5.

16. Nasr MB, Symeonidis C, Tsinopoulos I, Androudi S, Rotsos T, Dimitrakos SA. Spontaneous traumatic macular hole closure in a 50-year-old woman: a case report. J Med Case Rep. 2011;5:290.

17. Pichi F, Ciardella AP, Torrazza C, Morara M, Scano G, Mattana G, Nucci P. A spectral-domain optical coherence tomography description of ND: YAG laser hyaloidotomy in premacular subhyaloid hemorrhage. Retina. 2012; 32(4):861–2.

18. Tatlipinar S, Shah SM, Nguyen QD. Optical coherence tomography features of sub-internal limiting membrane hemorrhage and preretinal membrane in Valsalva retinopathy. Can J Ophthalmol. 2007;42(1):129–30.

19. F Kuhn, DJ Pieramici. Ocular trauma: principles and practice. Thieme Medical Publishers. 2002.

20. Kuhn F. Ocular traumatology. Springer. 2008.

4.4 FUNDUS FLUORESCEIN ANGIOGRAPHY IN TRAUMA

• Narayanan Raja

INTRODUCTION

Nonpenetrating or blunt ocular trauma, orbital trauma, and systemic trauma may cause various abnormalities of the posterior segment; vision can be unaffected or can be completely lost. Blunt trauma is the most common type of eye injury. Moreover, young people in the most productive stage of their life are the most common victims.[1]

Although no treatment exists for many of the manifestations of ocular blunt trauma, early diagnosis and prophylactic treatment may be important in some patients in order to prevent later visual loss. The mechanism of injury causing posterior-segment abnormalities can be direct or indirect—that is, systemic trauma away from the eye. The role of fluorescein angiography (FA) through limited, will be discussed in the following sections.

DIRECT INJURY

Commotio Retinae

Commotio retinae (Berlin's edema) is characterized by a transient, gray-white opacification at the level of the deep sensory retina occurring after blunt trauma.[2] Clinically, whitening or opacification that resolves within 4 to 5 days occurs at the level of the deep retina.[2] This opacification may be confined to the macula or may involve extensive areas of the peripheral retina.[3]

The overlying retina may show extensive preretinal, retinal, or subretinal hemorrhage, and choroidal rupture may be present.[3] Visual symptoms depend on the area of retinal involvement and on the accompanying ocular injuries.

On fluorescein angiography the areas of opaque retina block background choroidal fluorescence. In addition, the retinal vessels appear to be unimpaired with complete capillary filling, and in less severe cases these patients generally do not have associated leakage of dye into or under the retina (Fig. 4.4.1).[4]

Weeks later, because of degeneration of retinal pigment epithelial (RPE) cells, window defects are common. Less often, progressive patchy fluorescein staining at the level of the RPE without elevation of the tissue may be seen in cases of severe commotio retinae.

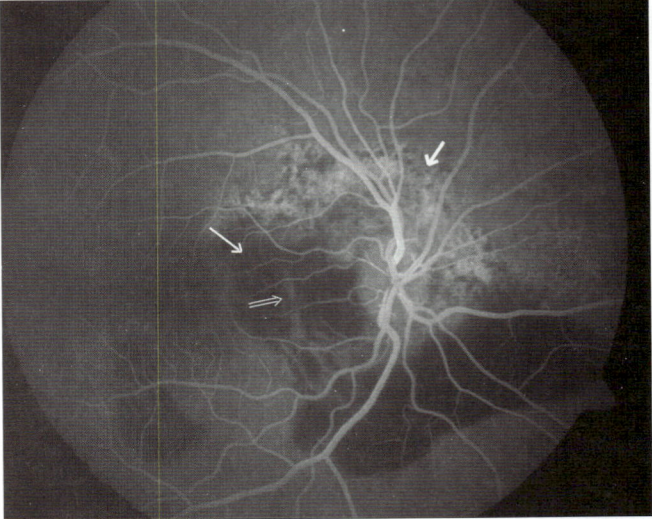

Fig. 4.4.1: Arteriovenous phase of FA, showing area of blocked fluorescence (thin →) corresponding to subretinal heme, linear streak of hyperfluorescence corresponding to choroidal rupture (empty →) and a peripapillary area of window defect (thick →) corresponding to retinal pigment epithelium

These findings were purported to represent acute pigment epithelial edema.[5] RPE abnormalities seen by early FA are associated with slower visual recovery.[6]

Macular Holes

Macular holes occur in 6.3% of eyes after blunt trauma.[1] Traumatic macular holes are associated in many cases with signs of severe blunt trauma, such as commotio retinae and choroidal rupture.

On FA, they will exhibit window defects, but RPE atrophy tends to have more residual pigment and consequently a more mottled appearance of the transmitted choroidal fluorescence. A pseudohole will not have a window defect.

Contusion Retinopathy

Direct or indirect blunt trauma may cause contusion of the RPE. The consequent functional damage results in an overlying serous RD.[3,5] FA shows patchy hyperfluorescence of the RPE.[5] Transmission defects of fluorescein dye are apparent later stages.

Choroidal Rupture

A choroidal rupture consists of a tear in the choroid, Bruch's membrane, or the RPE secondary to direct or indirect blunt trauma (Fig. 4.4.2).[2]

The retina is more elastic than is the choroid, so rupture limited to the choroid is the most common form. However, with severe injury, tears of the overlying edematous retina may occur. The diagnosis of choroidal rupture may be difficult immediately after injury because of subretinal hemorrhage. The relatively low incidence of secondary retinal detachment may be caused by the gliosis and RPE proliferation that are evident in the later stages and that act as a spontaneous retinopexy. Some posterior choroidal ruptures are subtle and diagnosed only with the aid of FA and indocyanine green angiography.[6] Early hypofluorescence associated with choriocapillaris injury and late hyperfluorescence in a curvilinear pattern concentric with the optic disk are characteristic.[7] As choroidal ruptures heal, fibrovascular proliferation, fibrous scar formation, and retinal pigment epithelial hyperplasia occurs (Figs 4.4.3 and 4.4.4).

Optic Nerve Avulsion

It is a devastating, although rare, cause of visual loss after blunt trauma. Patients typically describe a sudden loss of vision at the of time of orbital or ocular trauma. In cases of optic nerve avulsion, funduscopic examination immediately after the injury may reveal massive or minimal intraocular hemorrhage. A partial optic nerve evulsion may simulate an optic pit whereas the optic nerve may not be at all visible in a complete avulsion. FA may demonstrate either normal,[8] partial[4] or absent filling of the peripapillary retinal vasculature.

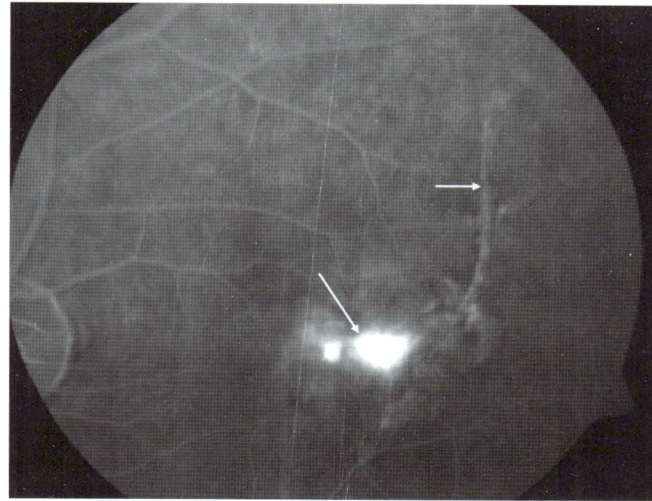

Fig. 4.4.3: Late phase of FA, area of hyperfluorescence suggestive staining corresponding to scar in color fundus photo with linear streak of hyperfluorescence corresponding to healed choroidal rupture

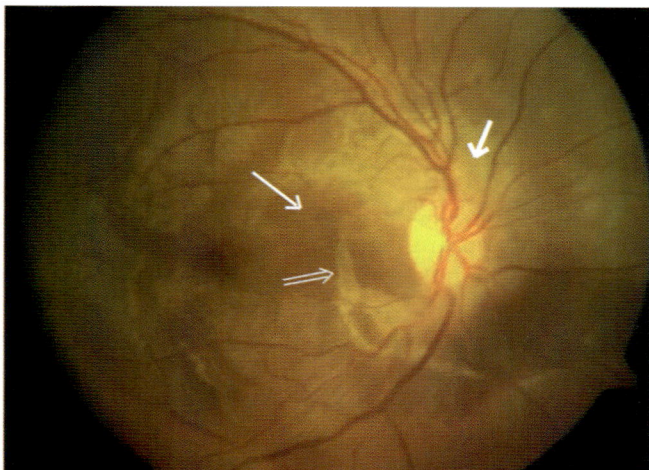

Fig. 4.4.2: Color photo showing subretinal heme (thin →) and choroidal rupture (empty →) with peripapillary retinal pigment epithelium atrophy (thick →)

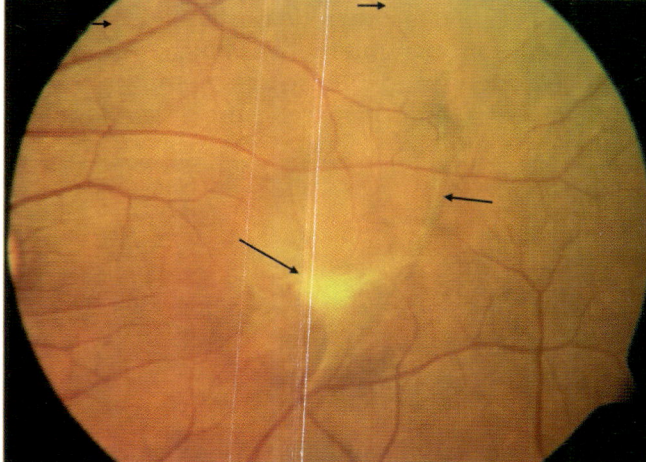

Fig. 4.4.4: Color fundus photo showing fibrous scarring (thin →) at the macula with linear choroidal rupture (thick →)

INDIRECT INJURY

Manifestations of Remote Trauma on the Posterior Segment

Posterior segment injury can occur when the body is injured in areas remote from the head and orbit. Acute macular neuroretinopathy, Purtscher's retinopathy, fat embolism syndrome, Valsalva's retinopathy, Terson's syndrome, battered child syndrome, and whiplash maculopathy occur without direct trauma to the eye. Because they are often overlooked by the trauma team, the ophthalmologist should be familiar with their recognition and natural history.

TRAUMATIC RETINAL VASCULAR OCCLUSION

Generalized retinal vascular constriction and actual occlusion of the central retinal vein and central retinal artery suggesting retinal vascular occlusion may be seen after blunt trauma.[5]

Possible mechanisms include generalized arteriospasm secondary to blunt injury and shearing of the central retinal vessels in the optic nerve secondary to extreme traumatic rotation of the globe. Angiography shows the typical picture of vascular occlusion as in nontraumatic cases (Figs 4.4.5a and b).

Purtscher's Retinopathy

The classic funduscopic findings in Purtscher's retinopathy consist of multiple patches of superficial retinal whitening and retinal hemorrhages surrounding a typically hyperemic optic nerve in patients who have sustained head trauma. FA may show leakage of dye from retinal arterioles, capillaries, and venules in the white retinal patches of patients with relatively mild Purtscher's retinopathy and arteriolar obstruction in more severe cases.[3] Although

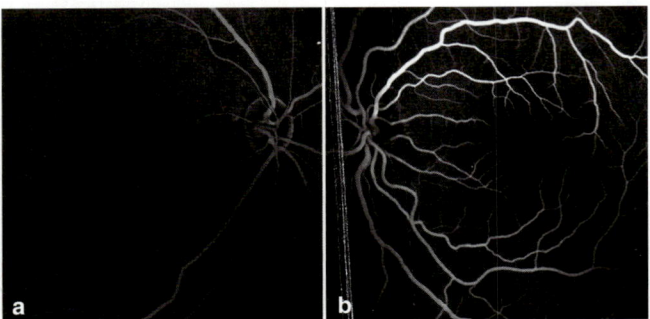

Figs 4.4.5a and b: Arteriovenous phase of FA of both the eyes, showing severe arterial attenuation of right eye with loss of perifoveal capillary network

hemorrhages and white retinal patches may eventually disappear, the patient may be left with a severe visual deficit because of optic nerve atrophy.[3]

The characteristic geographic distribution of ischemic patches can be explained by embolic occlusion of arterioles feeding the radial peripapillary capillaries. Granulocyte aggregates, or "leukoemboli", formed in response to complement activation, may cause this retinal arteriolar embolization.[9] No specific treatment is available.

Epiretinal Membrane Role of FA Window Defects d/t RPE Atrophy

FA is generally not necessary to confirm the diagnosis of ERM. Nevertheless, FA can demonstrate leakage from vessels that have become relatively incompetent owing to traction from the membrane. OCT examination is the gold standard for the study of the vitreoretinal interface. It not only demonstrates the presence of an ERM, but also helps in quantifying the degree of tractional neurosensory elevation and in differentiating an ERM from vitreomacular traction syndrome.

Sympathetic Ophthalmia

Sympathetic ophthalmia (SO) is defined as a bilateral granulomatous inflammation of the uvea that usually occurs as a complication of penetrating trauma or intraocular surgery. The classic clinical picture is that of a bilateral granulomatous panuveitis: "mutton fat" keratic precipitates, cells and flare in the anterior chamber, vitreous cells, isolated or confluent patches of yellow-white choroidal infiltrates and Dalen-Fuchs nodules.

Fluorescein angiography of active SO typically demonstrates multiple early hyperfluorescent or hypofluorescent RPE level lesions, both of which leak in the late phase. The optic nerve head may display hyperemia and angiographic leakage. Multiple early hyperfluorescent sites of choroidal leakage are also seen. These sites ("window defects") correspond to the Dalen-Fuchs nodules observed clinically. The less common appearance of SO is that of early hypofluorescent lesions on angiography. This appearance is similar to that seen in acute posterior multifocal placoid pigment epitheliopathy, in which the lesions block the choroidal fluorescence in the early phase and stain in the late phase. Presumably, the hyperfluorescent or hypofluorescent nature in the early phase is determined by whether the Dalen-Fuchs nodules have an intact or a disrupted overlying RPE. The angiogram of the eye with inactive SO characteristically has scattered multiple window defects. In addition to exudative detachment of the neurosensory retina and papillitis, patients with Vogt-Koyanagi-Harada disease as well as sympathetic ophthalmia may also develop serous detachment of the retinal pigment epithelium.

CONCLUSION

Trauma can induce a wide spectrum of alterations of the retina, RPE, and choroid. Most types of traumatic maculopathy, such as Purtscher's retinopathy, Berlin's edema, retinal contusion, traumatic macular hole, and choroidal rupture, are readily apparent on clinical examination. Choroidal rupture, although usually evident clinically, may be more obvious on FA. Contusion necrosis of the RPE may present clinically with an associated RPE detachment, an overlying neurosensory detachment, and a subtle change in RPE pigmentation. FA can demonstrate the site of leakage into the subretinal space, unless the RPE defect has healed over the natural course of the disease. In retinal contusion, a normal fluorescein angiogram indicates a good visual prognosis, wherease fluorescein leakage is associated with tissue damage, and nonperfusion carries a poor visual prognosis.[10]

FA is particularly helpful in differentiating retinal concussion (Berlin's edema), in which FA findings are normal, from retinal contusion, increased transmission of choroidal fluorescence on FA is seen.[10] In Purtscher's retinopathy, FA can document vascular closure, which accounts for the retinal infarctions.[11]

FOLLOW-UP

Most trauma-related conditions are followed clinically with serial evaluations of clinical appearance and visual acuity. Routine FA to follow trauma-related maculopathies is not necessary.

Patients with choroidal rupture through the fovea, which is generally obvious clinically, lose central vision. The outcome of Purtscher's retinopathy and of RPE contusion largely depends on the location of macular involvement.

REFERENCES

1. Cox MS, CL Schepens, et al. "Retinal detachment due to ocular contusion." Arch Ophthalmol 1966;76(5):678–85.
2. Williams D, Mieler WF, Williams GA. Posterior segment manifestations of ocular trauma, Retina 1990;10 (suppl):S35–S44.
3. Gass JDM. Stereoscopic atlas of macular diseases: diagnosis and treatment, e., St Louis, 1987, Mosby—Year Book.
4. Hart J. CSF Pilley. "Partial evulsion of optic nerve. Fluorescein angiographic study." Br J Ophthalmol 1970; 54(12):781–5.
5. Friberg TR. "Traumatic retinal pigment epithelial edema." Am J Ophthalmol 1979;88(1):18–21.
6. Arend O, RA Elsner AE. Indocyanine green angiography in traumatic choroidal rupture: Clinicoangiographic case reports. Ger J Ophthalmol 1995;4:257.
7. Hart J, Frank HJ. Retinal opacification after blunt non-perforating concussional injuries to the globe: a clinical and retinal fluorescein angiographic study, Trans Ophthalmol Soc UK 1975;95:94–100.
8. Chow AY, MF Goldberg, et al. "Evulsion of the optic nerve in association with basketball injuries." Ann Ophthalmol 1984;16(1):35–7.
9. Blodi BA, MW Johnson, et al. "Purtscher's-like retinopathy after childbirth." Ophthalmology 1990; 97(12): 1654–9.
10. Dean Hart JCD, Frank HJ. Retinal opacification after blunt non-perforating concussional injuries to the globe. Trans Ophthalmol Soc UK 1975;95:94.
11. Burton TC. "Unilateral Purtscher's retinopathy." Ophthalmology 1980;87(11):1096–1105.

4.5 ULTRASOUND BIOMICROSCOPY IN OCULAR TRAUMA

• **Ritu Arora** • **DK Mehta** • **Ritika Sachdev**

INTRODUCTION

Clinical UBM has shown significant potential as an aid in diagnosis of ocular trauma. However, the extent of associated injuries and the open nature of ocular injuries may preclude the manipulation necessary for such an examination. The resolution of probes with tranducers of 50 MHz is 50 μ while the depth of penetration is limited to 4–5 mm. It is a useful tool in the assessment of anterior segment structures especially in the presence of hazy media.[1]

ULTRASOUND BIOMICROSCOPY IN OCULAR TRAUMA

Berinstein et al described UBM as a safe and effective adjunctive tool for the clinical assessment and management of ocular trauma, especially when visualization is limited and multiple traumatic injuries are involved.[2,3]

Ozdal et al reviewed the indications for performing UBM examination in 109 patients.[4] UBM examinations were preformed for the evaluation of zonules before cataract surgery (49.5%), examination of the anterior segment in the presence of media opacity such as total hyphema or corneal scar (32.1%), detection of suspected ocular FBs (10.1%) and the evaluation of ocular hypotony (8.3%). The time course of imaging after trauma was variable and ranged from 1 day to 55 years.

In all, 61.5% eyes had a closed globe injuries whereas 38.5% had open globe injuries. The most common UBM findings in closed globe injuries were zonular deficiency (64.2%), angle recession (43.3%), iridodialysis (17.9%), dislocated lens (16.4%), hyphema in 13.4%, peripheral anterior synechiae (8.9%). The most UBM common findings in open globe injuries were zonular deficiency (54.8%), iridodialysis (26.2%), peripheral anterior synechiae (26.2%), angle recession (14.3% and ruptured anterior capsule (14.3%).

ASSESSMENT OF ZONULES

Pavlin and Foster were the first to describe the imaging of zonular fibers using UBM.[1] Zonular damage after closed globe injury is not uncommon and its significance is well known to the anterior segment surgeon. The loss of zonular fibers, in association with a traumatic cataract, might result in an unstable lens and with an increased probability of vitreous presentation and in the worst case scenario, loss of lens into the vitreous cavity.

Visualization of zonules requires a careful 360° scanning with the long axis of the transducer perpendicular to the zonules and has a significant learning curve. Zonular defects, when present, are seen as abrupt cessation of the bright reflective lines of zonular fibers associated with blunting of the ciliary processes.

The role of UBM in preoperative assessment of zonular status after trauma was evaluated by McWhae, et al.[5] 59 cases with no clinically visible zonular damage were examined by UBM with a 50 MHz probe. Occult zonular loss was identified in 42.9% of the patients. Referring surgeons found the information helpful in surgical planning and anticipating complications in these cases. This study concluded that UBM is an effective method for identifying occult zonular damage in patients with anterior segment trauma. They reported a significant learning curve in the examination technique. A similar study by Liu YZ, et al also established the the role of ultrasound biomicroscopy in delineating the presence and extent of zonular loss in subluxated lenses.[6]

FOREIGN BODIES

Foreign body detection rates reported are 36.5% by ultrasound, 88.9% by CT scan and 99.4% with UBM. The diagnosis of FB on UBM was based on high reflective echoes causing shadowing or reverberations.[7]

UBM is particularly valuable in picking up nonmetallic FBs. In cases with intracorneal and intrascleral FBs, UBM may be used to determine the depth of the visible FB.[8]

IRIS AND CILIARY BODY STATUS

Ocular trauma may result in diverse anterior segment pathologies such as hyphema, cyclodialysis and angle recession. Many of these anatomical disturbances can be detected and differentiated with UBM.

When hazy media or abnormal anterior segment architecture prevent or limit adequate visualization during gonioscopy, UBM can be used to differentiate cyclodialysis, angle recession and ciliary body detachment. In addition, the presence of supraciliary fluid and visualization of a connection from the anterior chamber (AC) to the supraciliary space confirms the diagnosis of cyclodialysis. Disinsertion of the iris root from its insertion into the ciliary body (iridodialysis), pupillary block and peripheral anterior synechiae in the presence of complete hyphema preventing visualization of the AC can also be identified with UBM.

The pathogenesis of transient high myopia after traumatic myopia has been evaluated in two patients using UBM by Ikeda et al.[9] UBM showed annular ciliochoroidal effusion with the ciliary body edema, anterior rotation of the ciliary processes, and disappearance of the ciliary sulcus and a myopia of 9.75 diopters was noted. The myopia and the UBM findings normalized in 11 days. In the second patient UBM revealed a partial cyclodialysis, shallowing of the AC and thickening of the crystalline lens. The resolution of these UBM findings and the normalization of the myopia was seen 17 days after trauma.

Our Study: Observations and Results (Pilot Study Done at Guru Nanak Eye Center 2005–2007)

We performed UBM evaluation of 30 cases of recent onset (less than 2 weeks) closed globe injuries reporting to Guru Nanak Eye Center, a tertiary eye care center at New Delhi. A summary of author observations is presented below.

Anterior Chamber

Central AC depth as assessed by UBM correlated well with the AC depth obtained using the A-scan. Hyphema was noted in 46.67% of author patients at the time of the initial UBM examination. It was seen as fine dispersed echogenic opacities in the AC.

Assessment of the Angle (Figs 4.5.1a and b)

Media opacity due to corneal edema or hyphema do not hinder the assessment of the angle by ultrasound biomicroscopy. All the 30 patients could thus be examined at presentation.

Angle recession was noted in 40% of the patients as widened ciliary body band behind the scleral spur with disinsertion of the iris from its root. Angle obliterations with iridocorneal adhesions as peripheral anterior synechiae (PAS) were also seen in 40% of the patients.

Gonioscopy and UBM—a Comparative Analysis

Though both are excellent methods for angle assessment, we found that the concomitant pathologies like hyphema often obscure the view of the angle by gonioscopy. Gonioscopy can be useful only after the media opacity resolves.

UBM however is not hindered by the presence of these media opacities and thus allows an earlier assessment of the angle.

Iris and Ciliary Body (Figs 4.5.1a and b)

The post-concussion vasodilatation and reactive hyperemia leads to iris and ciliary body edema. This

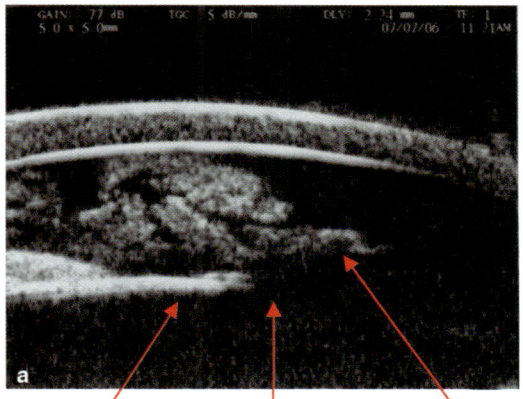

Intact capsule   Ruptured anterior capsule   Lens matter

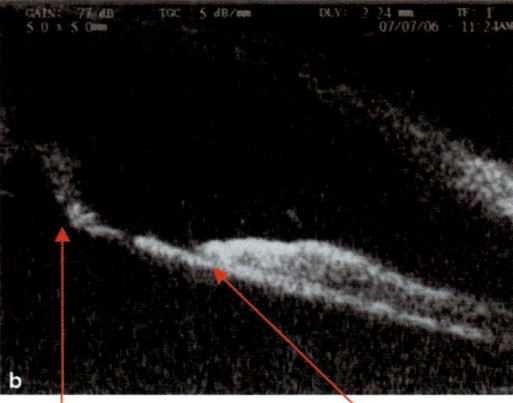

Ruptured anterior capsule   Intact capsule

Figs 4.5.1a and b: UBM for assessment of the anterior capsule

was well documented on UBM as thickening of the iris and the diffuse enlargement of the ciliary body with wide, often globular ciliary processes. Iris edema was seen in 6.67% of the patients and ciliary body edema was observed in 16.67% of the patients. Iridoschisis was clearly seen on UBM as splitting of the layers of the iris.

Lens and Zonular Assessment

Zonular assessment by direct visualization requires a careful and meticulous 360° scanning and has a significant learning curve. 43.33% of the patients in our study had zonular loss on UBM.

Though majority of the cases with zonular loss had clinically apparent subluxation, the extent of subluxation was not clearly defined. UBM examination not only confirmed the subluxation but also clearly delineated its extent. Morever, three cases which on clinical examination had no apparent subluxation were noted to have zonular loss of 1, 2.5 and 3 O'clock hours. Thus, while only 36.67% of the patients had zonular loss on clinical examination, UBM revealed zonular disruption in 43.33% of the cases. Zonular loss less than 3 O'clock hours was missed on clinical examination and UBM is a useful modality to pick up such occult zonular loss.

Zonular loss and associated UBM findings:
- Blunting of the ciliary processes
- Increased iridolenticular space
- Vitreous in the AC
- Localized deepening of the AC.

The presence of one or more of these signs often heralds the presence of zonular loss and warrants a careful UBM examination of the suspected area.

Blunting of the ciliary processes due to disruption of the zonular fibers which in the normal state keep these processes stretched has been noted by Pavlin et al.[23] All cases with zonular disruption in our series had associated blunting of the ciliary processes.

Increased iridolenticular space was seen in all cases with zonular loss in our series. Normally, the iris is apposed to the anterior surface of the lens and there is no iridolenticular gap. Iridolenticular space, seen in all patients with zonular loss, irrespective of the extent of involvement, was perhaps a manifestation of the tilting of the subluxated lens due to the loss of zonular support. Even a slight tilt which may escape notice in a detailed and comprehensive clinical examination will manifest as an increase in iridolenticular space on UBM. A highly significant relationship between iridolen-

ticular space and zonular loss was evident in our study. (p <.0000; Mann Whitney Test).

Vitreous herniation into the anterior segment was seen in all cases with greater than 3 O'clock hours of zonular loss.

Irregular deepening of the anterior chamber was seen in majority of the patients with zonular loss up to 9 O'clock hours. Patients with extensive zonular loss (more than 9 O'clock hours) also displayed a generalized deepening of the AC.

Capsular Status

The anterior capsular status is well delineated by the UBM examination. Anterior capsule rupture was clinically evident in 13.33% of the cases. The extent of capsular rupture was however well demarcated by UBM as the presence of loose lens matter often obscured the clinical examination of the capsule lying beneath it.

CONCLUSION

UBM has a well established yet only partly explored role in evaluating cases of ocular trauma and providing an insight to the pathology of the various manifestations of concussional injuries.

REFERENCES

1. CJ Pavlin, K Harasiewicz, MD Sherar, Foster FS Clinical use of ultrasound biomicroscopy. Ophthalmology 1991;98(3):287–95.
2. Berinstein DM, Gentile RC, Sidoti PA, Stegman Z, Tello C, et al. Ultrasound biomicroscopy in anterior segment trauma. Ophthalmic Surg Lasers, 1997;28:201–7.
3. Genovesi F, Rizzo S, Chiellini S, Romani A, Gabbriellini, et al. Ultrasound Biomicroscopy in the assessment of penetrating or blunt anterior chamber trauma. Ophthalmologica. 1998; 212 (Suppl 1):6–7.
4. Ozdal MP, Mansour M, Deschenes J. Ultrasound biomicroscopic evaluation of traumatized eye. Eye. 2003; 17(4):467–7.
5. Mcwhae JA, Crichton AC, Rinke M. Ultrasound biomicroscopy for assessment of zonules after blunt trauma. Ophthalmology. 2003;110(7):1340–3.
6. Liu Y Z, et al. Zhonqua Yanke Za Zhi. 2004; 40(3):186–8.
7. Guha S, Bhende M, Baskaran M, Sharma. Role of UBM in detection and localization of anterior segment foreign bodies. T Ann Acad Med Singapore. 2006;35(8):536–45.
8. Vincent A. Dermano, et al. Ultrasound biomicroscopy as a tool for detecting and localizing occult foreign bodies after ocular trauma. Ophthalmology.1999;106:301–05.
9. Ikeda N, Ideka T, Nagata M, Mimura O. Pathogenesis of transient high myopía alter blunt eye trauma. Ophthalmology. 2002;109(3):501–7.

4.6 ELECTROPHYSIOLOGY IN OCULAR TRAUMA

• JL Goyal • Jasneet Kang

INTRODUCTION

Ocular trauma is a major cause of preventable monocular blindness and visual impairment in the world. Management of traumatized eyes has dramatically changed over the years. The improved patient care is due to better understanding of the nature of injury and better diagnostic facilities available. In addition to clinical examination of the injured eye plain radiography, CT and USG are used for evaluation. Electrophysiological tests can also be done in cases of blunt and penetrating trauma to provide important information for ocular disease, diagnosis and treatment.

Visual electrophysiology diagnostic tests contain a family of noninvasive recordings which measure electrical signals that occur in the visual system in response to visual stimulation and reflect retinal, optic nerve and visual pathway function. Ocular electrophysiological tests consist of:
1. Pattern and flash ERG
2. Pattern and flash VEP
3. Electro-oculogram (EOG)
4. Multifocal techniques: mfERG and mfVEP.

In patients suffering from severe recent ocular trauma, it is important to know the extent of the retinal damage before assessing the possible recovery of visual function. Ophthalmoscopic examination of the fundus is often impossible because of opacities of the ocular media caused by the trauma.

In such cases, electrophysiological tests are of value in assessing the state of the retina and optic nerve function.

Indications

- Status of retina in presence of media opacities, e.g. post-traumatic corneal opacities, vitreous hemorrhage, etc.
- Objective assessment of extent of retinal detachment in media opacities.
- Diagnosis of optic nerve sheath hemorrhage, partial or complete optic nerve transaction, optic nerve compression.
- *Retained intraocular FBs:* For prognosis and progression of toxic changes, indications for intervention.

- Post-traumatic visual impairment. Routine testing of vision may be inaccurate or difficult to interpret following ocular trauma.
- Subtle optic nerve or cortical damage after head injury.

ELECTRORETINOGRAPHY

Electroretinography (ERG) is an action potential from the retina produced on stimulation by light.[1]

Method of Recording of Electroretinography

Electrodes: The ground electrode is placed on the forehead. The reference electrode is placed on the outer canthus. The active or the recording electrode can be placed on the:

- Cornea (contact lens electrode), e.g. JET electrode (Fig. 4.6.1)
- Conjunctival sac, e.g. gold foil electrode (Fig. 4.6.2)
- Surface electrode.
  1. In many contusions and in most cicatrized perforating wounds contact lens electrode can be used.

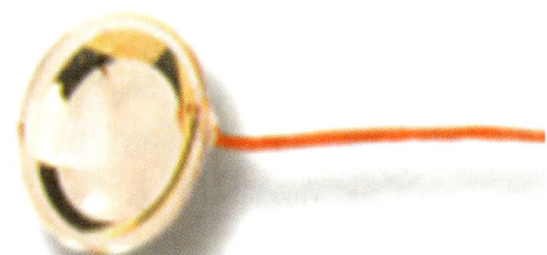

Fig. 4.6.1: ERG-JET electrode

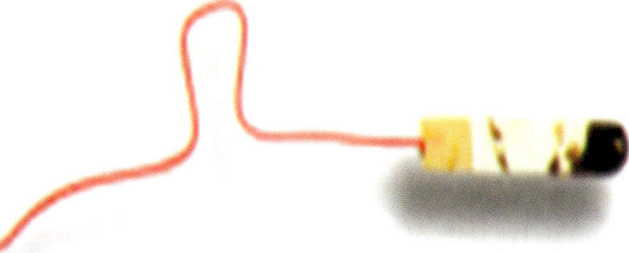

Fig. 4.6.2: Gold foil electrode

2. In very severe contusions and recently-sutured perforating wounds, it is impossible to use a contact lens electrode and non-contact electrodes, e.g. conjunctival sac/surface electrodes can be used.

The patient is dark adapted for 15 minutes before making the recording. The pupils are dilated. For flash ERG, the patient is seated in front of the hemispheric 40 cm diameter bowl facing the fixation target. For pattern ERG, the grating or the checkerboard pattern is displayed on a TV screen (Fig. 4.6.3). The test is first done with a bright red flash (**Red filter dark adapted trial**), followed by a series of blue flashes (**Blue filter dark adapted trial**). Lastly the test is repeated with a series of white flashes (**White light dark adapted trial**). After the results of each flash are averaged and stored, the patient is light adapted for 2–3 minutes and the process is repeated.[2]

WAVEFORMS OF ERG

Flash ERG: The normal ERG curve under mesopic illumination is shown in Fig. 4.6.4. It is biphasic with a cornea negative a-wave, a cornea positive b-wave, multiple wavelets on the ascending limb of the b-wave known as oscillatory potentials (Fig. 4.6.5).

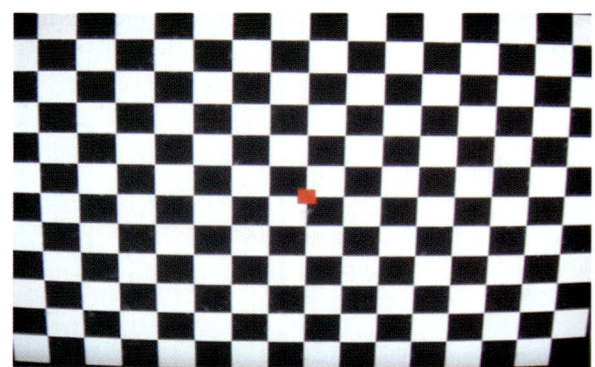

Fig. 4.6.3: Checkerboard pattern of ERG

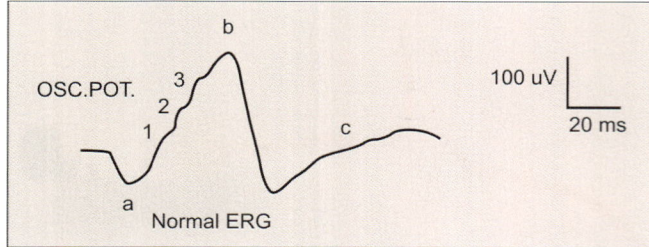

Fig. 4.6.4: Normal waveform of flash (ERG)

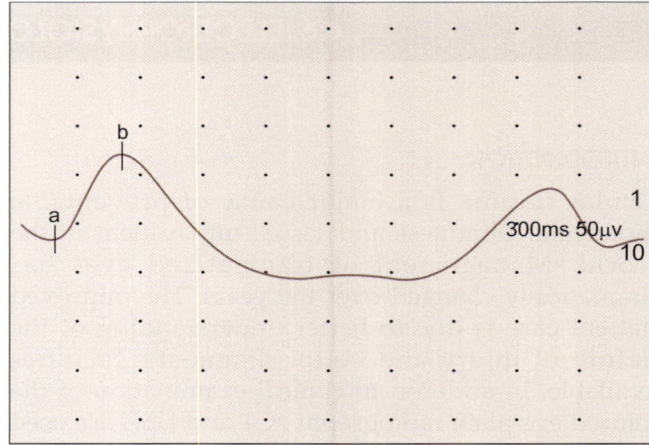

Fig. 4.6.5: Flash electroretinography (ERG) of right and left eye in a patient showing normal waveforms

The a-wave originates from the inner segment of the photoreceptors.

Positive b-wave was originally thought to arise from the Müller's cells but more recent studies suggest that it is actually a result of bipolar cell activity.[1,2]

In mesopic conditions, b-wave has twice the amplitude of a-wave. The positive c-wave may be rarely seen and is believed to originate from the pigment epithelium.[3]

Normal Values

a-wave latency: 25–30 msec
b-wave latency: 40–70 (average 50 ms)
c-wave amplitude: $\geq 100\ \mu V$ (jet electrode).

PATTERN ELECTRORETINOGRAM

Pattern electroretinogram (PERG) is the response of the central retina to an isoluminant stimulus, usually a reversing black and white checkerboard. It allows both a measure of central retinal function and in relation to its origins, an evaluation of retinal ganglion cell function. It is of great value in the electrophysiological differentiation between the optic nerve and the macular dysfunction.[3]

The PERG consists of the following three components (Fig. 4.6.6):

1. N35 negative wave at approx 35 msec (N_1)
2. P50 positive wave at approx 50 msec (P_1)
3. N95 negative wave at approx 95 msec (N_2)

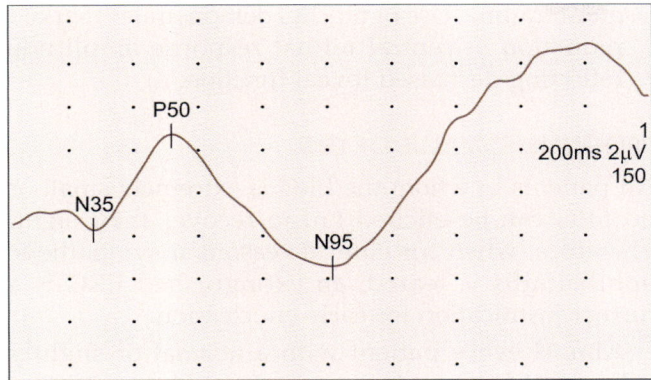

Fig. 4.6.6: Normal waveform of pattern ERG

Normal Values

- 1–8 µv normal amplitude
- Less than 1 µv definitely abnormal.
- Ratio N2/P1 amplitude > 1.1
- Ratio less than 1.1 is abnormal.

RESPONSES

Types of abnormal ERG (Fig. 4.6.7):

i. *Subnormal ERG:* When the amplitude is < 2SD beneath the normal mean a-wave or b-wave.

ii. *Negative ERG:* If the b-wave is small, it will not counter the a-wave downward slope, making the a-wave look like a deep V (b/a ratio less than one).

iii. *Minimal ERG:* A scotopic response < 100 mV or a photopic response < 50 mV.

iv. *Extinguished ERG:* Very small waveforms, indistinguishable from the background noise.

v. *Supernormal ERG:* Amplitude > 2SD above the mean b-wave or both a-wave and b-wave.

CLINICAL APPLICATIONS

1. *Retinal detachment:* The value of electrodiagnostic tests is greater in those cases where due to opacities in the media ophthalmoscopic examination is either difficult or not possible. The ERG can be used to estimate the extent of functional retina in cases of RD. In retinal detachment, the amount of ERG reduction is related to the size of detachment and degree of dysfunction of the detached retina. Both rod and cone responses may be reduced and prolonged with similar effects on a-wave and b-wave. The ERG is likely to be severely reduced in chronic, large RD.[4]

In general ERG b-wave amplitudes correspond to the amount of attached healthy retina, although the detached retina may function for some time. In cases of RD there is immediate marked reduction of b-wave amplitude. The b-wave amplitude also gives prognosis after RD surgery.[4, 5]

2. *Retained IOFBs:* The ERG is useful to assess cases of retinal FBs and trauma to estimate the extent of retinal dysfunction. FBs affect retinal function depending on the extent of tearing of the retina, the location and composition of the object. ERG is used to assess the level of retinal degeneration in cases of chronic metallic intraorbital FBs.[6]

Ocular siderosis develops secondary to the intraocular retention of an iron-containing foreign body and may result in progressive retinal degeneration. To avoid this, early FB extraction is recommended, but, depending of the location of the FB, the risk associated with surgical removal may outweigh the risk of siderosis.[7]

The ERG in such cases can document the functional changes that may occur in the course of iron toxicity, and thus influence management.

The electrophysiological findings in siderosis have been well characterized. There may be a transient supernormal response in the initial stages (Fig. 4.6.8a). If the FB is not removed, the ERG b-wave decreases with preservation of the a-wave (Fig. 4.6.8b). Rod

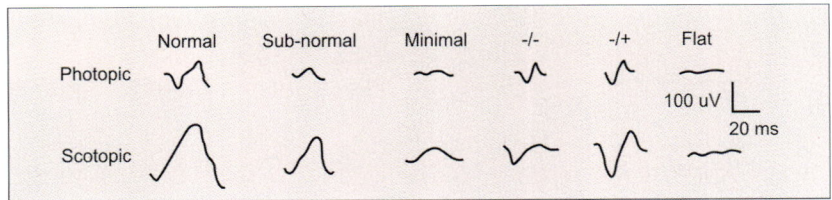

Fig. 4.6.7: Different patterns of normal and abnormal photopic and scotopic ERG

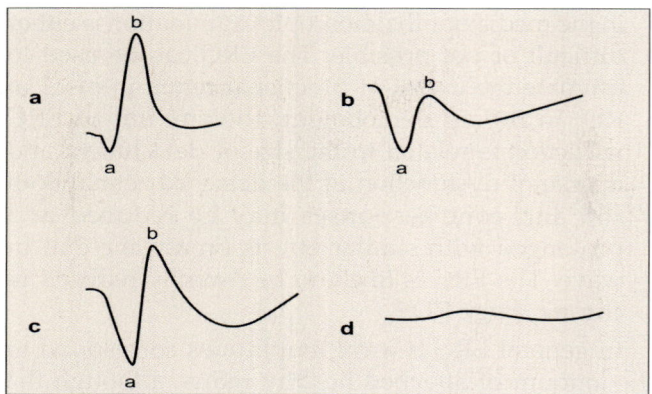

Figs 4.6.8a to d: Electrophysiological findings in ocular siderosis

ERGs are classically more impaired than cone ERGs. At this stage, extraction of the metallic body may still normalize visual function. Without the removal of the intraocular FB, the ERG deteriorates further with increased attenuation of the b-wave and later reduction of the a-wave (Fig. 4.6.8c). In end stage disease, the ERG becomes undetectable (Fig. 4.6.8d).[8]

In ocular siderosis, a preoperative EOG reduction in amplitudes of as much as 40% may be reversible after IOFBs removal. **In general if b-wave amplitudes are reduced to 50% or greater compared to the fellow eye, it is unlikely that the retinal physiology will recover unless the FB is removed.**[8,9]

3. Commotio retinae and traumatic macular hole may occur after blunt trauma and mfERG has been used to evaluate the central retinal damage following blunt trauma. Use of mfERG demonstrates marked reduction in central retinal response amplitude reflecting decreased foveal function.

PROGNOSTIC VALUE OF ERG

All patients in whom the ERG is extremely small or no ERG can be elicited fail to recover their sight. Therefore, when for clinical reasons a sympathetic ophthalmitis is feared, an extinguished ERG is a further justification for early enucleation.

Almost every patient with a normal or slightly subnormal ERG achieve a good recovery of vision, even after very serious trauma.[10]

The ERG recorded soon after severe ocular trauma has therefore an important prognostic value. However, a normal ERG soon after the trauma does not preclude the occurrence of a late RD which can be diagnosed by a decrease in the amplitude of repeat ERGs.

Extinguished bright flash ERG in traumatic vitreous hemorrhage is a poor prognostic sign.[4,11]

VISUALLY-EVOKED POTENTIAL (VEP)

The recording of the electrical activity of the occipital cortex in response to a stimulus of light from electrodes placed on the scalp is known as VEP (Fig. 4.6.9). It is an averaged and amplified record of action potential. Since foveal representation in the striate cortex is thousand times more than extra-foveal retina, VEP mainly determines the integrity of the foveal part of the visual system.[12]

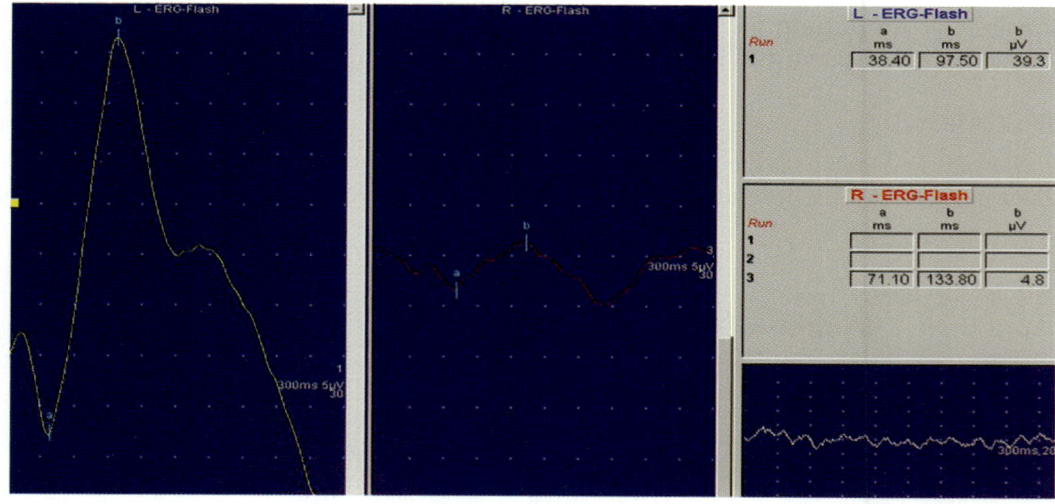

Fig. 4.6.9: Patient of siderosis showing decreased b-wave amplitude in the affected right eye with normal waveform in the left eye

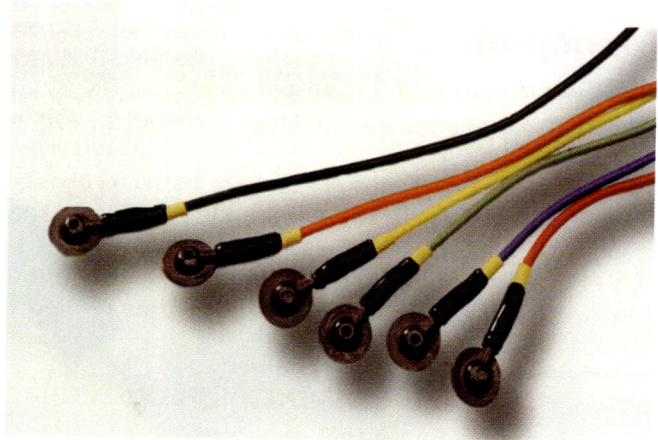

Fig. 4.6.10: Standard silver-silver chloride for recording (VEP)

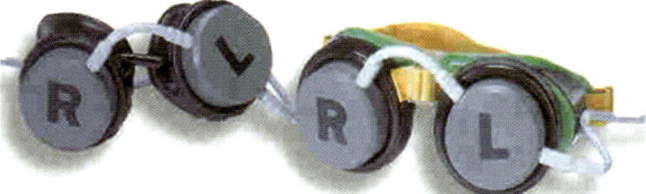

Fig. 4.6.11: LED glasses for flash VEP in children

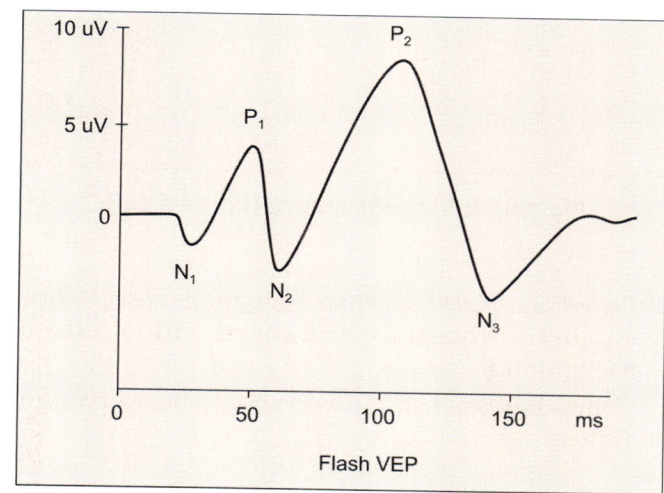

Fig. 4.6.12: Normal waveform of flash VEP

ELECTRODES

Standard silver-silver chloride (Fig. 4.6.10) or gold disk surface electrodes are recommended for recording VEPs. The electrodes are placed as follows:

- *Recording electrode:* On the scalp over the visual cortex; 1 inch above inion
- Reference electrode at forehead, vertex, mastoid, earlobe
- Ground electrode at forehead.

Based on types of the stimulus used, two types of VEP recording can be taken.

Flash VEP

A short duration, markedly supra-threshold, diffuse flash of light is used either with strobe flash lamp or Ganzfeld stimulator at the rate of 1–4 stimuli per second. 64–128 stimuli are averaged. The flash should subtend a visual field of at least 20° and the stimulus is presented in a dimly illuminated room. In children light emitting diodes (LED) goggles are used to give flash stimuli (Fig. 4.6.11). Here, LEDs are present in the goggles itself so that even if the child moves its head, it will give proper flash stimulus.

A flash VEP merely indicates the perception of light by the visual cortex and is used in case of media opacities (corneal opacity/vitreous hemorrhage) or for anxious patients and uncooperative children, where author want to know whether any vision is present or not.

Normal waveform of flash VEP: The most common components are N_2 and P_2 around 90 and 120 msec latency, respectively (Fig. 4.6.12). N_1, P_1, N_2, P_2 and N_3 nomenclature of waves is given to differentiate flash VEP from PVEP. N_1, N_2, N_3 are the negative waves while P_1, P_2 are the positive waves.

Normal Values of VEP

Latency of P_2 = 100 msec +/−10 msec
Amplitude > 5 μv.

Pattern VEP

The stimulus used here is a projector or TV screen generating the image of a checkerboard pattern. The recommended patterned stimulus is a black and white checkerboard. All checks are square and there are equal numbers of light and dark checks. There are further two types of stimulus:

1. *Pattern reversal stimulus:* The pattern reversal stimulus consists of black and white checks that change phase (i.e. black to white and white to black) abruptly and repeatedly at a specified number of reversals per second with no change in the overall luminance of the screen.

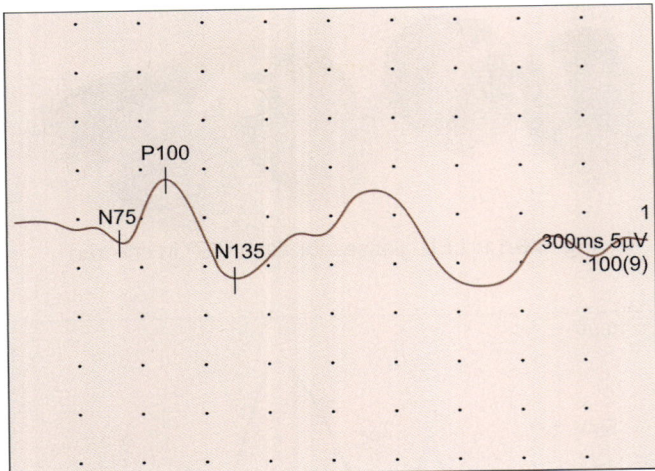

Fig. 4.6.13: Normal waveform of pattern VEP

2. *Pattern onset/offset stimulus:* For pattern onset/offset a pattern is abruptly exchanged with a diffuse background.

Commonly used stimulus is checkerboard pattern stimulus.

Normal Values

Normal value of PVEP

- *Amplitude of P100:* Normal ≥ 5 uv, non-specific, voluntarily affected.
- *Latency of P100:* Normal: 90–110 msec

CLINICAL UTILITIES

The VEP recording shows interindividual variability. However, when recording from two eyes of the same person are compared, the variability is less than 10%. In normal persons, the response from the two eyes are symmetrical, hence an asymmetry in the recording from two eyes is indicative of an abnormality in the visual pathway (Fig. 4.6.13).

VEP testing is helpful to determine whether optic neuropathy or more posterior visual pathway defect is present.

VISUAL POTENTIAL ASSESSMENT IN OPAQUE MEDIA

In cases of post-traumatic corneal scars and opacities, VEP can be done prior to penetrating keratoplasty to know the visual potential in the traumatized eye (Figs 4.6.14 to 4.6.16).

Traumatic optic neuropathy: There are only a few studies which have dealt with VEP in the evaluation of post-traumatic blindness.[13,14]

Aggarwal et al assessed the prognosis for recovery of vision in patients with blindness due to head injury, and to analyze the predictive value of VEP and concluded that recovery of VEP from no response to abnormal wave or abnormal wave to normal VEP are indicators of relatively good visual prognosis.[15]

COMPRESSIVE OPTIC NEUROPATHIES AND ISCHEMIC RETINAL LESIONS

Compressive optic neuropathy and ischemic lesions may show a decrease in amplitude on pattern VEP.

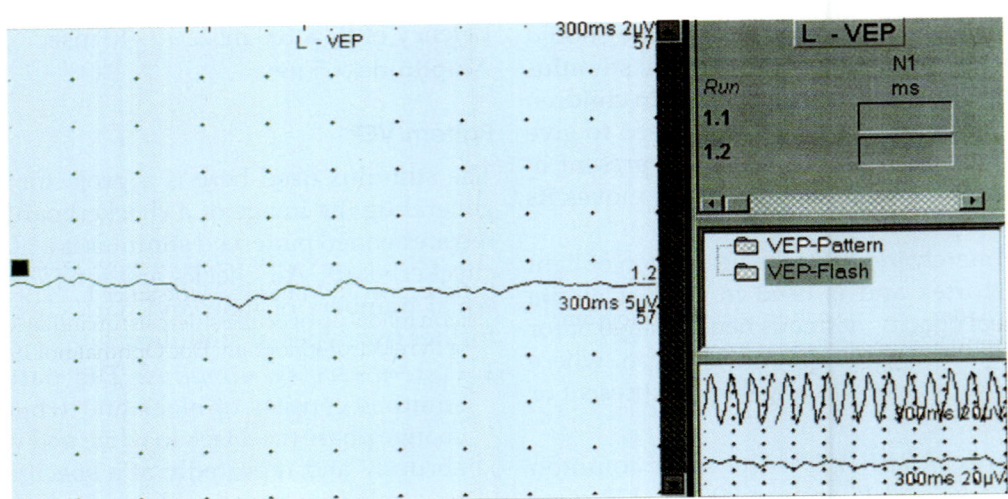

Fig. 4.6.14: Flat VEP in a patient of post-traumatic corneal scar indicating poor visual potential

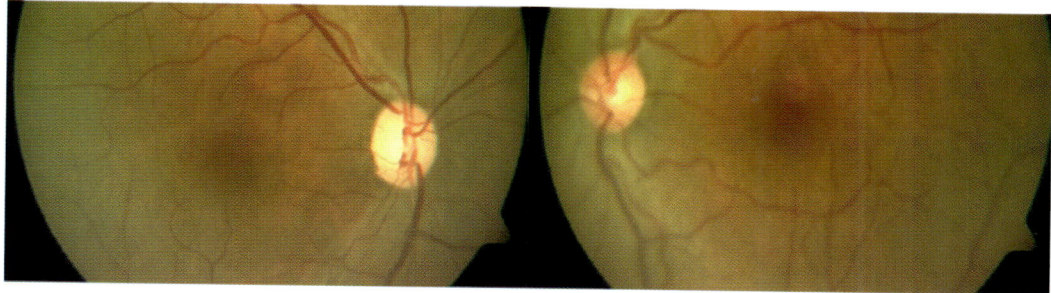

Fig. 4.6.15: Fundus photograph of the same patient showing right-sided traumatic optic neuropathy and left eye normal fundus and below (VEP) of right eye showing non-specific waveforms and normal waveform in left eye indicating poor visual potential and the affected eye

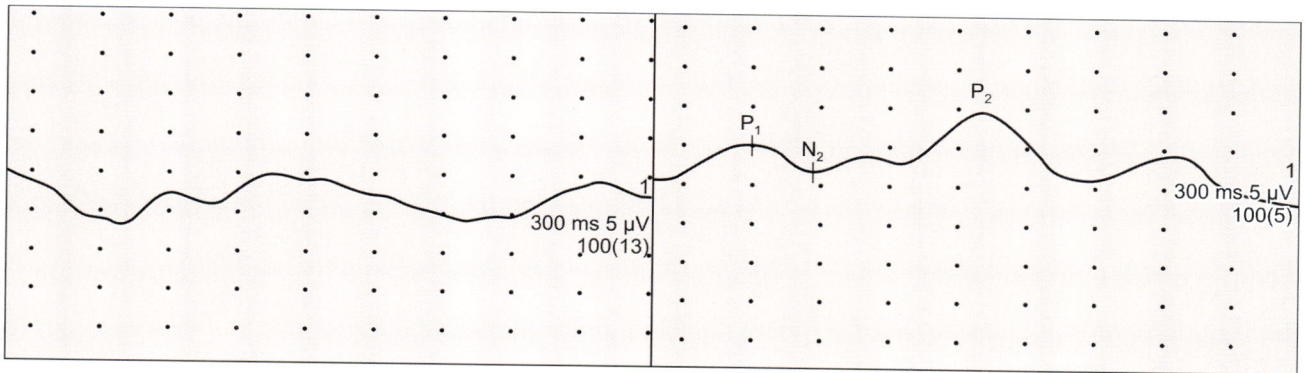

Fig. 4.6.16: Right eye showing no specific wave, left eye with normal wave pattern on FVEP

Flash VEP might be normal in some of these cases. PVEP is more reliable than flash VEP as a diagnostic or prognostic indicator.

In conclusion, electrophysiologicals tests should be done in traumatized eyes to gauge the visual potential of the injured eye. In opaque media standard ERG, bright flash ERG and flash VEP are done to assess the visual potential.

ERG and VEP are important diagnostic and follow-up electrodiagnostic parameter for optic neuropathies.

REFERENCES

1. Berninger TA, Arden GB. The pattern electroretinogram. Eye 1988;2 (Suppl):S257–83.
2. Marmor MF, Zrenner E: Standard for clinical electrophysiology. International Society for Clinical Electrophysiology of Vision. Arch Ophthalmol 1993;111:601–4.
3. Marmor MF, Zrenner E. Standard for clinical electroretinography (1994 update). Doc Ophthalmol 1995;89:199–210.
4. Zrenner E, Ziegler R, Voss B. Clinical applications of pattern electroretinography: melanoma, retinal detachment and glaucoma. Doc Ophthalmol 1988;68:283–92.
5. Gahlot DK, Khosla PK, Tewari HK. Value of electrophysiological investigations in retinal detachment. Indian J Ophthalmol 1979;27:174–7.
6. Knave B. Eelectroretinography in eyes with retained intraocular metallic foreign bodies. Acta Ophthamol 1969;100(Suppl):3–63.
7. Imaizumi M, Matsumoto CS, Yamada K, et al. Electroretinographic assessment of early changes in ocular siderosis. Ophthalmologica 2000;214:354–9.
8. Kuhn F, Witherspoon CD, Skalka H, et al: Improvement of siderotic ERG. Eur J Ophthalmol 1992;2:44–5.
9. Schechner R, Miller B, Merksamer E, Perlman I. A long term follow up of ocular siderosis: quantitative assessment of the electroretinogram. Doc Ophthalmol 1990;76:231–40.
10. Jayle GE, Tassy AF. Prognostic value of the electroretinogram in severe recent ocular trauma BJO 1970;54:51–8.
11. Harding GFA. Evaluation of ocular trauma, opaque media. In: Heckenlively JR, Arden GB, eds. Principles and Practice of Clinical Electrophysiology of Vision. St. Louis, Mosby Year Book, 1991:567–72.

12. Harding GF, Odom JV, Spileers W, et al. Standard for visual evoked potentials 1995. The international society for clinical electrophysiology of vision. *Vision Res.* 1996;36:3567–72.

13. Mahapatra AK, Bhatia R. Predictive value of VEP in unilateral optic nerve injury. Surg Neurol 1989;31:339–42.

14. Nau HE, Gerhad L, Focrster M, Nahser HC, Reinhardt V, Joka TH. Optic nerve trauma: clinical electro-physiological and histological remarks. Acta Neurochir 1987;89:16–27.

15. Agarwal A, Mahapatra AK. Visual outcome in optic nerve injury patients without initial light perception. Indian J Ophthalmol 1999;47:233–6.

5

Orbital and Adnexal Injuries

5.1 ORBITAL TRAUMA

• Usha Kim

INTRODUCTION

Orbital trauma is one of the few true emergencies which an ophthalmologist faces in his or her daily practice. A good understanding of the risk factors along with timely intervention cannot only prevent irreversible loss of vision, but can also mean the difference between life and death of the patient. The increasing frequency of road traffic accidents and consequently the increasing number of patients who present to the ophthalmologist with history of trauma necessitates a good understanding of this condition.

ANATOMY

But before going into details of orbital trauma, a thorough knowledge of the structures forming the orbit is mandatory (Fig. 5.1.1).[1]

The orbit, in simplified terms, can be described as a four-sided pyramidal compartment with the base facing forward and apex projecting medially toward optic foramen. Each orbital cavity has a volume of

about 30 cc.[2] In addition to the eyeball and the extra-ocular muscles, the orbital cavity contains vessels and nerves supplying not just the eye, but also areas surrounding the orbit.

Although easy to understand, the simplistic pyramidal description of the orbit fails in two obvious places. As the bony cavity essentially forms around the globe, the dimensions of the cavity are largest not at the base, but approximately 15 mm behind it, corresponding to the equator of the eyeball. Also the floor of the orbit does not reach the apex, making the cavity triangular in section in the region.[3] Added to this description is the fact that the boundaries between the four walls are poorly defined and rounded. Perhaps a better description of the orbital cavity was the one given by Whitnall,[4] who compared the orbit to a pear with the optic canal being the stalk.

The base, or the orbital rim, is outlined by strong bony margins: the supraorbital arch of frontal bone above, the zygoma and maxilla below, the zygoma laterally, and the frontal process of maxilla medially. Though this orbital rim provides a strong and efficient protective barrier to the orbital contents, it is weakened at the junction of its constituent bones, described as suture lines. These include the fronto-zygomatic suture along the lateral wall, the infraorbital suture along the floor and the fronto-ethmoidal suture along the medial wall. An injury at or near these suture lines can cause displacement of the bones, giving rise to the typically described 'step' deformity.

The four orbital walls can be described as the roof, medial wall, floor, and the lateral wall of the orbit.

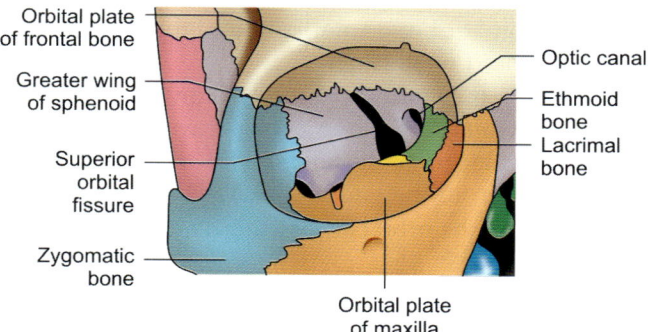

Fig. 5.1.1: Bones forming the orbital walls

Orbital plate of frontal bone
Greater wing of sphenoid
Superior orbital fissure
Zygomatic bone
Optic canal
Ethmoid bone
Lacrimal bone
Orbital plate of maxilla

ROOF OF THE ORBIT

- Formed by the orbital plate of frontal bone anteriorly and posteriorly lesser wing of sphenoid.
- The roof is extremely thin and fragile except posteriorly where it is formed by the lesser wing of sphenoid.
- It includes the lacrimal gland fossa for the orbital lobe of the lacrimal gland and the fovea, which is a small depression about 5 mm behind the superior orbital rim for the tubercle of the superior oblique muscle.
- An injury to the roof of the orbit, most commonly due to a penetrating injury through the lids, is extremely dangerous as it lies adjacent to the anterior cranial fossa and frontal sinus.

MEDIAL WALL

- It is formed by four bones:
  1. Frontal process of maxilla
  2. Lacrimal bone
  3. Orbital plate of ethmoid
  4. Body of sphenoid
- The thinnest parts of the medial wall are the lamina papyracea, which overlies the ethmoidal sinus, along with the maxillary bone.
- The superior oblique muscle lies in the angle between the roof and medial wall, and the medial rectus muscle runs along the medial wall. The medial wall, at its weakest points, is most commonly fractured in an indirect blow out fracture and these muscles are vulnerable to entrapment (Figs 5.1.2a to c).

ORBITAL FLOOR

- The triangular orbital floor is formed by three bones:
  1. Orbital plate of the maxilla
  2. Orbital surface of zygomatic bone
  3. Orbital process of palatine bone.
- This floor forms the roof of the maxillary sinus. Tumors of the maxillary sinus often invade the orbit and present as proptosis. Similarly, in a blowout fracture, orbital contents may prolapse into the maxillary sinus.
- The inferior rectus muscle lies along the floor of the orbit near the apex. Anteriorly, the inferior oblique passes below the inferior rectus.

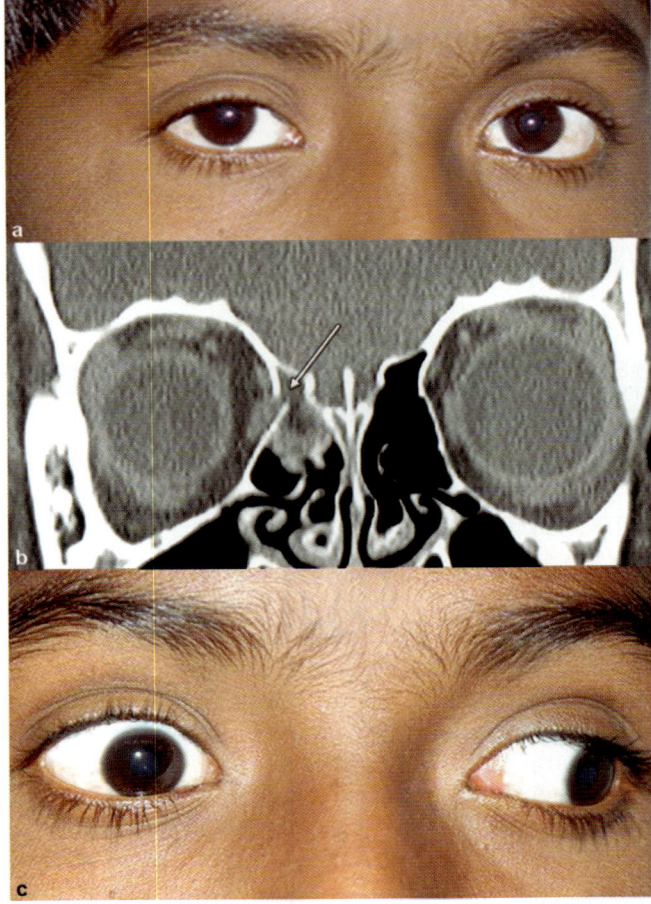

Figs 5.1.2a to c: This child presented with history of blunt trauma to the right eye. The only presenting feature was a left face turn (a); CT scan revealed a medial wall fracture of the right orbit (b) with medial rectus entrapment, which resulted in restricted adduction of the right eye (c)

LATERAL WALL

- Lateral wall is composed of the orbital surface of the zygomatic bone anteriorly, and the greater wing of sphenoid posteriorly.
- Although the lateral wall is the strongest of the four orbital walls, the globe projects well beyond the anterior margin of the lateral wall and is vulnerable to injury from the lateral aspect.

Trauma to the orbit can be broadly distributed into three categories:
1. Blunt trauma to the orbit
2. Lid and canalicular injuries
3. Orbital fractures.

Although there lies no sharp demarcation between them and a patient may present with features of more than one of these categories, a broad distribution helps us understand the presenting features of various types of injuries and their management, which will in turn help us formulate an organized, stepwise approach when presented with such a patient. In the following pages, we shall go over the principles of examination and management of these patients.

ORBITAL SOFT TISSUE INJURIES

The bony perimeters of the orbit offer the greatest defense against blunt trauma. In some instances, the orbital bones are bypassed by relatively small objects such as a ball or a small projectile, thereby resulting in direct injury to the globe, lids, extraocular muscles and orbital soft tissue. Severe trauma by larger objects can cause soft tissue injury along with orbital fractures (Fig. 5.1.3).

Examination

A majority of patients with orbital injuries have coexisting injuries elsewhere in the body. A lot of times the ophthalmologist may be the first doctor to attend to these patients. In such cases, the priority is to render first aid on an emergency basis in the form of medical or surgical treatment. The TABC rule of checking for trachea, airway, breathing and circulation should never be forgotten. Next step is to fully document the nature and history of the injury.

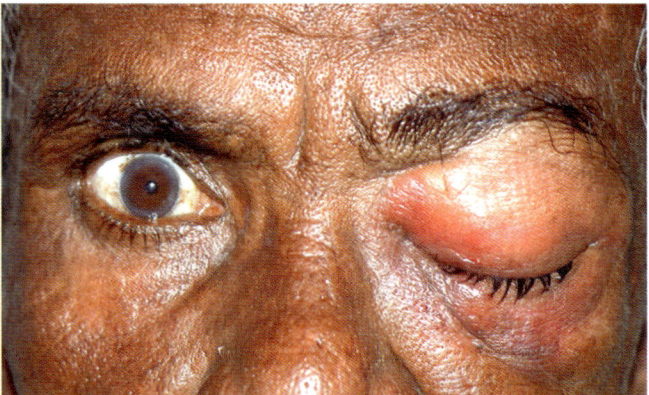

Fig. 5.1.3: Blunt trauma to the left orbit presenting with severe edema of the left upper lid. The anterior segment evaluation was within normal limits

Questioning should be Directed toward Determining

- The amount of energy transferred to the globe and orbit
- The physical characteristics of the object
- In addition, the location of the impact area may be important in estimating potential damage to the orbital bony structures and visual system.

The general guidelines include:
- Visual acuity, visual fields, color vision should be tested.
- Pupil shape, size and reaction are recorded.
- Ocular motility and displacement of the globe is looked for.
- Orbital rim is palpated for tenderness, crepitus and bony irregularity.
- Ultrasonography (USG) B-scan, X-ray and computed tomography (CT) scan orbit should be considered whenever necessary.[5]
- Photographic documentation of all injuries is useful.
- History of pre-existing ocular abnormalities as well as other systemic diseases should be elicited.

The examination can be divided into four basic parts:
1. The ocular examination
2. Soft tissue adnexal examination
3. Orbital evaluation
4. Examination of face.

Ocular examination must be performed first to rule out an injury of the globe. Above documented points should be looked for. For some cases, especially pediatric patients, evaluation under anesthesia may be necessary.

The adnexal examination should delineate the extent and depth of lacerations, and whether septum, canaliculus or lid margin are involved. Lid position and levator function should be assessed. If there is any possibility of canalicular laceration, involved canaliculus should be probed.

The orbital evaluation includes testing of extraocular muscle function including range of motion and diplopia in all gazes. Testing for hypoesthesia over cheek, side of nose, upper lip and gum should be looked for. Orbital rim is palpated for tenderness, crepitus and bony irregularity. If a foreign body or fracture is suspected, X-ray or CT scan should be done. However, when optic nerve compression or injury is suspected, magnetic resonance imaging (MRI) is the investigation modality of choice.

As adnexal injuries are often associated with facial trauma, a thorough examination of head and neck should be done. Help of an ENT specialist or neurosurgeon, as and when required, can be taken. It is important to have photographic documentation of all injuries.

Treatment

Patients with ocular adnexal trauma can have associated multisystem injuries. So, an appropriate treatment protocol is mandatory which includes ensuring adequate airway and controlling excessive bleeding and stabilizing the patients cardiovascular status. Injury to cervical spine should be ruled out and in case of the slightest suspicion of cervical injury, there should be total immobilization of the patients neck. Once other systemic injuries are ruled out, focus can be directed toward ocular examination and priority should be given to preserve the vision.

Medical Management

Ice Packs

Topical ice packs applied over a cotton gauze not only help to reduce edema, but also provide mild superficial anesthesia. Ice packs applied as frequently and continuously as possible for up to 1 week will diminish periorbital swelling and help to stay the spread of ecchymosis.

Antibiotics

Infection following blunt adnexal injuries is most often due to skin disruption with subsequent periorbital cellulitis or infected hematoma. Topical antibiotic ointment should be considered for prophylaxis when the integrity of skin has been violated. If periorbital cellulitis occurs, culture should be obtained and hot fomentation applied. Drainage of any abscess, debridement of necrotic tissue, and topical and systemic antibiotics should be considered.

Intraocular Pressure Management

A close monitoring of intraocular pressure (IOP) should be done. The urgency with which measures are undertaken to reduce IOP depends upon the degree of imminent risk of irreversible visual loss. Non-perfusion of the central retinal artery demands immediate intervention to prevent irreversible retinal ischemia.

Corticosteroids

Corticosteroids hasten the resolution of orbital edema and return of ocular motility. Corticosteroids are also useful to prevent sympathetic ophthalmitis when uveal tissue has extruded into orbit, in preventing an IOP rise due to orbital congestion, and definitely in decreasing preoperative and postoperative orbital swelling. Pulse methyl prednisolone therapy is useful in visual recovery when optic nerve is compromised.

Surgical Management

Lateral Canthotomy[6]

The most common situations warranting a lateral canthotomy include an orbital hematoma or hemorrhage with

- Elevated IOP
- Nonperfusion of the central retinal artery
- Central visual loss
- Afferent pupillary defect
- Cherry-red spot.

This procedure helps by an immediate release of orbital pressure. Fundus should be re-examined to determine whether perfusion has been re-established.

Peritomy

Conjunctival peritomy is useful in relieving tense, sight-threatening, subconjunctival or tenons space hematoma. Under topical anesthesia, direct incision over a subconjunctival clot may allow adequate anterior escape of hematoma and lower the orbital pressure. Tenons space hematoma requires a more formal limbal peritomy and subtenon dissection to decompress the clot.

Orbital Decompression[7]

Orbital decompression may be necessary when there is vision loss due to orbital edema, hematoma, congestion or emphysema that is unresponsive to medical management. A determination must be made regarding which orbital compartment is involved—subtenon's, intraconal, extraconal, subperiosteal, optic nerve sheath or diffuse. Radiologic imaging (ultrasound or CT scan) is helpful in this determination. Diffuse orbital hemorrhage unresponsive to lateral canthotomy may require decompression of the bony orbit.

LID AND CANALICULAR TRAUMA

Due to the functional importance of the close apposition of the lids and puncta to the globe, trauma to the lids presents a unique challenge. This chapter delineates the basic principles involved and describes the surgical methods of repair currently applied. Aim of management of eyelid trauma is to:

- Maximize the results of primary treatment
- Minimize the need for secondary reconstruction.

The type of injury can be assessed from the mechanism of injury. The focus of this chapter will be on the injuries caused by mechanical energy.

A preliminary history and bedside evaluation of the involved eye enables the surgeon to assess the extent and nature of the injury. The eye should be carefully covered and protected after a preliminary examination, until a full evaluation and repair can be done in an operating theater (this subject is dealt in details in following chapters 5.2 and 5.3).

Suturing Techniques[1,8]

Good approximation of the wound edges with minimal tension and no residual wound gape is the most important requisite in the successful repair of eyelid defects. This can be achieved by meticulous closure of the wound in layers.

Different suturing techniques are applied for the three important sites of lid repair, namely:

1. Deeper tissues
2. Skin
3. Lid margin.

An absorbable suture, preferably 6-0 vicryl or plain/chromic catgut is used for the closure of deeper layers. This repair of the deeper tissues should be done in as many anatomical layers as required, as an underlying wound gape here can lead to a depressed scar and leaves a potential space for collection of fluid or hematoma formation. To avoid subsequent corneal abrasions, care is taken that the sutures do not pierce the conjunctiva.

Nonabsorbable interrupted or continuous sutures are used for skin closure, while absorbable sutures are preferred in children. The bite should include full thickness of dermis, equally placed on each side, to prevent a two level scar (Figs 5.1.4a and b). The needle should enter and exit at right angles, which will result in pouting of the wound edges and prevents a sunken scar.

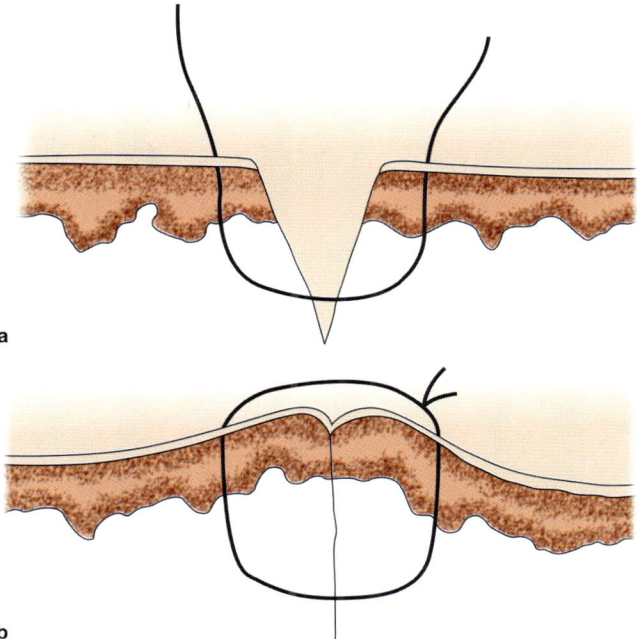

Figs 5.1.4a and b: Technique of skin suturing. Note the inclusion of the full thickness of dermis in the bite, right angled entry and exit of the needle and equal thickness of the bite on either side

Undermining the skin on either side of the wound is a useful technique to reduce tension across the suture line. A bolster may me used in cases of extreme wound tension, or when the tissue is expected to heal poorly. A continuous suture is a fast and effective technique for closure of skin wounds not under tension (Figs 5.1.4a and b). A running interlocking suture provides additional wound strength and stability.

Before we begin repair of the lid margin, wound edges should always be made parallel, clean and regular. The placement of a 6-0 absorbable suture in the gray line with a bite 2 mm from the lid margin is followed by closure of remaining wound. As in skin defects, a pouting effect achieved over the gray line produces a straight lid margin after healing.

The ends of the gray line suture are kept long and buried under the superficial skin suture to avoid rubbing over the cornea (Figs 5.1.5a and b).

Management of Lid Lacerations

Trauma to eyelids can be divided according to whether the lid margin is involved or not, and also

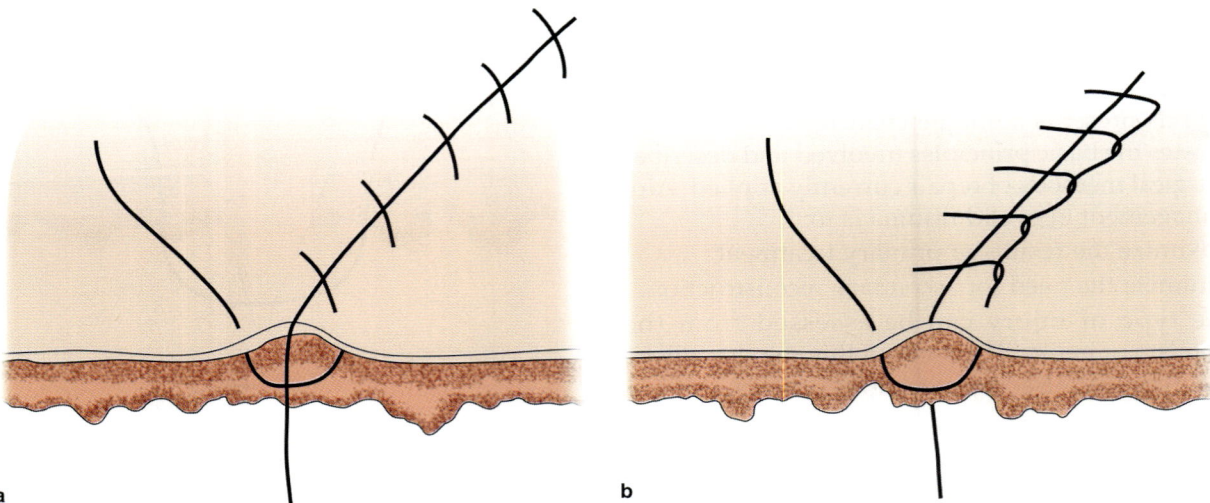

Figs 5.1.5a and b: Skin suturing using continuous sutures (a), and continuous interlocking sutures (b)

into injuries with or without associated tissue loss. The location and severity of lid laceration dictates the approach to repair.

Lid repair can be described under the following headings:
- Lid lacerations not involving lid margin
- Lid lacerations involving lid margin
  – Direct closure
  – Rotational flaps
  – Lid sharing procedures
  – Grafts
- Canthal injuries
  – Medial canthal injuries
  – Lateral canthal injuries
- Canalicular injuries.

Lid Lacerations Not Involving Lid Margins

Basic principles of suturing in a case of lid laceration not involving the margin remain the same as described above. Direct closure of the wound can be attempted as long as the eyelid margin is not distorted. A meticulous closure in multiple layers is important, taking care not to injure the conjunctiva.

In cases where direct closure of the wound without significantly distorting the lid margin is not possible, advancement or transposition of local skin flaps can be attempted (Figs 5.1.6a to c).

Full thickness skin grafts, from the preauricular or postauricular region, are best suited for the repair of anterior lamellar eyelid defects. A graft from the contralateral eyelid has also been described for upper lid defects, as it provides better motility.

Lid Lacerations Involving Lid Margins

Surgical correction of eyelid defects involving the lid margin are broadly classified into three categories, depending upon the extent of tissue loss:

1. Small defects ($\leq 33\%$)
2. Medium defects (33–50%)
3. Large defects (> 50%).

Small Defects

Direct closure of the wound can be attempted in lid defects with loss of less than one-third of lid margin, provided there is no tension over the sutured wound. Lateral canthotomy or cantholysis may be done if additional mobilization of the wound edges is required (Fig. 5.1.7).

Medium Defects[9]

A modification of the Tenzel's semicircular rotation flap is the most common procedure used to repair medium sized defects (Fig. 5.1.8). Lateral cantholysis is done and a semicircular skin flap is made curving opposite to the involved lid to mobilize the lateral edge of the wound, facilitating closure. Tarsal sharing procedures can also be attempted for these defects.

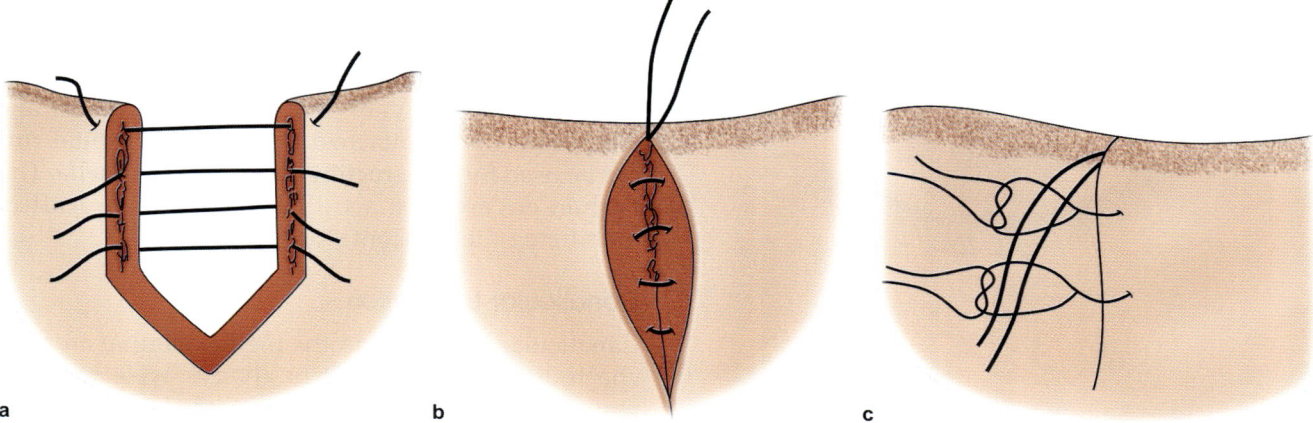

Figs 5.1.6a to c: The lid margin and deeper tissues are sutured using interrupted absorbable sutures (a). The ends of the marginal suture are kept long (b) and sutured along with the superficial skin (c) to avoid rubbing against the cornea

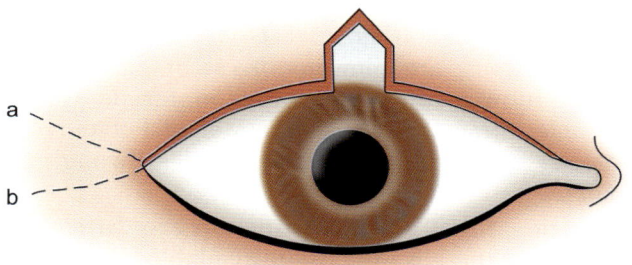

Fig. 5.1.7: Mobilization of lateral wound edge by performing a lateral cantholysis (a) or a lateral canthotomy (b)

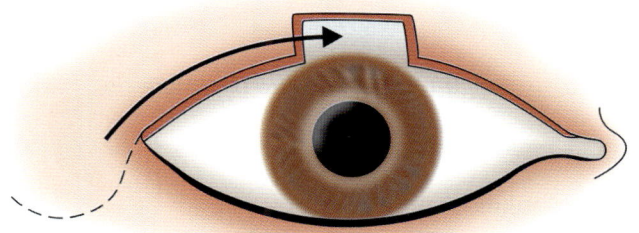

Fig. 5.1.8: Tenzel's rotation flap

Large Defects

a. Upper lid defects
b. Lower lid defects

a. Upper Lid Defects[10]

Large defects require advancement of adjacent tissues. Cutler Beard procedure involves creating a full thickness lower eyelid flap, approximately 5 mm from the lid margin and mobilizing this flap into the upper eyelid defect beneath the remaining lower eyelid margin (Fig. 5.1.9).

The posterior lamella can alternatively be reconstructed by a free tarsoconjunctival graft from the contralateral upper eyelid. This is then covered by a full thickness skin graft or by mobilizing the surrounding skin and muscle, if adequate redundant skin is present.

b. Lower Lid Defects[11]

The lower lid equivalent of the Cutler Beard procedure, is the modified Hughes procedure. But, one major difference between the two procedures is that here only the tarsoconjunctival flap is mobilized from the upper eyelid. The flap is then covered by a full thickness skin graft taken from the pre/post-auricular region. Lid sharing techniques should however be avoided in children due to risk of deprivational amblyopia.

A large lower lid defect can also be repaired using the Mustardé cheek rotation flap (Fig. 5.1.10).[12] The posterior lamella then has to be constructed using either a free tarsoconjunctival autograft, hard palate mucosa, auricular cartilage or a Hughes flap.

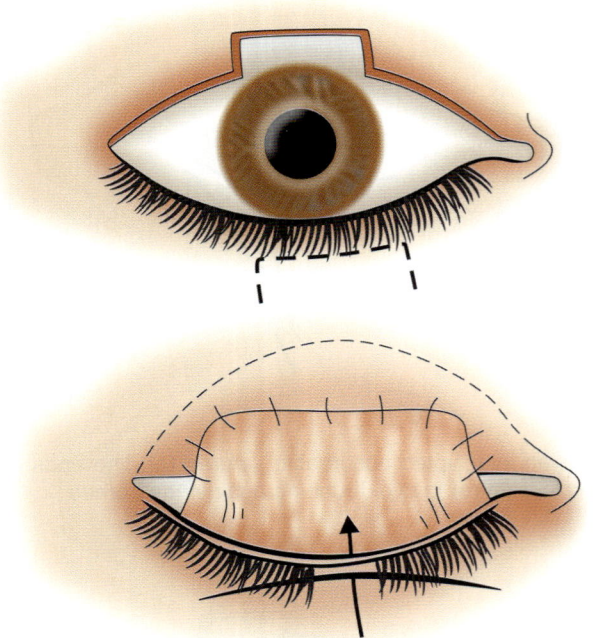

Fig. 5.1.9: Cutler Beard procedure

Canthal Injuries

Medial Canthal Defects

Small defects at the medial canthus can be repaired by direct closure of the wound. Large defects can be managed by anchoring the medial canthal tendon or the tarsus to the periosteum using a 4-0 prolene suture. Care has to be taken to fully cover the prolene suture in two layers using an absorbable suture.

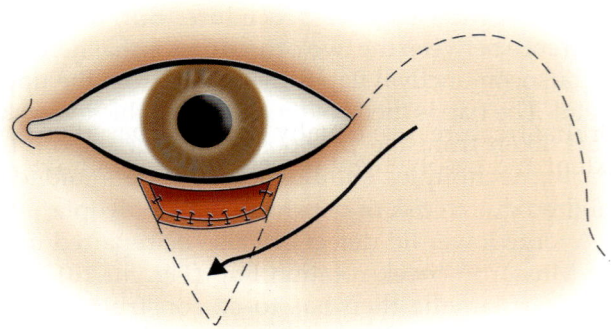

Fig. 5.1.10: Mustardé cheek rotation flap

Lateral Canthal Defects

Tarsal sharing procedures or semicircular rotation flaps can be used to repair defects at the lateral canthus. Alternatively, a strip of periosteum and temporalis fascia, attached at the lateral orbital rim, can be used for constructing the posterior lamella. This is then covered by a full thickness skin graft or mobilizing the adjacent skin.

Canalicular Laceration

Canalicular laceration in the medial canthal area is a challenging problem. It is always wise to use a magnifying loupe or even an operating microscope during examination, as lacerations of canalicular system are often missed. An attempt should be made to repair both upper and lower canaliculus.

A stent placed between the torn canaliculus stabilizes the wound margins sufficiently for an end-to-end anastomosis (Fig. 5.1.11).[13] Various stents used for this purpose are mini-monoka stent, placement of silastic tubing, and when other materials are not available, intracath can be used as a stent. Polyethylene material is avoided, because it erodes through the tissues.

Injuries directly at the punctum are difficult to repair since there is little tissue available for suturing around the punctum without placing sutures directly through the canaliculus. Monocanalicular or bicanalicular intubation may be useful for such repairs. If the area is badly damaged, the development of an auxillary punctum or opening into the canaliculus may be attempted, as for excision of tumors in the punctal area (*see* also in chapter 5.3).

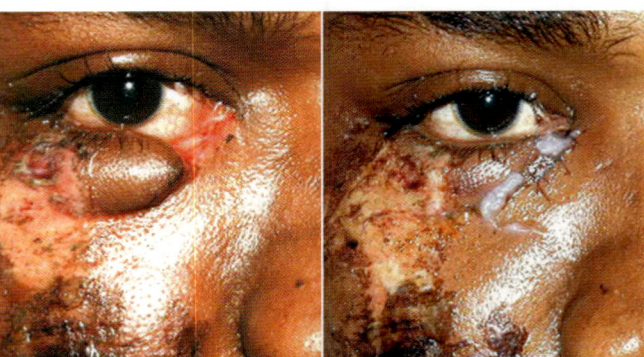

Fig. 5.1.11: Lower lid laceration involving the canaliculus repaired with stenting of the inferior canaliculus

Levator Muscle Trauma

Laceration of levator muscle/aponeurosis, results in drooping of upper lid. Even in the presence of severe lid edema, levator function can be detected by a dimpling of upper eyelid crease when patient looks superiorly. If this is absent, trauma to the levator muscle or its nerve supply is suspected, in which case exploration and repair should be done as early as possible, once soft tissue signs has resolved. Delayed repair is difficult as anatomical details of muscle and surrounding structures becomes obscured.

Best surgical approach of a lacerated levator muscle repair, is through an anterior eyelid crease incision. This approach allows easy dissection, along the levator aponeurosis up to the orbital septum. Exploration is carried out until the proximal cut edge of the levator muscle is identified. This is then reattached to the distal end, if identified, or to the tarsal plate.

Traumatic disinsertion of levator aponeurosis, which is characterized by acute onset of ptosis with good levator function and a high upper lid crease, is managed by exploration and reattachment of aponeurosis to the tarsal plate (*see* also in chapter 5.2).

Delayed Repair of Eyelid Injuries

Delayed repair of eyelid injuries is challenging due to formation of scar tissue, which results in distortion and contracture. If initial repair had been attempted and tissues were anatomically aligned, contracture can be treated simply by scar excision and repeat approximation of tissue or by a full thickness skin graft (Figs 5.1.12a and b).

However, if initial repair was not undertaken or tissues were not anatomically aligned, meticulous dissection is required to correctly identify tissue structures and achieve proper alignment. This, however, may not be possible in all cases.

Having said this, if wound has already healed and the eye is sufficiently protected, it is advisable to avoid any surgical intervention till the scar has fully developed, which usually takes a period of 3–6 months.

ORBITAL FRACTURES

Orbital fractures are most often associated with acute ocular and adnexal injuries.

The surgeon must be able to not only properly evaluate the patient but also understand and use

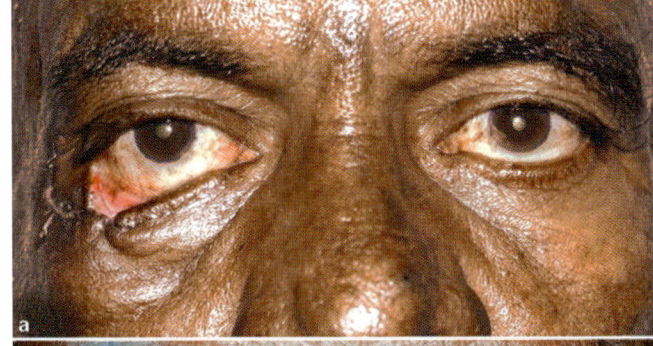
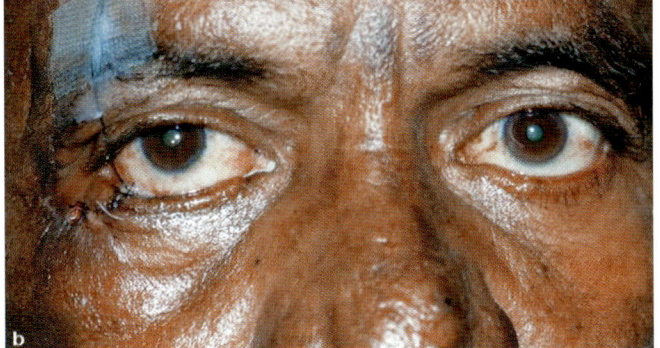

Figs 5.1.12a and b: Lower lid laceration repair by direct apposition

appropriate diagnostic techniques to help to determine whether or not surgical intervention is necessary.

It is not unusual for orbital fractures to involve the globe, eyelids, sinuses and brain. It is therefore essential that a complete ophthalmic examination be performed to detect direct or indirect injury to the globe, optic nerve or its blood supply. A CT scan and neurosurgical evaluation should be done if there is any suspicion of concomitant intracranial injury.

In general, orbital fractures may be divided into two broad categories: a fracture of the orbital bones without involvement of the orbital rim is termed as a pure blowout fracture, while if the orbital rim is also involved, it is called an impure blowout fracture.

Classification of Orbital Fractures

Orbital fractures are usually classified based on their extent and involvement of periorbital structures.

LeFort Classification

Midfacial injuries are an important group of orbital fractures that extend beyond the orbit. LeFort classification divides midfacial fractures into three groups (Fig. 5.1.13).

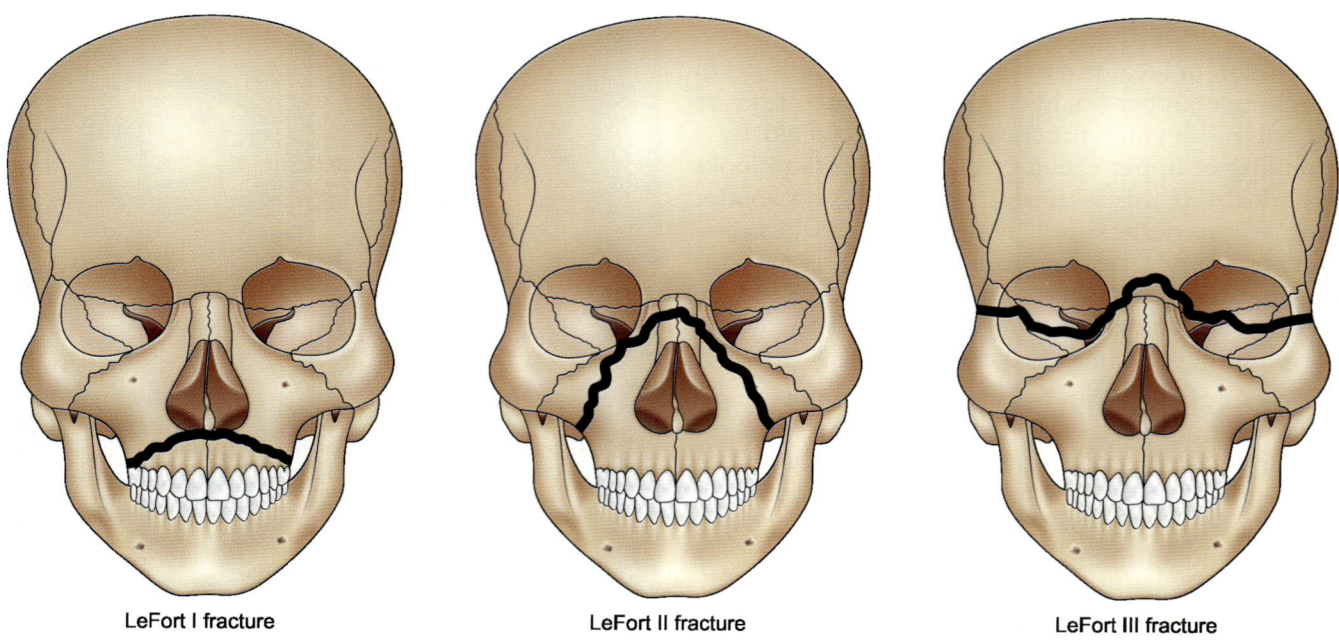

LeFort I fracture   LeFort II fracture   LeFort III fracture

Fig. 5.1.13: LeFort classification of midfacial fractures

LeFort Type I Fracture

Also known as Guerin's fracture, it is a relatively inferior transverse fracture within the body of the maxilla in the region above the teeth without true involvement of the orbit.

LeFort Type II Fracture

It is a pyramid shaped maxillary fracture extending to the medial floor and wall of the orbit. This fracture typically involves the nasal and lacrimal bones in addition to the maxillary bone.

LeFort Type III Fracture

This subtype is a complex, extensive, midfacial fracture also known as craniofacial dysjunction or "free floating" maxilla, since the midface is essentially detached from the skull and is suspended in place by soft tissues alone. This fracture extends through the ramus of the mandible, in addition to the lateral wall, floor and medial wall of the orbit.

Orbital Roof Fractures

Orbital roof fractures occur most frequently due to a penetrating injury through the upper lid, and may represent a threat to life due to its close proximity to the anterior cranial fossa. Besides direct central nervous system (CNS) injury, orbital roof fractures may also be associated with an intracranial foreign body, or the presence of a dural tear with cerebrospinal fluid leakage.

Fracture and involvement of the nasofrontal duct or frontal sinus can also accompany an orbital roof fracture. Bony fragments from orbital roof fractures can cause mechanical restriction of the superior muscle complex, but this situation is unusual.

Naso-orbital and Medial Wall Fractures

Fracture of the lamina papyracea that serves as the lateral wall of the ethmoid sinus is relatively common in naso-orbital and medial wall fractures. Sudden increase in intraorbital pressure due to transmission of hydraulic forces when an individual receives blunt trauma or a blow to the globe or anterior orbit is postulated as the mechanism of such fractures.

In a large number of these cases, signs and symptoms are limited to epistaxis or orbital emphysema. In most cases, asking the patient to avoid blowing their nose until symptoms have resolved is sufficient, as these fractures generally heal without any long-term sequelae. In some cases however, naso-orbital fractures may contribute to the development of post-traumatic enophthalmos (Figs 5.1.14 and 5.1.15),

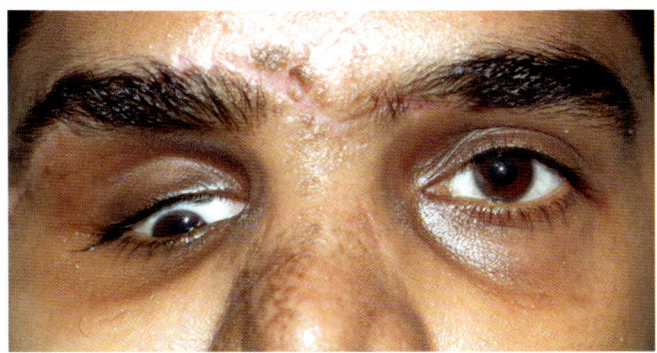

Fig. 5.1.14: Orbital floor fracture presenting with gross enophthalmos with downward displacement of the globe

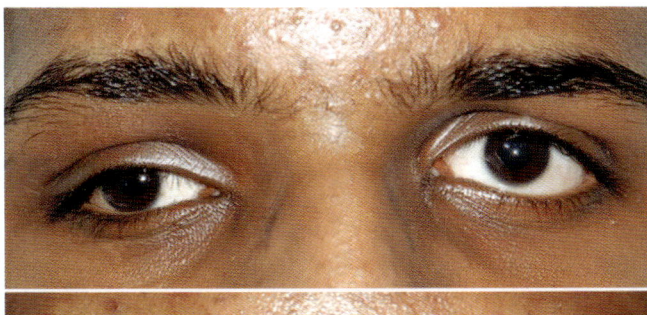
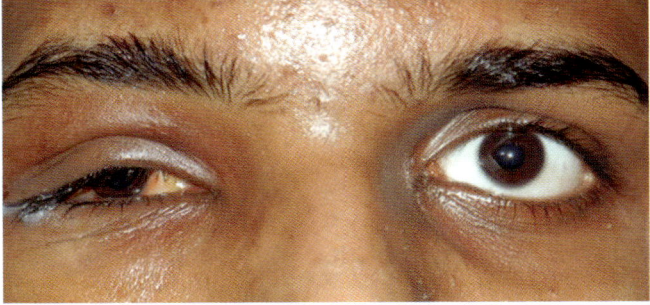

Fig. 5.1.15: Preoperative and postoperative pictures of orbital floor fracture repair with prolene mesh

which results from orbital tissues and fat prolapsed into the ethmoid air cells.

A frequent association of these fractures is direct or secondary injury to the medial canthal tendon with subsequent functional or cosmetic problems such as medial lid or canthal angle malposition, punctual eversion and telecanthus. Medial fractures may interfere with normal globe motility by tethering the medial rectus muscle, which warrants surgical exploration to prevent or minimize permanent limitation of motility due to fibrosis and scarring.

Orbital Floor and Tripod Fractures

Orbital floor fractures are the most common group of fractures which warrant surgical correction. Depending upon the mechanism of injury, these fractures may be classified as direct or indirect.

Trauma to the inferior rim of sufficient force may directly fracture the relatively thick bones that make the orbital rim. The fracture usually occurs along the proximal aspect of the zygoma or at its articulation with the medial or maxillary portion of the inferior rim. Forceful or crushing trauma may result in multifocal zygomatic fractures, often involving the zygomatic arch or its posterior articulation in addition to its lateral and inferior orbital rim articulation.

This three part zygomatic fracture is referred to as a tripod fracture. When nondisplaced, these fractures often require no reduction or fixation. However, displaced, depressed or rotated tripod fractures result in loss of the normal prominence of the cheek and may limit the normal excursion of the mandible. Fractures causing cosmetic or functional sequelae should be repaired primarily by open or closed reduction or by open reduction and internal fixation.

Orbital floor fracture presenting with gross enophthalmos with downward displacement of the globe.

The best diagnostic imaging modalities for confirming the presence of a blow out fracture are the X-ray and CT scan. The most important plain film radiograph for evaluating a blow out fracture is the Water's view. CT scan is confirmatory, especially in terms of soft tissue details. For evaluation of the orbital floor, finely cut (1.5–2 mm), direct, coronal views are most helpful.

Examination

While examining a patient of orbital trauma, certain important features have to be looked for which can give a clue towards the presence of orbital fractures.

Globe Displacement

After assessing the integrity of the globe and the status of the optic nerve, symmetry of globe position should be properly evaluated. The globe can be axially malpositioned or dystopic, and should be compared with the opposite eye. Any asymmetry of the globe position should be documented and quantified for future comparison.

The presence of axial displacement is usually easily apparent. This anterior or posterior deviation can be accurately quantified by use of a Hertel or Leudde exophthalmometer. When the lateral orbital rim is not intact, it can be measured with the help of Mutch exophthalmometer.

Palpation of the Orbital Rim

Palpating the orbital rim is a quick and important technique for evaluating the integrity of the bony orbit. Features to look for include a breach in continuity of the orbital rim, or the classically described step-deformity, which occurs due to displacement at the suture lines. Severe tenderness in a localized area cues the examiner to the presence of subtle rim fractures, especially if the deformity is masked by overlying soft-tissue swelling.

Intercanthal Distance

Expansion of the distance between the medial canthal angles of both eyes is termed telecanthus. This change in intercanthal distance is sometimes seen in midfacial fractures and in cases involving soft-tissue injury with severing or disinsertion of the medial canthal tendon.

Such changes are readily apparent in unilateral cases but less so in bilateral cases. In such cases, it can be assessed by comparing a straight edge measurement of the interpupillary distance with the intercanthal distance. A ratio of less than 2:1 in a setting of orbital or midfacial trauma is usually indicative of telecanthus.

Nasolacrimal Drainage System

The lacrimal drainage system is frequently disrupted in patients with orbital or naso-orbital trauma because of its close proximity to the medial canthal structures. Evaluation and repair of the system is usually deferred until soft tissue swelling has subsided, except in cases where immediate repair of laceration of the canalicular system is required.

Infraorbital Nerve Sensation

Since the floor of orbit serves as the roof of the canal carrying the infraorbital nerve, a decreased sensation along the distribution of this nerve is a subtle but priceless clue in the diagnosis of orbital floor fractures.

This nerve is sensory in nature, transmitting sensation from:

- Skin and conjunctiva of the lower lid
- The skin and subcutaneous tissues of the side of nose
- The skin and mucous membrane of the upper lip, gum and labial glands.

In general, fracture of the orbital floor can be suspected in the presence of diminished sensation along the distribution of this nerve.

Orbital Emphysema

Crepitus in the periorbital tissues is a clear clinical sign of an orbital fracture since this occurs only in the presence of a communication between the orbital tissues and the periorbital sinuses. Orbital emphysema is frequently encountered with medial orbital fractures due to the close proximity of the ethmoid sinus.

Ocular Motility

Ocular motility should be evaluated in all cardinal fields of gaze. Post-traumatic limitation of ocular motility or lid elevation can result from a number of causes, including direct injury to muscles or their innervation, mechanical restriction due to muscle entrapment, and central nervous causes including increased intracranial pressure.

The distinction between true entrapment and neuromuscular limitation of motility can be made by the forced-duction test and force generation test. While large fractures are more likely to cause enophthalmos, small orbital floor fractures are more likely to cause muscle entrapment due to a trap-door effect, and less likely to cause enophthalmos. True mechanical restriction or significant enophthalmos is an important indication for surgical correction.

Forced-duction Test

Entrapment of inferior rectus and possibly the inferior oblique muscles and their adventitial attachments are the usual cause of true mechanical restriction associated with orbital floor or blowout fractures. The forced-duction test is helpful in determining whether mechanical restriction is the actual cause of limited eye movements.

Local anesthesia and vasoconstriction of the superficial vasculature of the globe are obtained by placing a 4% xylocaine-soaked pledget over the inferior surface of the globe. A toothed forceps is used to grasp the inferior rectus muscle insertion or the perilimbal tissue between the 6 o'clock limbus and the inferior rectus insertion. The globe is then passively moved in the vertical meridian. Limitation of forced duction test can also occur in the presence of significant orbital edema, extraocular muscle swelling due to hematoma or edema and also in cases with coexisting atraumatic restrictive myopathies, as in thyroid orbitopathy.

Management of Orbital Fractures

Indications for Surgery

Indications for and timing of surgical repair of orbital fractures always remains a controversial topic for contention. Indications for surgical intervention include:

- Diplopia accompanying ocular motility limitation
- Positive forced-duction test
- Gross enophthalmos
- Hypo-ophthalmos along with radiographic evidence of a blow out fracture.

Simple radiographic presence of a blow out fracture is not an indication for surgical repair.

Most important presenting complaint of patients with post-traumatic enophthalmos is often cosmetic and not functional. This consideration should be taken into account as appropriate for each patient.

Timing For Surgical Repair

The timing for surgical intervention depends upon the presence of associated injuries, the degree of impairment, and the patient's age.

Surgical intervention, when appropriate, is technically easier in terms of scarring and fibrosis and may have a better functional result if performed within first 10 days after injury. It is often better to wait a few days after the injury to allow for some resolution of soft tissue swelling and hemorrhage before considering surgical intervention. This is true even when true entrapment is evident clinically or verified by forced duction testing, because of the greater technical ease of repair and the possibility of more accurate estimation of secondary or delayed enophthalmos development.

A short course of systemic corticosteroids helps to speed the resolution of diplopia when present, unmask enophthalmos more quickly and reduce patient discomfort and disability. However, corticosteroids carry the potential risk of sino-orbital infections, particularly in cases with hemorrhage and stagnant fluid in the sinuses. Such patients should be followed up closely.

However, in cases where acute surgical intervention is not appropriate for any reason and delayed repair is ultimately warranted, it is preferable to wait more than six weeks after injury. At this time, inflammation of the orbital tissues is usually resolved and accurate assessment of globe, ptosis or enophthalmos can be made.

Repair of Orbital Floor Fracture

A number of surgical approaches for repair of the orbital floor fracture have been described, including translid-inferior orbital rim, subciliary, Caldwell-Luc and inferior fornix or transconjunctival incisions. An inferior forniceal-lower limb lateral canthotomy approach gives excellent exposure (Fig. 5.1.16).

A lateral canthotomy is done, followed by passage of stay sutures through lower lid. This suture is used to retract the lid for exposure during the fracture repair. The conjunctiva and lower lid retractors are then incised, the incision being deep up to the periosteum overlying the orbital rim. Care should be taken to remain within the inferior orbital rim to avoid buttonholing the lower lid or traumatizing the infraorbital nerve. Globe is protected using a malleable ribbon retractor, and the periosteum is elevated using a periosteal elevator. With help of ribbon retractor, orbital contents are elevated superiorly. This aids in excellent exposure of fracture site and any entrapped tissues, which are bluntly separated, taking care not to traumatize infraorbital neurovascular bundle. Once all the tissues are separated, implant material is then placed over the fracture site.

The type and amount of implant depends upon the size of fracture and surgeon's preference. Various autologous and alloplastic material are available.

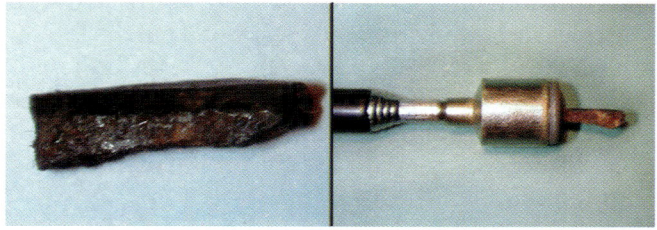

Fig. 5.1.16: Metallic foreign bodies removed from the orbit

Autologous material may be harvested from iliac crest, rib or calvarium, while alloplastic material can be bone cement, silicon, teflon, silastic, supramid, titanium mesh or medpore implant.

The globe should be passively moved after placement of implant, to check for any residual muscle or soft tissue entrapment. The conjunctiva is closed with 6-0 absorbable suture, usually vicryl. The lower lid retractors and deeper tissues need not be sutured, to avoid postoperative lid retraction. Stay sutures are removed and a lateral canthoplasty is done.

INTRAORBITAL FOREIGN BODY

Ocular trauma, especially when caused by a projectile, is often complicated by the presence of an intraorbital foreign body (FB). Though the principles of approach and removal of the FB remain similar to orbital fractures, it is important to note that not all FB necessitate removal. Due consideration must be given to the indications for and possible complications of embarking upon surgery.

Imaging

It is important to understand the principle behind the choice of imaging modality when an intraocular or intraorbital FB is suspected. An incorrect choice may not only lead to the clinician missing the FB thereby causing unnecessary delay, but can also gravely aggravate the injury as we shall see in the following discussion.

The three most common groups of intraorbital FB include:
1. Vegetable matter[14]
2. Glass
3. Metallic FB[15]

Glass and metallic FB are radio-opaque, hence can be easily picked up on plain radiographs or CT scan. Though the CT scan has the obvious advantage of better localization of the FB,[16] the cost factor and widespread availability makes the plain radiograph a priceless screening modality, especially in the Indian setup.

Ferromagnetic FB, when suspected, are an absolute contraindication to MRI. Magnet induced movement of the FB can lead to trauma to the orbital tissues along with migration of the FB.

Imaging modality of choice when a wooden FB is suspected remains a topic of great debate. Both fresh

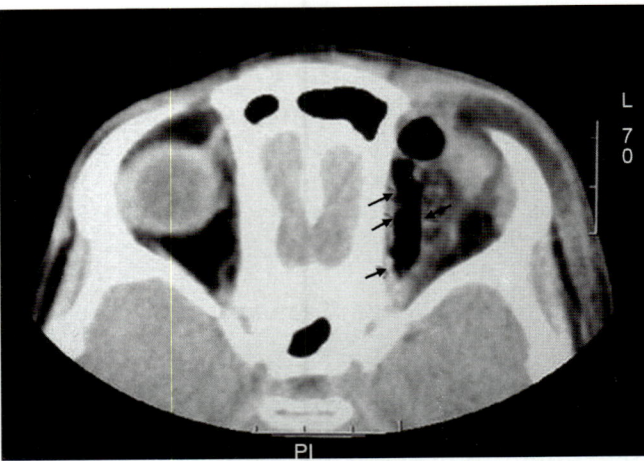

Fig. 5.1.17: An intraorbital wooden foreign body appearing hypodense on CT scan

and old wooden FB appear hypointense on an MRI,[17] due to the high air content in fresh wood and high moisture content in old wooden FB as they imbibe fluid from surrounding tissues. T1-weighted images are preferred over proton density and T2-weighted images, because they provide better contrast between fat and wood. However, an MRI scan cannot differentiate between a recent and an old wooden FB.

Presentation of a wooden FB on CT scan varies from an area of low attenuation in the initial stages due to high air content, to an area of high attenuation in the later stages due to high water content (Fig. 5.1.17). Recently, introduced wooden FB may be missed on a CT scan. However, the use of contrast and proper windowing can better differentiate wood from air and bone fragments, thus better identifying any coexisting fractures. This, along with the fact that CT scan is safer in case of a metallic FB and is far less expensive, faster and easily accessible than an MRI, makes CT scan the modality of choice. Fish hook injuries are common in coastal areas (Figs 5.1.18 and 5.1.19a to c). Removal of these FB poses a special problem and needs to mention the type of hooks and retrieval route may have to be decided according to structure of the fishing hook (Fig. 5.1.20).

Management

As already mentioned, not all orbital FBs warrant surgical removal. In addition to the difficulty in approaching and isolating an orbital FB, there is

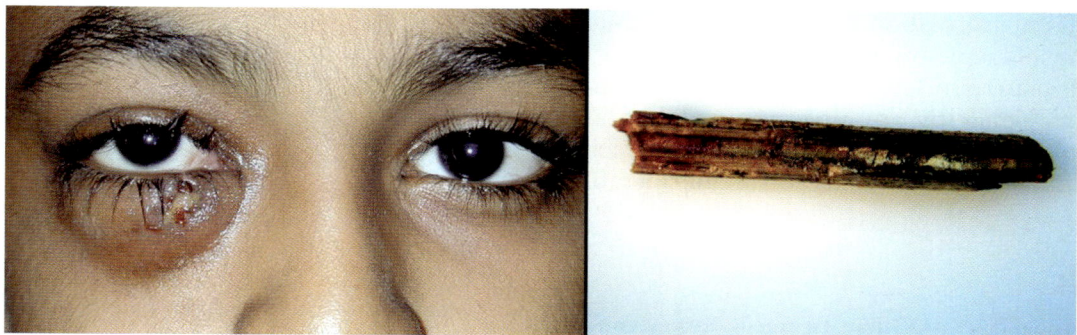

Fig. 5.1.18: Wooden foreign body removed from the inferomedial aspect of right orbit

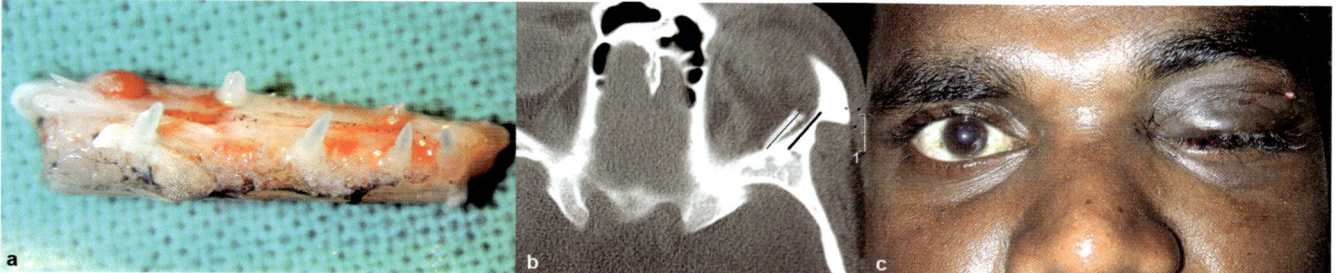

Figs 5.1.19a to c: The teeth of a swordfish (a) removed from the left orbit of a fisherman (b, c)

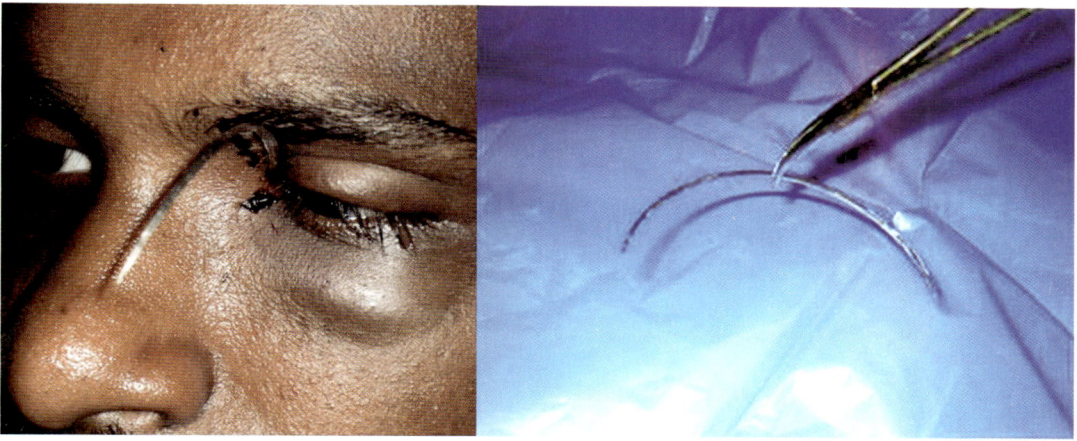

Fig. 5.1.20: A fishing hook removed from the superomedial aspect of the left orbit

always the risk of damage to adjacent tissues during surgery.

Inert ceramic or metallic FBs with smooth edges lying in the posterior orbit may be observed if they are nonmobile, nonreactive and not causing functional deficit due to direct pressure or mass effect.

FBs lying in the anterior orbit or those which cause functional restriction and inflammation of surrounding tissues must be removed. Vegetable matter is especially prone to causing bacterial as well as fungal infection which is resistant to conservative management.

The wound and the FB, if removed, should be cultured and appropriate antibiotics must be administered regardless of whether surgery is planned.[18] Chronic orbital infection along with an abscess or fistula formation following minor trauma should arouse suspicion of an underlying FB.[19] A vegetable FB surrounded by intense inflammation is difficult to isolate by any imaging modality, and clinical features along with a high index of suspicion may be all that can guide the surgeon on the operating table.

REFERENCES

1. John J Woog, Peter AD Rubin, George B. Bartley volume 3 section 12 – oculoplastics. Albert&Jakobiec's principles and practice of ophthalmology, 3rd ed.

2. Duke-Elder S, Wybar KC. The anatomy of the visual system. In: Duke-Elder S, ed. System of ophthalmology, St Louis: CV Mosby; 1961.

3. Last RJ. Eugene Wolff's Anatomy of the Eye and Orbit: The orbit and paranasal sinuses, 6th edn. HK Lewis & Co.Ltd, London pp. 1–29.

4. Whitnall SE. The anatomy of the human orbit and accessory organs of vision. OXford Press, New York 1921.

5. Fina C Barouch, Kathryn A Colby Chapter 373 – Evaluation and Initial Management of Patients with Ocular and Adnexal Trauma Albert: Albert & Jakobiec's Principles and Practice of Ophthalmology, 3rd edn.

6. Linden JA, Renner GS. Trauma to the globe. Emerg Med Clin North Am 1995;13(3):581–605.

7. Visual Recovery Following Emergent Orbital Decompression in Traumatic Retrobulbar Haemorrhage Kelvin YC Lee

8. Nerad JA. Eyelid and Orbital Trauma. In Oculoplastic surgery: the requisites in ophthalmology, St. Louis: Mosby; 2001;320–326.

9. Tenzel RR. Reconstruction of the central one half of an eyelid. Arch Ophthalmol. 1975;93(2):125–6.

10. Cutler NL, Beard C. A method for partial and total upper lid reconstruction. Am J Ophthalmol. 1955 jan;39(1):1–7.

11. Hughes WL. Total lower lid reconstruction: technical details. Trans Am Ophthalmol Soc. 1976;74:321–9.

12. Mustardé JC. Major reconstruction of the eyelids: functional and aesthetic considerations. Clin Plast Surg. 1981 Apr;8(2):227–36.

13. Anastas CN, Potts MJ, Raiter J. Mini Monoka silicone monocanalicular lacrimal stents: Subjective and objective outcomes. Orbit. 2001;20(3):189–200.

14. Zenter J, Hassler W, Petersen D. A wooden foreign body penetrating the superior orbital fissure. Neurochirurgia 1991;34:188–90.

15. Duke elder SS. Text Book of Ophthalmology Vol, VI, Henry Kimpton, London 1954.

16. Fulcher TP, McNab AA, Sullivan TJ. Clinical features and management of intraorbital foreign bodies. Ophthalmology. 2002;109(3):494–500.

17. Ho VT, McGuckin JF Jr, Smergel EM. Intraorbital wooden foreign body: CT and MR appearance. AJNR Am J Neuroradiol. 1996;17(1):134–6.

18. Kuhn, Pieramici. Ocular Trauma: Principles and Practices. In: John A Long and Thomas M Tann, eds. Chapter 36, orbital trauma; 383–90.

19. Michon J, Liu D. Intraorbital foreign bodies. Semin Ophthalmol. 1994;9(3):193–9.

5.2 EYELID TRAUMA

• AK Grover • Shaloo Bageja • Shilpa Taneja

INTRODUCTION

Eyelid injuries are on the rise primarily because of the increasing incidence of road traffic accidents, industrial mishaps and intentional assaults on the human body. Injury to the eyelids, lacrimal system or orbital wall may be isolated or may occur in association with mid-facial injuries.

HISTORY

An accurate history is essential to assess the severity of injury. However, sometimes the ophthalmologist can anticipate the extent and severity of injury from the mechanism of injury. It is important to elicit the mode of injury, whether it is with sharp or blunt objects or due to thermal or chemical injury or due to dog bites. In cases of animal bites, a complete tetanus immunization history is obtained and if required proper immunization should be given. The contaminated wound due to dog bite should be washed thoroughly.

PATIENT EVALUATION

Patient's injury must be dealt according to the priority. Before proceeding to the management of localized injury the basic "ABC" (Airway, Breathing, Circulation) must be evaluated. Repair of globe takes precedence over repair of eyelid laceration (Fig. 5.2.1). In adnexal injury, the decision whether to repair the wound immediately or to delay repair depends on the degree of tissue edema or the presence of hematoma or infection. In certain situations, it may be required to involve the plastic surgeons.

OPHTHALMOLOGICAL EXAMINATION

The ocular examination should be performed very delicately and meticulously. Whenever, there is an eyelid injury, the globe must be thoroughly examined. Attempt should be made to determine the visual acuity. Conditions where in visual system evaluation is difficult, optic nerve and retinal functions may be tested by assessing the pupillary reactions. A confrontation visual field examination should also be

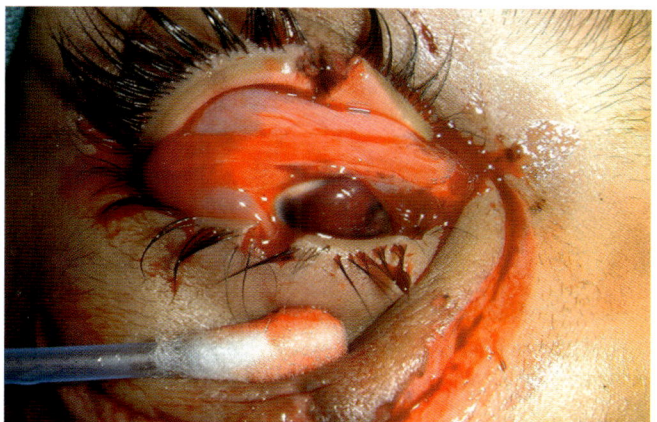

Fig. 5.2.1: Marginal lacerations involving upper and lower lid with open globe injury

done for any field loss. Observation of ocular adenxae is done before manipulating the injured eye. In the absence of signs of penetrating ocular injury a thorough anterior segment examination, IOP measurement and fundus evaluation must be performed. One should look for the presence of exophthalmos, since this may indicate a retrobulbar FB or hemorrhage. Subcutaneous emphysema, anesthesia of infraorbital skin or bony step offs of orbital rim all indicate orbital bone damage. Presence of marked lid edema may necessitate use of a Desmarres lid retractor.

EVALUATION OF THE LID INJURY

1. *Duration:* The time lapsed since the patient suffered injury is important to decide the approach to wound repair.
2. *Mode of injury:* Whether it is a blunt or penetrating injury. Dog bites are contaminated wounds and one need to take preventive measures. Chemical and thermal injuries necessitate a delayed secondary wound repair.
3. *Site of injury:* It is important to know whether the lid margin is intact or lacerated. Injuries in the region of medial canthus may be associated with lacrimal injuries (Fig. 5.2.2).

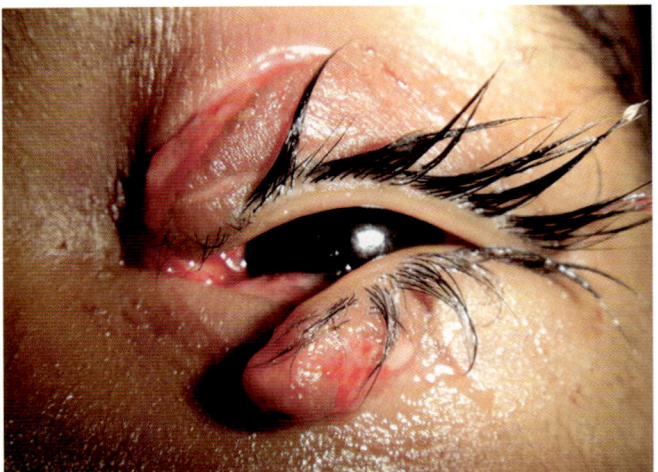

Fig. 5.2.2: Medial canthal injury with avulsion of lower lid and bicanalicular laceration

4. *Tissue loss:* It is essential to note whether there has been any tissue loss because it may necessitate the mobilization of adjacent tissue or skin flaps from adjacent areas or free skin grafts (Figs 5.2.3a to c).

5. *Infection:* If infection is present, the wound repair may be postponed for a few days till the infection subsides.

6. *Injury to the levator aponeurosis:* Full thickness lid defect or exposed orbital septum suggests injury to levator muscle or aponeurosis (Fig. 5.2.4). It may be diagnosed if possible by asking the patient to look up as his frontalis muscle is blocked by pressing on the forehead. Inability to look up or absence or any wrinkling of the upper lid skin suggests injury to levator complex.

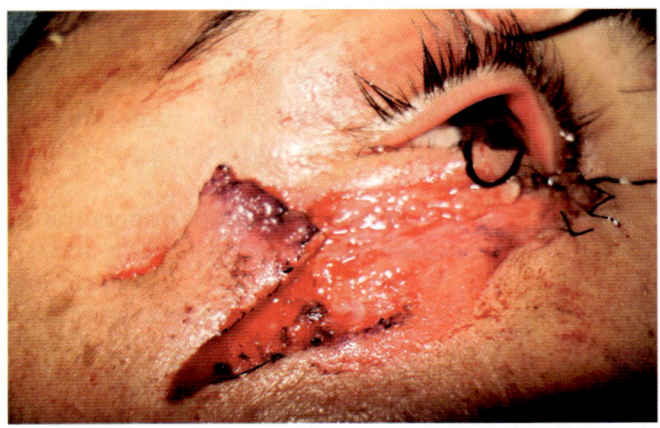

Fig. 5.2.3a: Lower lid injury with tissue loss

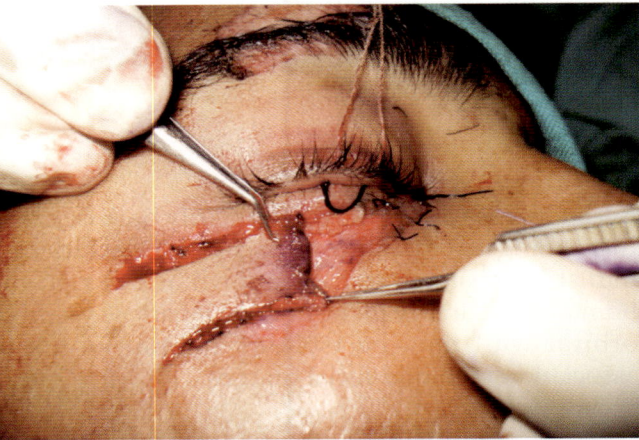

Fig. 5.2.3b: Repair using an advancement flap

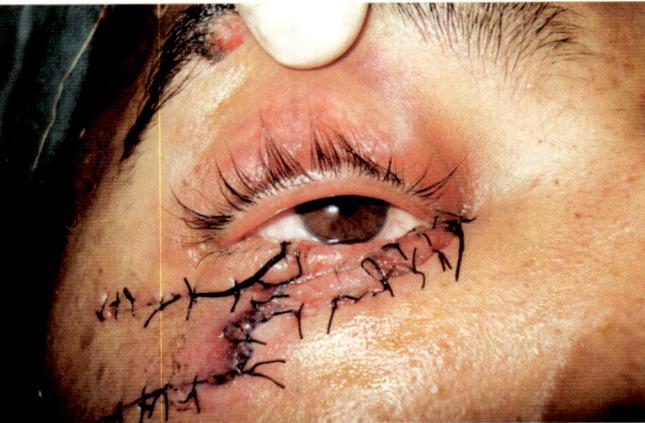

Fig. 5.2.3c: Repair using an advancement flap at the completion of the procedure

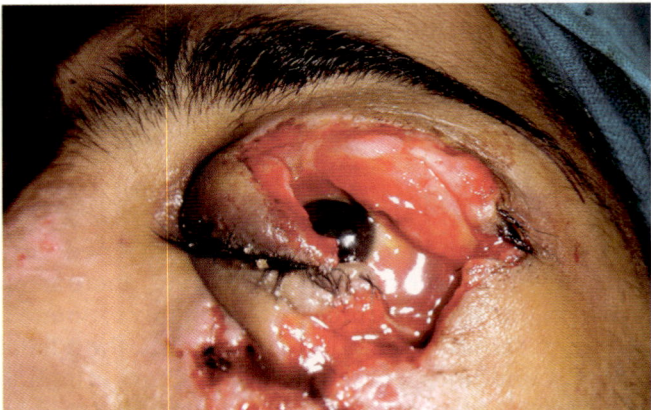

Fig. 5.2.4: Full thickness upper and lower lid laceration. Showing the transected levator aponeurosis

LABORATORY AND RADIOLOGIC EVALUATION

An appropriate laboratory evaluation is performed in an emergency department. A complete blood count and necessary blood chemistry analysis is carried out. Radiologic evaluation is advised when indicated.

MEDICOLEGAL DOCUMENTATION

All injuries must be documented in detail with drawings and if possible photographic documentation.

GOALS OF EYELID REPAIR

1. To re-establish anatomical configuration.
2. To restore physiological function.
3. To provide better cosmetic appearance.

TIMING OF SURGERY

Primary repair: In patients presenting within 24 hours of injury, primary repair of the wound is undertaken immediately. The primary repair affords the chance for best cosmetic and functional results.

Delayed primary repair: In cases where patient presents more than 24 hours after injury or where there is marked lid edema or infection, a delayed primary repair is performed after 3–4 days. During this waiting period, cold saline compresses, anti-inflammatory drugs and antibiotics are administered to reduce tissue edema and to control infection.

Secondary wound repair: In cases, where the patient presents a long time after injury or in cases of chemical and thermal burns, healing by second intention must be allowed to take place. In such cases, one must wait for a minimum of 5–6 months before planning a secondary wound repair.

REPAIR OF EYELID INJURIES

Principles to be followed for repair:
1. Local/general anesthesia.
2. Sustained hemostasis with infiltration of 2% xylocaine with adrenaline.
3. Thorough examination (with a focus on special structures such as the canaliculi, the canthal tendons and the levator function).
4. Cleansing the wound.
5. Removal of foreign material from the wound.
6. Debridement of only that tissue that is conclusively devitalized.
7. Repair of special structures like the canaliculi, canthal tendons and levator aponeurosis.
8. Closure in layers.

PRIMARY WOUND MANAGEMENT

Primary wound management may be discussed under the following heads:
1. Repair of lid margin laceration:
   a. With minimal loss of tissue
   b. With moderate loss of tissue
   c. With severe loss of tissue.
2. Lid laceration involving injury to levator muscle or aponeurosis.
3. Injuries involving medial canthus.
4. Injuries involving lateral canthus.
5. Total avulsion of an eyelid.
6. Management of canalicular laceration.
7. Thermal and chemical injury.

REPAIR OF NONMARGINAL LID DEFECTS

Simple Lacerations

Smaller linear defects can be sutured without any undermining as they involve only skin and underlying muscle. But, the round defect should be converted into an elliptical shape. There should be no tension or vertical pulling effect on the lid margins. Eyelid skin is usually sutured with 6-0 silk or nylon or prolene suture. Nonabsorbable skin sutures should be removed in about 5 days. The vertical linear wounds may be broken into multiple Z-plasties in order to improve the scar.

If the laceration in the upper lid extends upward to involve the eyebrow, it is essential to align the eyebrow first.

Deep Lacerations

Deep nonmarginal lacerations require careful layer by layer inspection of the wound to assess the integrity of the orbital septum, levator aponeurosis, rectus muscles, and globe. It requires careful closure in layers (Fig. 5.2.5). Subcutaneous closure is done with 5-0 vicryl.

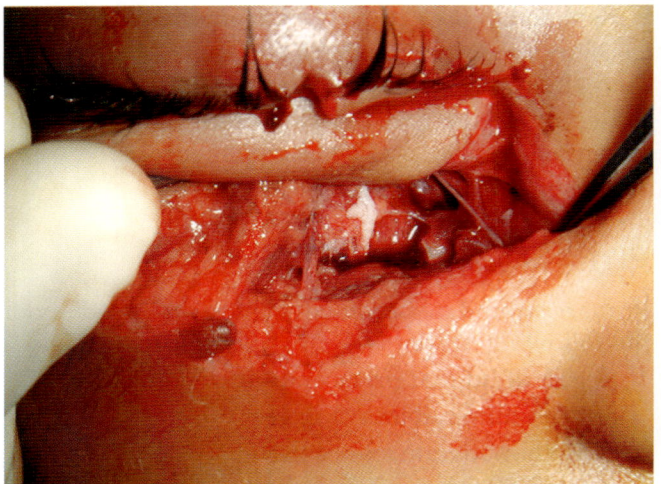

Fig. 5.2.5: Deep lower lid laceration requiring repair in multiple layers

REPAIR OF LID MARGIN LACERATION

i. With Minimal Loss of Tissue

Repair of marginal injuries can be difficult due to swelling. Although the lid margins should be freshened if devitalized tissue is present, to form straight, smooth surgical edges, sacrificing, as little tarsus as possible. Meticulous closure of eyelid margin is crucial to achieve acceptable cosmetic results and minimal postoperative complications. Inadequate closure can lead to lid notching, lagophthalmos and exposure keratopathy.

The margin is repaired using the three-suture technique. Use of magnification helps the repair.

Lid margin sutures are passed first. A 6-0 silk suture is passed through the gray line 3 mm from the edge of the tear, to a depth of 3 mm. This is brought out of the wound and reinserted into the other side of the laceration 3 mm deep to the lid margin and emerging through the gray line 3 mm from the edge of the wound (Fig. 5.2.6a). The same suture is then passed back into the gray line on the same side, 1 mm from the edge of the tear, to a depth of 1 mm (Fig. 5.2.6b). The needle is brought out and reinserted into the opposite edge of the tear 1 mm deep to lid margins and emerging through the gray line 1 mm from the margin of the wound. Two more vertical mattress sutures are passed exactly in the same way through the posterior lash line and in the plane of the meibomion gland openings. These three sutures are triply tied and ends left long (Fig. 5.2.6c).

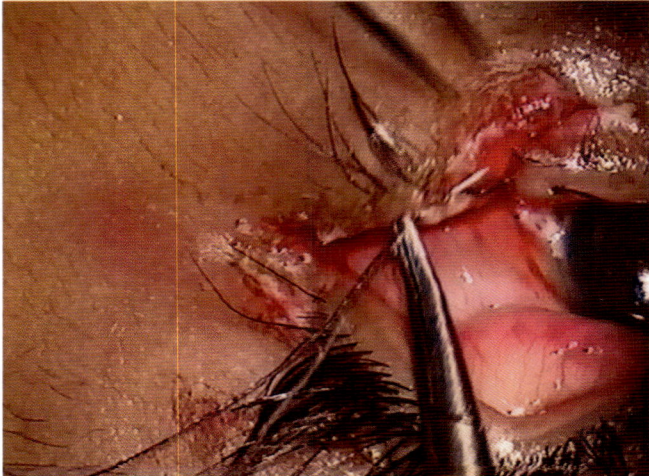

Fig. 5.2.6a: A 6-0 silk suture is passed through the gray line 3 mm from the edge of the tear, to a depth of 3 mm and is being reinserted into the other side of the laceration 3 mm deep to the lid margin

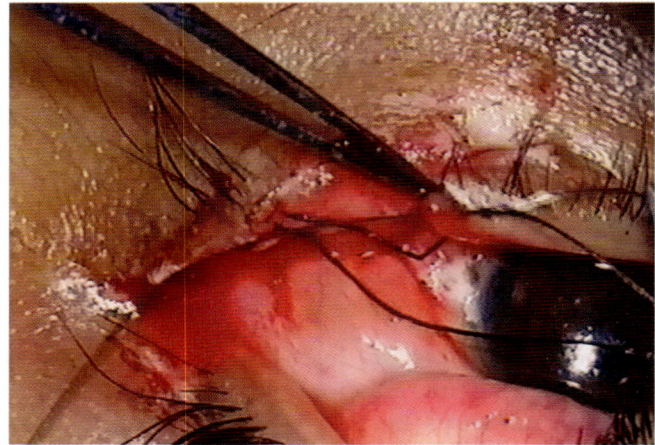

Fig. 5.2.6b: The suture is then passed back into the gray line on the same side, 1 mm from the edge of the tear, to a depth of 1 mm

5-0 polyglactin sutures are used to reapproximate the tarsus. There is no need to place sutures on the conjunctival surface since it will heal with the approximated tarsal edges. Skin sutures are removed in 4–5 days. Lid margin sutures are left *in situ* for 10–14 days.

Undue tension should be avoided on the marginal laceration as this may lead to wound dehiscence. Whenever there is tension on the wound, one can use the sliding or advancement flaps.

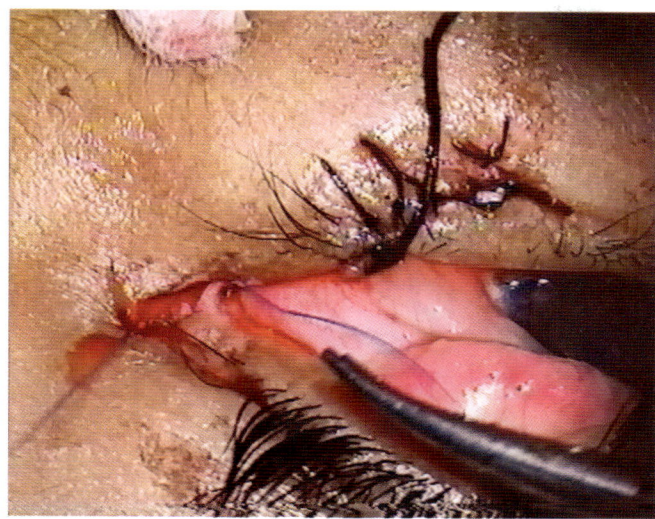

Fig. 5.2.6c: Three marginal sutures are passed and ends are left long

ii. With Moderate Loss of Tissue (From One-fourth to One-half of Eyelid)

When there is moderate loss of tissue with involvement of one-fourth to one-half of the eyelid horizontal relaxation of the eyelid is required. This can be achieved by lateral canthotomy and cantholysis of either the upper or lower limb of the lateral canthal tendon, depending on the eyelid involved. The cantholysis can be graded according to the size of the defect. 5-0 prolene suture is used to fixate tarsus to the lateral rim periosteum. Subcutaneus closure is done with 5-0 vicryl.

In case, the defect is too large to be closed with canthotomy and cantholysis, a tenzel semicircular flap can be raised. For upper lid defect, the arc of the semicircle is downward and for the lower lid the arc is above the canthus.

Surgeon may also use transconjunctival flap, or free transconjunctival graft or Mustarde's marginal pedicle rotation flap for reconstruction.

iii. With Severe Loss of Tissue (More Than Half of Eyelid)

For very large defects grafts from the opposite eyelid or surrounding tissue are used for repair. The commonly used techniques are Cutler Beard procedure, Hughes tarsoconjunctival advance-ment flap, Mustarde's cheek rotation flap or free transconjunctival graft and mucocutaneous advancement.

TRAUMA TO LEVATOR MUSCLE OR APONEUROSIS

Patient presenting with ptosis should be observed for atleast 6 months as spontaneous resolution may occur with time.

Whenever, the orbital fat is exposed, it indicates disruption of the orbital septum and the wound should be adequately explored (Fig. 5.2.7a). The levator palpebrae superioris (LPS) fibers are identified by their vertical orientation, in comparison with the orbicularis muscle fibers, which run circumferentially. The levator aponeurosis or muscle should be repaired if possible at the primary stage. If the aponeurosis has been disinserted from the tarsus, the cut edge is drawn forwards and reinserted by placing three 5-0 double arm vicryl sutures through the tarsus. Both arms of the suture are then passed through the aponeurosis. If surgery is being performed under local anesthesia, the level of aponeurosis can be adjusted by having the patient look in the straight-ahead gaze. If the orbital septum has been opened due to injury, it should not be sutured since this could result in lagophthalmos. If the laceration is at the level of the lid fold, the eyelid crease is recreated by placing 2–3 sutures. The sutures are passed through the skin muscle layer and include a superficial bite of the levator aponeurosis with 6-0 silk or separately with 5-0 vicryl (Figs 5.2.7b and c).

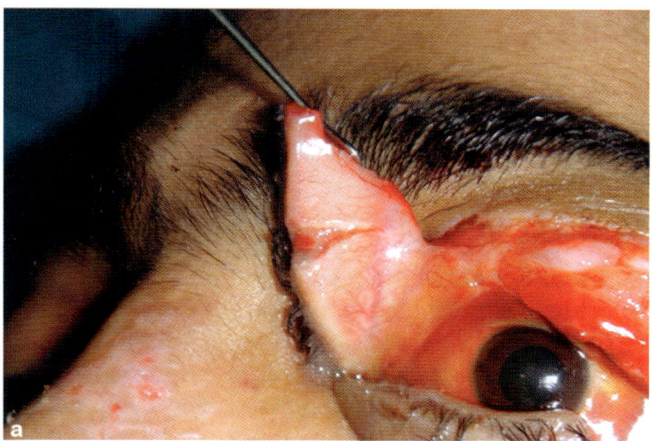

Fig. 5.2.7a: Full thickness upper lid defect with exposed orbital septum with injury to the levator aponeurosis

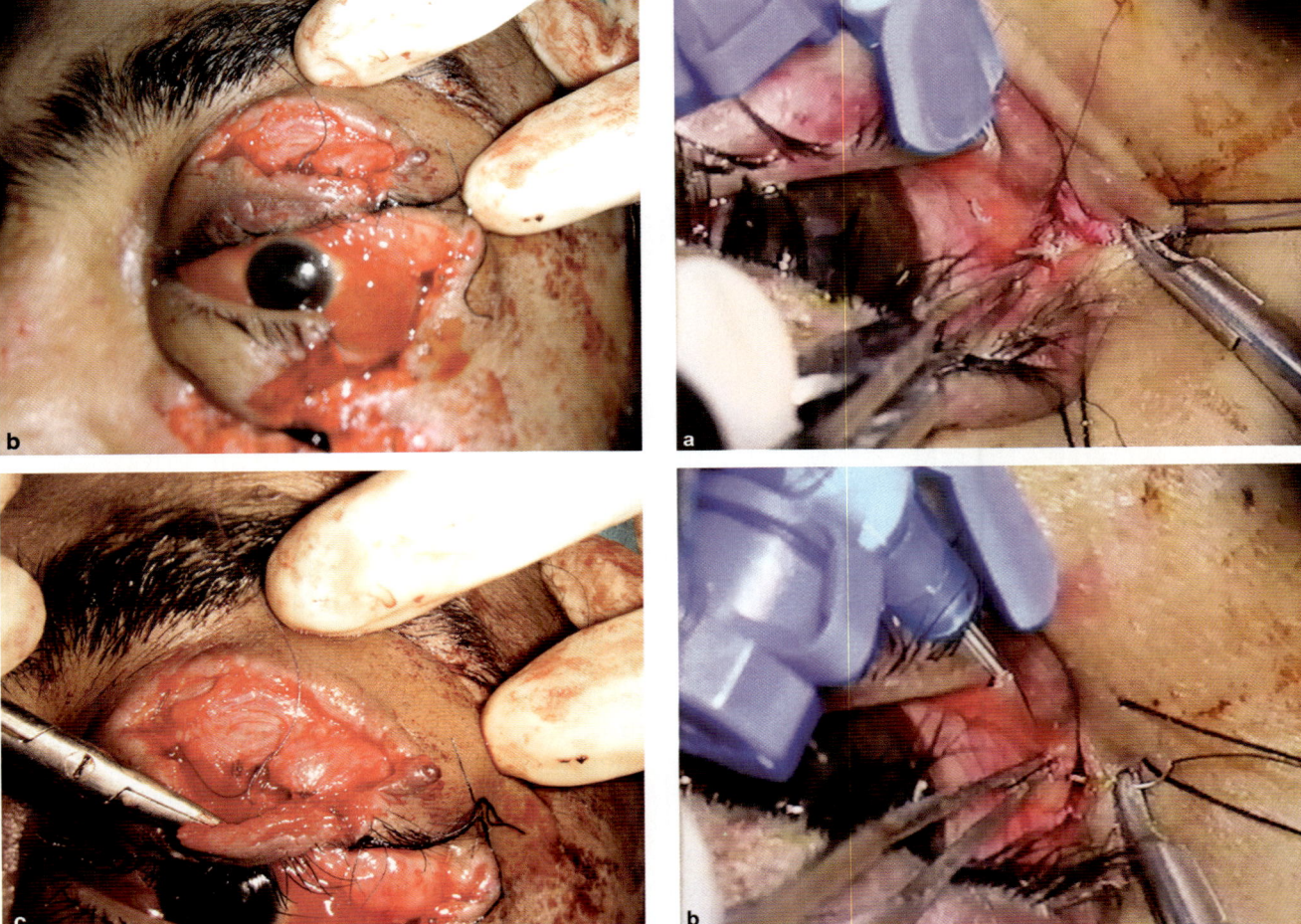

Figs 5.2.7b and c: Suturing of the levator aponeurosis with 5–0 vicryl

Figs 5.2.8a and b: Medial canthal tendon sutured with 5–0 vicryl

INJURIES INVOLVING MEDIAL CANTHUS

Avulsion of the lid at the medial canthus mostly involves the lower lid. Medial canthal injuries are usually associated with canalicular injury (Figs 5.2.8a and b). Intubation of the canaliculus should be performed prior to canthal repair. The surgeon should assess whether the anterior or posterior limb is avulsed. Repair of the posterior limb is more critical to achieve proper lid positioning.

One should assess whether there is soft tissue injury alone or bone is also fractured. In case of soft tissue injury, if both ends are visualized, the distal cut end is identified and sutured to its proximal part. If the proximal portion is not identified, then the horizontal mattress suture is passed through the distal avulsed

end and then the needle is passed through the periorbita in the region of posterior lacrimal crest. with 4-0 prolene suture. If there is no periorbita, then microplating is used to fixate medial canthal tendon. This ensures it is anchored adequately, so that the puncta are turned inward and ectropion does not result. In case of fracture, it is important to stabilize the fracture and then fixation or transnasal wiring can be performed to repair medial canthal tendon.

INJURIES INVOLVING LATERAL CANTHUS

If the lateral canthal tendon (LCT) is found to be severed, it is repaired by passing 4-0 nonabsorbable prolene mattress sutures through both ends which should be anchored to the periorbita on the inner aspect of the lateral orbital tubercle (Whitnall's tubercle). One should aim for overcorrection as the healing tends the canthus inferiorly.

TOTAL AVULSION OF EYELID

In this condition avulsed segments should be found and the avulsed tissue placed in a sterile container containing antibiotic solution and stored in a refrigerator until it can be surgically reimplanted.

MANAGEMENT OF CANALICULAR LACERATION

Avulsion of lid at the medial canthus or lacerations in this region will result in complete severance of the canaliculi. Various techniques of surgical repair of canalicular lacerations have been described in the past by various authors. The basic principle in the repair of the lacerated canaliculus is re-establishing of the drainage function. The development of fine sutures, refinement in surgical technique and the use of the microscope have contributed to a better prognosis.

Stents

Monocanalicular or bicanalicular stenting may be done. Monocanalicular have the advantage of not disturbing the normal canaliculus. Silicone is the most commonly used material. Mini-manoka stent is one of the options. However to overcome, the cost factor and difficult availability we have been using an alternative technique.

The first step is to identify the two cut ends of the canaliculi. The lateral cut end is identified by passing a lacrimal probe through the punctum. To identify the medial cut end, the wound is examined under magnification, preferably an operating microscope. The tiny opening of the cut canaliculus is rather paler than the surrounding tissues. However, if the cut end is not obvious, it is identified by pooling sterile saline in the wound and then watching for bubbles while injecting air from the upper canaliculus. The use of a pigtail probe to identify the medial end of the lacerated canaliculus should be avoided because of the risk of creating false passages and trauma to the intact canaliculus.

Once the two cut ends are identified, a mini-manoka tubing or a 22 gauge cannula (venflon) sleeve after removing the sharp tip of the stillete is introduced up

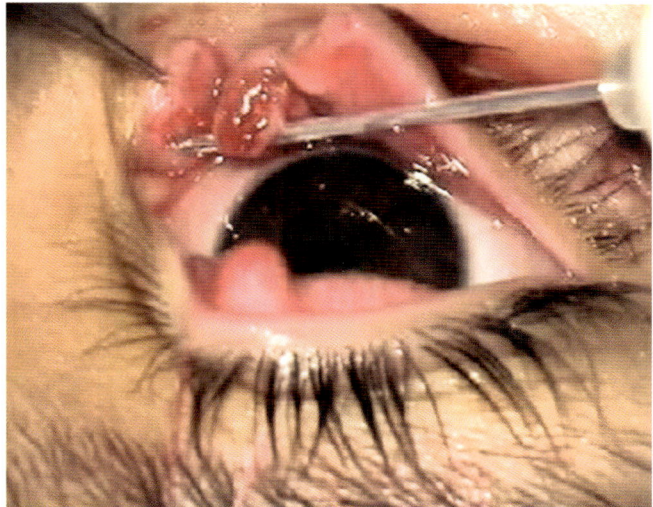

Fig. 5.2.9a: Lacrimal probe is passed through the cut ends of the lower canaliculus

to the medial sac wall (Fig. 5.2.9a). Four pericanalicular bites are then taken with 8–0 vicryl or nylon sutures, two posterior and two anterior (Fig. 5.2.9b).

The lid margin wound is closed by the technique of marginal repair, as described. It is of paramount importance that the medial canthal tendon (MCT) should be repaired when it has been disrupted. The silicone tubing or sleeve is left in place for at least 3 months.

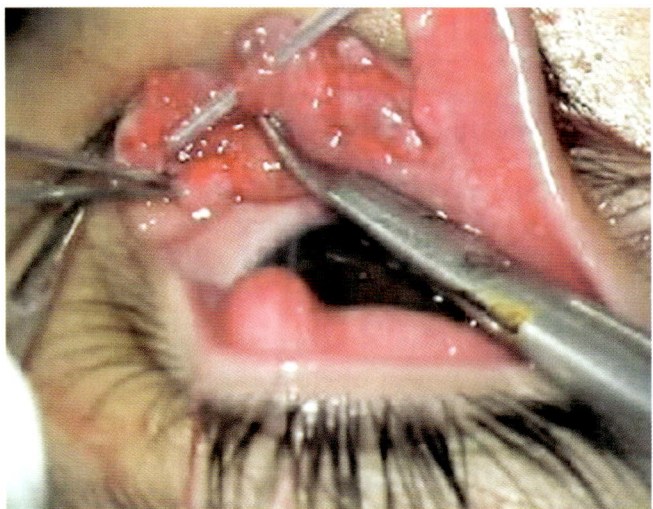

Fig. 5.2.9b: Pericanalicular suture applied posteriorly with 8–0 vicryl suture

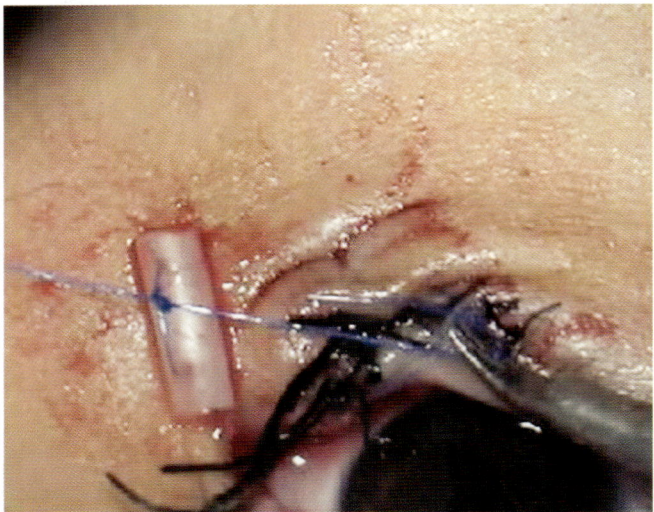

Fig. 5.2.9c: Fixation of tube by passing double arm prolene through the tube and then through the skin and emerging towards the medial canthus and fixed to the polythene bolster

When not using a mini-manoka stent, one of the common most problems encountered is extrusion of the tube from the intubated canaliculus. To retain a monocanalicular stent, fixation sutures (double arm) are passed through the tube and eyelid skin over a peg. These sutures are then carried subcutaneously upwards and medially and tied again over a peg (Fig. 5.2.9c). These sutures provide an upward and inward traction to the tube preventing its extrusion. Alternatively, to aid in its retention, the silicone tubes may be passed into the nose by using Quickert-Dryden probing system wherein the silicone tube is fixed to a malleable probe which is passed into the inferior meatus through nasolacrimal duct and recovered from there. The other end of the tube is also passed into the nose from the opposite punctum (bicanalicular intubation). This ensures retention of the probe for the required period of time.

THERMAL AND CHEMICAL INJURIES TO THE LIDS

Emergency treatment of chemical burns consists of immediate, copious, prolonged irrigation with water or saline. No time should be wasted in looking for a specific neutralizing agent. Irrigation must be continued for a minimum of 30 minutes. Local debridement of necrotic tissue and foreign particles should be done.

Burns of the medial canthal area can cause closure of the punctum and canaliculi. So a daily dilatation may be done. Tubing may be passed into the canaliculus to help to maintain patency of these structures.

As the swelling decreases, lagophthalmos may develop, with resultant exposure of the cornea. At this stage tarsorrhaphy may be performed to protect the globe. During the healing phase in severe burns, cicatricial ectropion may develop due anterior lamellar contraction. Skin grafting is the usual treatment for these eyelid malpositions caused by wound contracture.

SECONDARY REPAIR OF LID INJURIES

Secondary repair is necessary for esthetic as well as functional improvement.

Timing of Repair

Scars should be left for 5–6 months before any secondary surgery is carried out. Though in cases of severe lagophthalmos and exposure keratopathy, one may need to intervene early.

The objective of surgical reconstruction is to release contractures by removing all scar tissue and replacement of the defect with skin.

Secondary repair may be required for following underlying conditions:
- Eyebrow deformity
- Marginal misalignment
- Canthal malposition
- Cicatricial ectropion
- Traumatic ptosis
- Traumatic coloboma
- Traumatic epicanthal fold
- Symblepharon.

Eyebrow Deformity

Eyebrow deformity in see Figs 5.2.10a to d.

Marginal Misalignment

Nonrepair or faulty repair of the full thickness lid laceration involving the lid margin, results in excessive scar formation and misalignment.

When the scar tissue is limited to the lid margin, the scar tissue is excised and resuturing of the margin gives sufficiently good results.

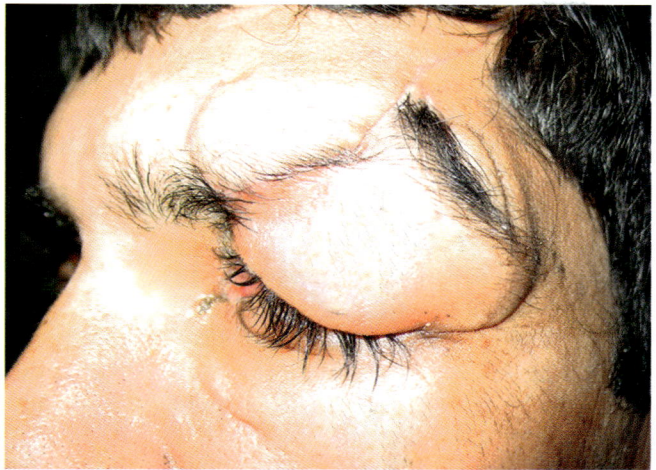

Fig. 5.2.10a: Left eyebrow deformity and traumatic ptosis

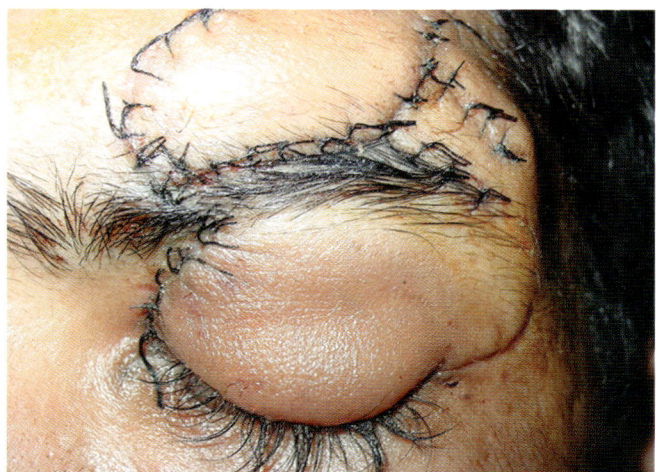

Fig. 5.2.10c: Wound edges sutured back to restore original anatomy

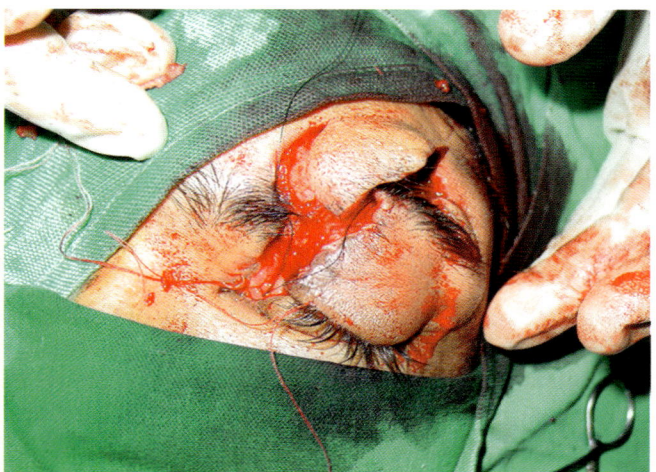

Fig. 5.2.10b: Scar edges incised to restore alignment

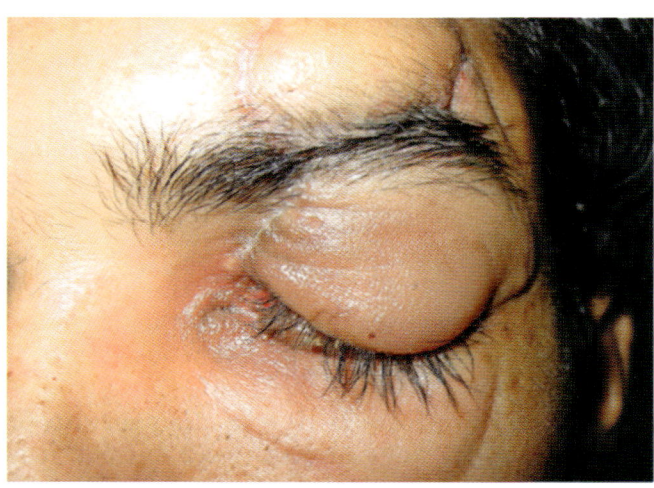

Fig. 5.2.10d: Result following repair

When the scar extends beyond the lid margin, excision of all scar tissue must be combined with a Z- or V-Y plasty. If the scar is very long, multiple Z-plasties can be prepared to achieve-lengthening of the tissue.

Z-plasty is a transposition of triangular shaped skin flaps. It serves to lengthen or changes the tension on an antecedent scar or wound defect (Fig. 5.2.11).

V-Y plasty

A V- shaped incision is given on the line of scar with the apex of the V centered in it. The surrounding tissue lateral to it is undermined. This results in release of the V in one direction thus lengthening the base of the V. The areas is then closed by suturing the former base of the V in a linear fashion with interrupted 6-0 silk. The arms are thus converted into Y.

Canthal Malposition

Canthal malposition may involve the medial canthus or the lateral canthus. Medial canthus may show either a vertical displacement or a shift laterally. Traumatic telecanthus requires shortening of the medial palpable ligament by tucking to the periosteum at the posterior lacrimal crest. Transnasal wiring is necessary where the problem is more severe.

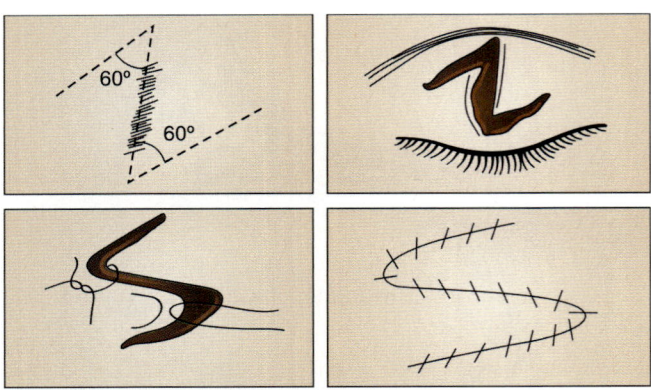

Fig. 5.2.11: Diagram showing the principle of Z-plasty

Rounding of the lateral canthus follows a long standing division of the canthal tendon. This may be repaired by recreation of the original injury and suturing the divided tendon. The exposed cut edges of the tarsal plate is sutured with 5-0 prolene to the periorbita of the orbital margin or to the periosteum. If the rounding is marked, the junction of the two lids is divided completely and resutured in an acutely angled fashion.

Traumatic Ptosis

A traumatic ptosis should be observed for at least 6 months or until no further spontaneous return of function occurs.

If traumatic ptosis is due to disinsertion or laceration of the levator palpebrae muscle, it is important to identify the levator muscle, so that its tendon can be returned to the upper margin of the tarsus during the surgery.

In other cases, choice of procedure may be made on the basis of evaluation as for any other case of acquired ptosis. A Fasanella Servat procedure, levator shortening procedure, or frontalis sling procedure will be required depending upon the levator action. If there is associated lid deformities like notch, they must also be tackled at the same sitting.

Cicatricial Ectropion

Cicatricial ectropion usually occurs after injuries, particulary extensive burns of the face due to contracture of the anterior lamella of the lid. Medical management with lubricants may be effective in minor cases. Localized scars can be benefited by Z- or V-Y

plasty. A partial or full thickness skin graft is usually required for correction of generalized scar (Figs 5.2.12a to g). Recently, nonsurgical injection of hyaluronic acid filler and autologous fat graft is believed to stretch the tethered skin and act as a tissue expander to correct the lid.

The basic principles for skin grafting for ectropion are:
1. Upper eyelid should be repaired first. Preferably one eyelid at one time.
2. Hairless and color matched skin is taken for grafting. Skin graft may be taken from the upper lid, postauricular region, supraclavicular fossa and the upper inner arm.
3. Scar tissue should be excised fully.
4. The graft should be at least a 30% over correction of the defect created by the lysis of the scar to allow for postoperative graft contraction.

When the ectropion is excessive, a horizontal lid shortening procedure like wedge resection or lateral tarsal strip may be required.

EYELID DEFECTS

Extensive laceration with loss of tissue generally lead to traumatic colobomas. It may be either a partial or a full thickness defect of the lid margin.

Management is determined by the size of the defect and the state of the corneal epithelium. Initially, it is possible to manage most of the defect with conservative measures, i.e. topical lubricants and bandage contact lenses. In general, colobomas of the lower lid are better tolerated than those of the upper lid. Trichiasis is frequently associated and is often the precipiting factor in the decision to operate. Small defect (< 30%) can be repaired by direct layer closure. Moderate defects (30–50%) of the upper and lower lid should be converted to a pentagonal lid defect by freshening the margins and closed with or without a lateral cantholysis and a semicircular flap as described by Tenzel. Large defect (> 50%) are better repaired using a bridging procedure.

However in the pediatric age group, one needs to avoid using bridging flaps, which occlude the pupillary axis and may induce amblyopia.

Traumatic Epicanthal Fold

Traumatic epicanthal fold may result from facial injuries, where one or both canthi are displaced

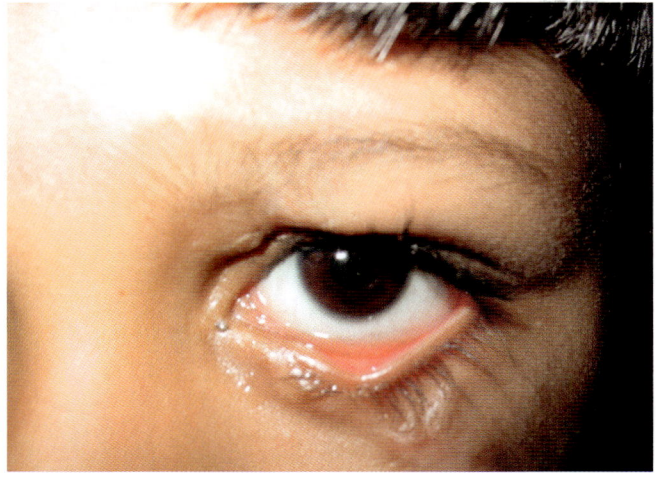

Fig. 5.2.12a: An 11-year-old boy with cicatricial ectropion involving left upper and lower lid

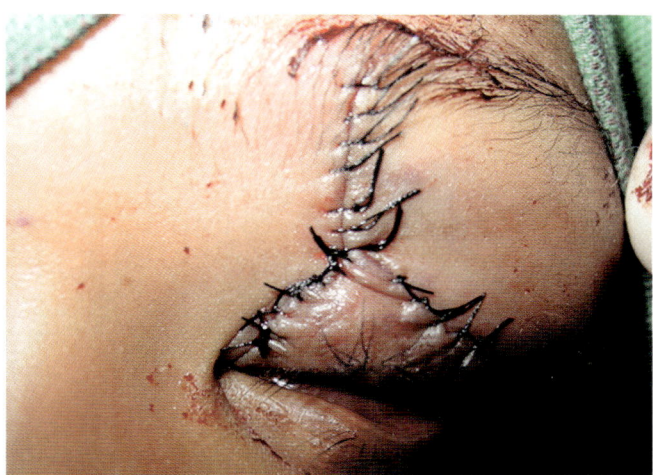

Fig. 5.2.12d: Closure as Y

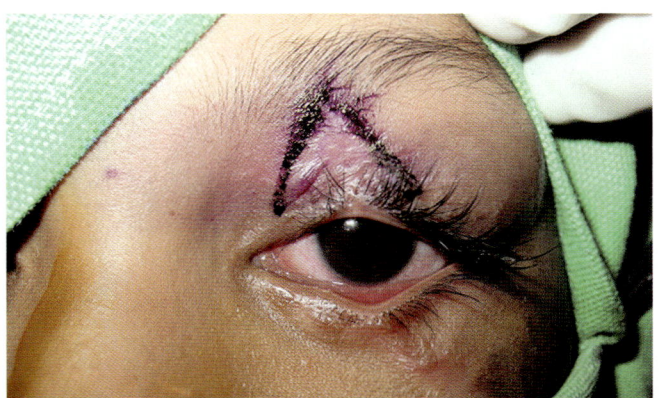

Fig. 5.2.12b: Marking for V-Y plasty of upper lid

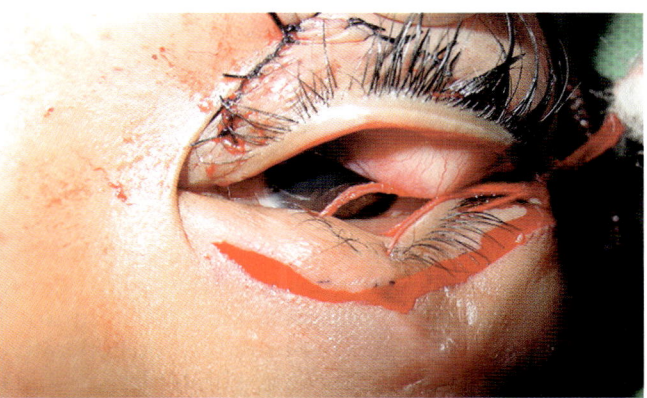

Fig. 5.2.12e: Skin incision given 3 mm below the eyelid margin and in the lower eyelid for skin grafting

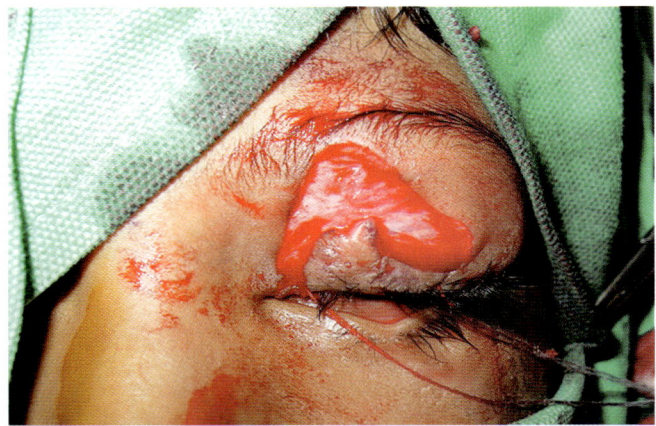

Fig. 5.2.12c: Subcutaneous dissection and scar excision

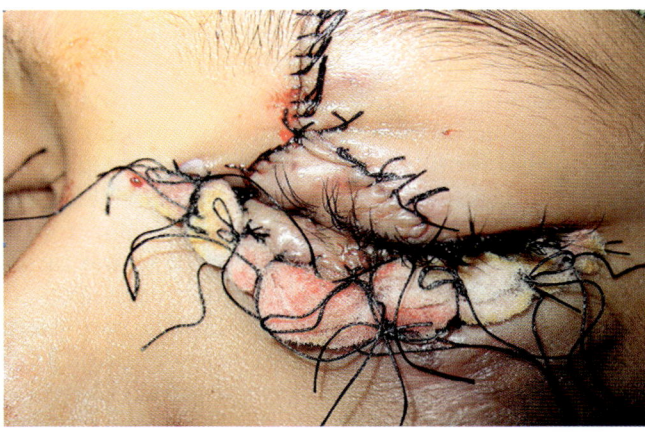

Fig. 5.2.12f: Bolster applied over the skin graft in lower lid

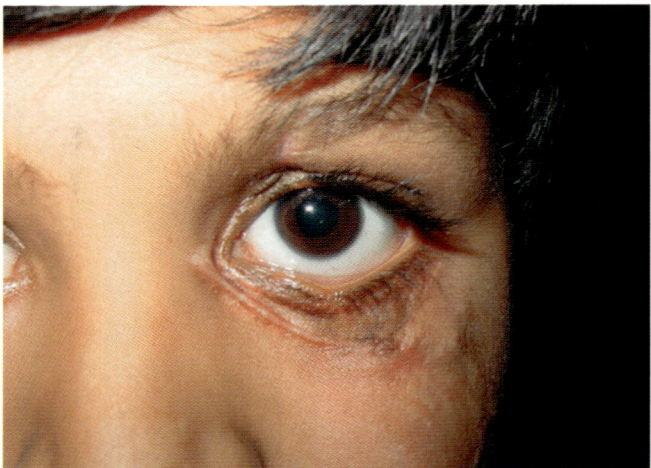

Fig. 5.2.12g: Postoperative appearance. Marked improvement in upper and lower lid ectropion

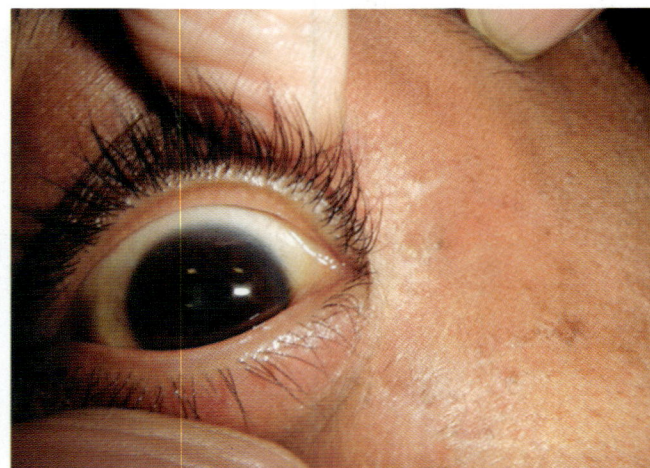

Fig. 5.2.13a: Showing post-traumatic epicanthal fold

medially. On examination, there is a vertical fold in the medial canthal or lateral canthal area. It may develop in any vertical or near vertical scar which exist in the skin around either the medial or the lateral canthus.

The traumatic epicanthal fold is generally corrected by Y-V technique or a Z-plasty may be used (Figs 5.2.13a to c). It is important to carefully dissect the orbicularis from the transposition flap in order to flatten the medial canthal area. Meticulous suturing of the skin edges is needed to reduce postoperative scarring. It may be ameliorated with topical steroids.

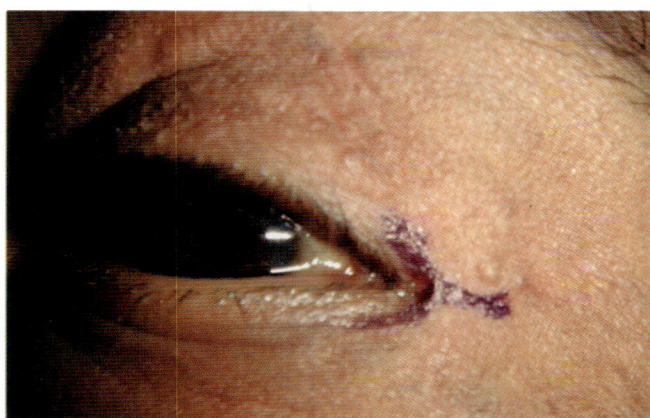

Fig. 5.2.13b: Y-shaped incision marked over the epicanthal fold

Traumatic Symblepharon

Traumatic symblepharon occurs when there is adhesion between the bulbar and the palpebral conjunctiva of the eyelid due to trauma. These condition may arise after penetrating injury of the eyelid, lacerated injury or burns, which lead to a bridge of mucosa running from the lid to the globe with normal fornix lying peripheral to it (deep).

Treatment consist of operative seperation of the lid. Incision is given to the conjunctiva parallel to the border of symblepharon from its end to the tarsal border. After dissecting the conjunctival flap, it is secured to the internal aspect of the lid. The bare sclera is then covered with conjunctival flap or mucosal graft and symblepharon ring is kept *in situ* for 8–12 weeks. Once the graft is vascularized after 1–2 weeks a topical steroid is applied.

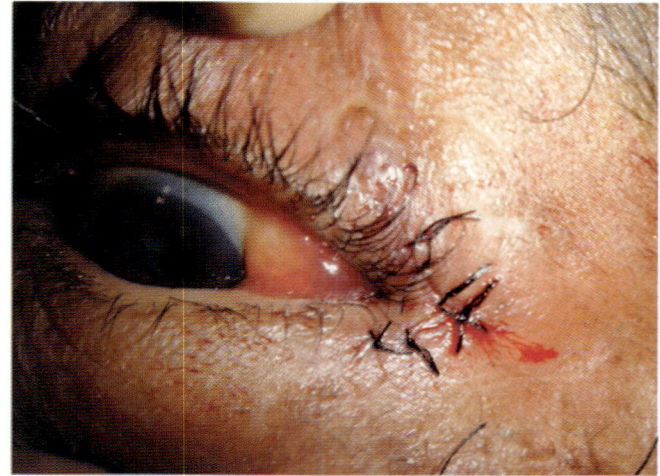

Fig. 5.2.13c: Undermining and closure as V

CONCLUSION

Adequate primary repair of the lid injury gives the most satisfactory results and meticulous repair is mandatory for lid injuries. However, where it becomes necessary, a secondary repair gives reasonably good correction, both functional and cosmetic.

BIBLIOGRAPHY

1. Caviggioli F, Klinger F, Villani F, Fossati C, Vinci V, Klinger M. Aesthetic Plast Surg. 2008;32(3):555–7.
2. Committee on Trauma of the American College of Surgeons : Advanced trauma life support course, Chicago, 1984, Amercian College of Surgeons.
3. Conlon MR, Smith KO, Cadera W, Shun D, Allen LH. An Animal model studying construction techniques and histopathologic changes in repair of canalicular a lacerations. Can J Ophthalmol 1994:29:3d.
4. Crowford JS. Lacrimal intubation seet with suture in the lumen. Ophthal Plast Reconstr Surgery 1988;4:249.
5. Fezza JP. Plast Reconstr Surg. 2008;121(3):1009–14.
6. Goldberg MF, Tessler HH. Occult intraocular perfora-tions from brow and lid lacerations, Arch ophthalmol 1971;86:145.
7. Gossaman DM, Berlin JA. Management of acute adenexal trauma. In surgery of eye lid , orbit and lacrimal systems. American Acad Ophthalmol, 1993.
8. Grover AK, Bhatnagar A. Trauma to Eyelids, Canalicular lacerations and its management. JKSOS, 1991;3(2):135–46.
9. Grover AK , Kaur S. Principles of Oculoplastic Surgery : CME Series No.5, In: AK Grover, eds.
10. Grover AK, Kaur S. Principles of Oculoplastic Surgery: CME Series No.5. In: AK Grover, ed.
11. Gupta VP. Basic Principles of eye lid reconstruction: CME Series No.5, In: AK Grover ed.
12. Kennedy RH May J, Dailey J, Flanagan JC. Canalicular laceration: an 11 years epidemiologic and clinical study. Ophthalmic Plasticand Reconstructive Surg. In: Loft HJ. Wobig JL, eds. Daily RA, The bubble test: an atraumatic method for canalicular laceration repair. Ophthalmic Plastic ann Reconstructive Surg 1996;12;61–64.
13. Levine MR, Buckmn G. Semicercular flap revisited.Arch Ophthalmology 1986;104:915–17.
14. Long JA. A method of monocanalicular silicone intubation. Ophthalmic Surg 1988;19:204–205.
15. McLeish WM, Bowman B, Anderson RL. The pigtail probe protected by silicone intubation a combined approach to canal icul ar reconstruction. Ophthalmic Surg 1992;23:281–283.
16. Mustarde JC. Repair and Reconstruction in the Orbital Region. Edinburgh: Churchill Living stone: 1971, Chap 7–8.
17. Reifler DM. Management of canalicular laceration. Surv Ophthalmol 1991;36:11.
18. Ritleng Peirre. A simplifed technique for lacrimal intubation. Ocular surgery news. Vol 14, No 7.
19. Tenzel RR. Reconstruction of the central one half of an eyelid. Arch Ophthalmol 1975;93:125–126.

5.3 MANAGEMENT OF CANALICULAR TRAUMA

• VP Gupta • Pragati Gupta • Rigved Gupta

INTRODUCTION

Canalicular injuries remain the most common form of lacrimal system injury. Eyelid/periorbital injury near medial canthus lacerates one or both canaliculi. Eyelid margin is conventionally divided into:

1. *Ciliary portion:* Three-fourths eyelid lateral to puncta having cilia at lid margin.
2. Nonciliary portion about one-fourth eyelid from puncta to the medial canthus without any cilia at lid margin. Any injury to nonciliary part of lid margin damages canaliculi. Superficial location of canaliculi along the lid margins predisposes canalicular injury. Canalicular/nasolacrimal system injuries may go undetected in multisystem trauma patients. As a general rule, canalicular laceration must be suspected in any injury involving medial part of eyelid or medial canthal region. We have encountered canalicular lacerations in the age range of 1–58 years including children and young adults. Males are more frequently involved than females.
   - *Causes of canalicular lacerations:* Canalicular injuries are caused by direct or indirect eyelid or facial trauma including nasoethmoidal fractures. Both sharp and blunt objects have been encountered in canalicular injuries. Sharp objects can directly cut or severe the nonciliary portion of eyelid involving the canaliculi. Sharp objects commonly implicated in canalicular injuries include knife, hooks (even blouse hooks in young children), glass, coat hangers, finger poke/fingernails scratches, etc. Animal bite such as dog bites and cat claws are common causes of these injuries in children. Direct trauma resulting in avulsion of medial part of lid lacerates the canaliculus from common canaliculus. Various blunt injuries to the ocular adnexa causing canalicular lacerations include fist fights, fall from height on blunt object, glancing blows to the face, wooden stickiron rod injury, cycle handle, road side accidents, etc.
   - Canalicular trauma may be in the form of isolated canalicular laceration or may be the part of eyelid and periorbital injuries. The injury may involve single canalicular laceration (Fig. 5.3.1), both upper and lower canaliculi (Fig. 5.3.2) or severe the common canaliculus.

Incidence

Although only few cases of facial trauma may have canalicular injuries, canalicular injuries have been reported in 16% of eyelid lacerations. The inferior canaliculus is involved in majority of cases (> 50–75%). A survey of eye surgeons in the United Kingdom found that 83% of 92 surgeons repaired fewer than 5–10 canalicular lacerations per year.

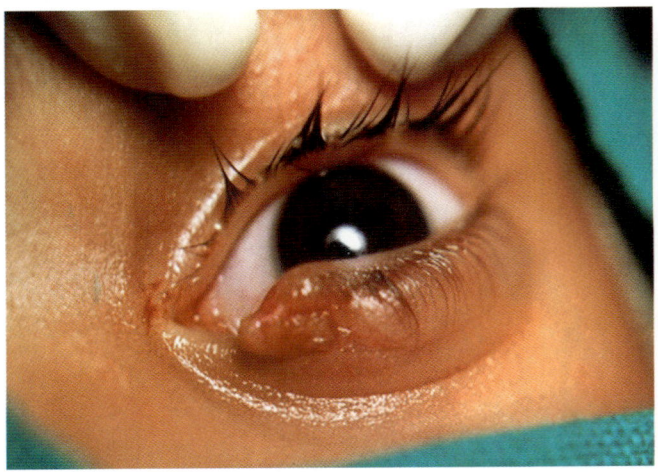

Fig. 5.3.1: Lower canalicular laceration left eye

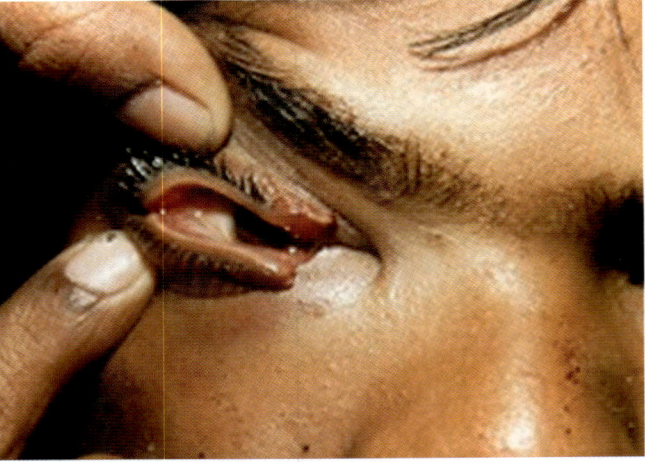

Fig. 5.3.2: Bicanalicular laceration right eye

MANAGEMENT OF CANALICULAR LACERATION

The need to repair monocanalicular laceration: The repair of monocanalicular laceration is controversial because it is believed by many surgeons that one canaliculus may be sufficient for tear drainage. Others believe that lower canaliculus was more important than lower for tear drainage. Werb was of the opinion that conservation of lower canaliculus was for tear drainage and upper canaliculus for the ophthalmologist. It has been suggested that a single canaliculus may be adequate for tear drainage to prevent epiphora. However, many patients develop tearing with only single functioning canaliculus. It would be impossible to predict which patient would be symptomatic with one functional canaliculus. Several studies have demonstrated that superior canaliculus is sufficient to keep the patient symptom free in case of lower canaliculus injury whereas other surgeons suggested that lower canaliculus is more important in tear drainage. Occlusion of upper canaliculus was followed by epiphora. Upper canaliculus may take the function of lower canaliculus in case of its blockage. Jones et al studied the conduction time of fluorescein dye from the eye to the nasal cavity of nursing students after occluding one punctum with polyethylene plugs. They concluded that:

i. 14 of 36 (39%) eyes showed greater tear drainage through upper than the lower canaliculus

ii. 5 (14%) eyes showed equal tear elimination through upper and lower canaliculi

iii. 17 (47%) eyes had elimination through lower canaliculus.

Linberg and Moore evaluated symptoms of epiphora after occlusion of one and both ipsilateral puncta using hydroxypropyl cellulose plugs. It was noted that 50% of upper and lower occlusions produced mild symptoms. They also concluded that a single functioning canaliculus was usually sufficient to drain basal or minimally stimulated tear secretion; however, it was not sufficient to eliminate reflex tears in 50% of cases. One clinical study of 57 canalicular injuries it was concluded that upper or lower monocanalicular obstructions did not cause epiphora in a normal warm indoor environment, however these patients were symptomatic in adverse environmental conditions due to reflex tear secretions. Canalicular repair performed by experienced lacrimal surgeon with proper instrumentation and appropriate technique yields very high success rate. Tear drainage studies show that both upper and lower canaliculi play a role in tear drainage. Therefore, repair of all monocanalicular lacerations (upper or lower) appears to be a valid approach.

Diagnosis

Correct diagnosis and appropriate management of canalicular lacerations is essential to prevent post traumatic scarring and subsequent epiphora. One should have high index of suspicion for canalicular lacerations even in trivial injuries within 6 mm medial to punctum and lacerations in the medial eyelid and medial canthal area. The 00 lacrimal probe should be passed after dilating the punctum to confirm. The probe emerges from lacerated end of distal canaliculus (Fig. 5.3.3).

Timing of Repair

There is no need to repair canalicular lacerations immediately. Immediate repairs in emergency set-up should be avoided because of nonavailability of experienced lacrimal/oculoplasty surgeon, trained assistants/staff, proper magnification/operating microscope. Stents and appropriate sutures. Most of the repairs should be performed within 24–48 hours. Author has performed successful repairs even up to 5–7 days after injury for canalicular lacerations missed at the time of initial examination. Even late repairs are worth trying.

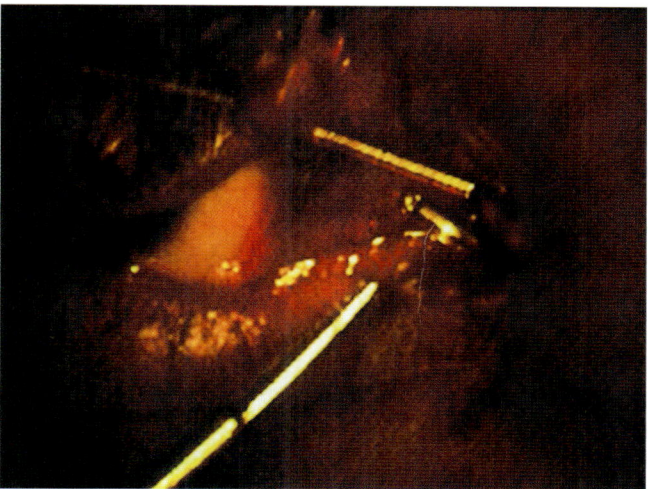

Fig. 5.3.3: Probe emerges from upper canalicular laceration

Location of Repair

All canalicular repairs should be performed in major operation theater which is well-equipped with operating microscope or magnification and proper illumination, stents, 6, 8-0 vicryl and 6-0 polypropylene sutures, suction apparatus and trained assistants. It is thus obvious that such repairs should never be done in minor operation theater.

Preoperative evaluation: All patients with such injuries should undergo preoperative clinical evaluation which includes detailed history taking, general, systemic and ocular examination including detailed evaluation of lid and canalicular injuries.

The goal of repair: Management of canalicular lacerations varies widely. The goal of repair is to "reunite torn edges of canalicular mucosa in proper anatomic alignment". This goal is achieved by:

- Detection of cut ends of distal and proximal canaliculi
- Stenting of the canaliculi is a must for proper healing of torn edges and prevention of stricture during maturation of wound edges
- Canalicular/pericanalicular suturing
- Layered closure of lid margin and medial canthus.

Anesthesia

- *Children:* General anesthesia
- *Adults:* Local anesthesia/general anesthesia.

Local Anesthesia

The anesthetic agents for local infiltration consists of a 50:50 mixture of 2% lidocaine with 1:200,000 epinephrine and 0.75% bupivacaine (marcaine) and 150 units of hyaluronid. Topical proparacaine/xylcaine with adrenaline 2% eye drops are additionally instilled in the conjunctival sac and at the lacerated canaliculus and puncta. Infraorbital nerve block: 1 mL of local anesthetic is injected about 1 cm below the middle of inferior orbital margin. Nasociliary nerve block: anterior ethmoidal and infratrochlear branches of nasociliary nerve that supply sensory innervations to medial eyelids, canaliculi and lacrimal sac can be blocked by injecting 2–3 mL above the MCT and then passing the needle along the medial wall of the orbit for 2 cm posteriorly.

General Anesthesia

For bicanalicular silicone intubation (BCSI) down the, nasolacrimal duct (NLD) throat pack along with endotracheal tube is a must to prevent aspiration of blood, in case of brisk bleeding from nasal structures during BCSI.

The surgical techniques to repair canalicular laceration:
1. Bicanalicular silicone intubation down the NLD also known as BCSI with nasal fixation.
2. Bicanalicular annular silicone intubation (BCASI).
3. Monocanalicular intubation.

Materials of Stents

Stent materials—thick hair, absorbable/nonabsorbable sutures, bone, metallic wires, rubber polyethylene, silicone, teflon. Silicone is the best stent material as it is inert, soft, pliable, stable and biocompatible.

Types of Stents

- *Monocanalicular stents:* Vier's rod, Johnson's rod, Beyer's rod, polythene/silicone/teflon tubing
- Mini-monoka silicone stent
- Ritleng monocanalicular stent (Fig. 5.3.4)
- Bicanalicular stents:
  - Silicone intubation sets with lacrimal probes (Figs 5.3.5a to c)

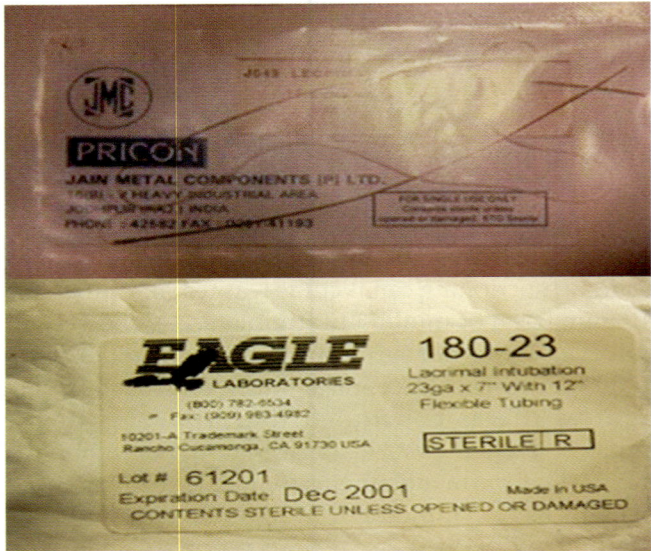

Fig. 5.3.4: Prepackaged, sterile, malleable, stainless steel, lacrimal probes with swaged silicone tubes

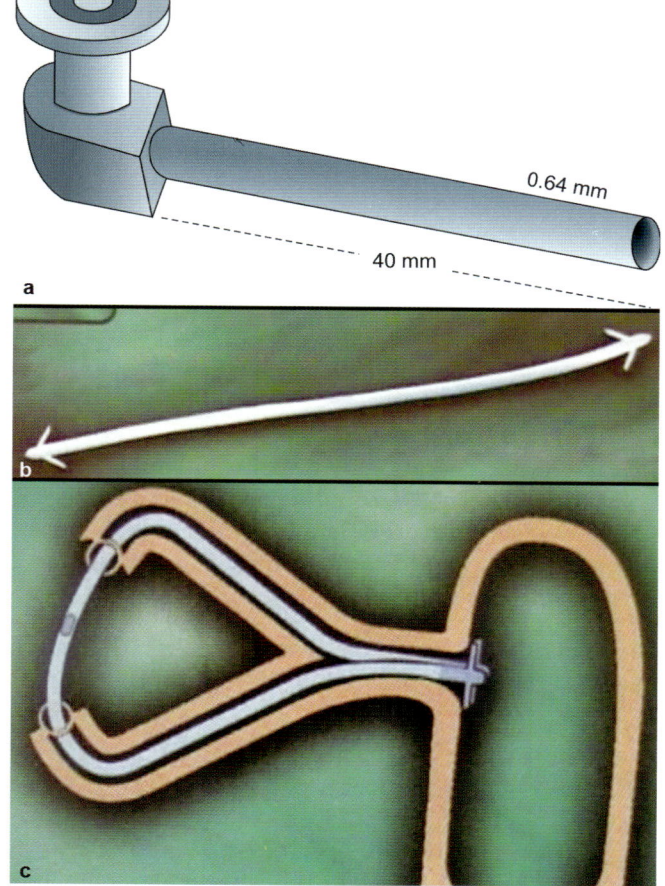

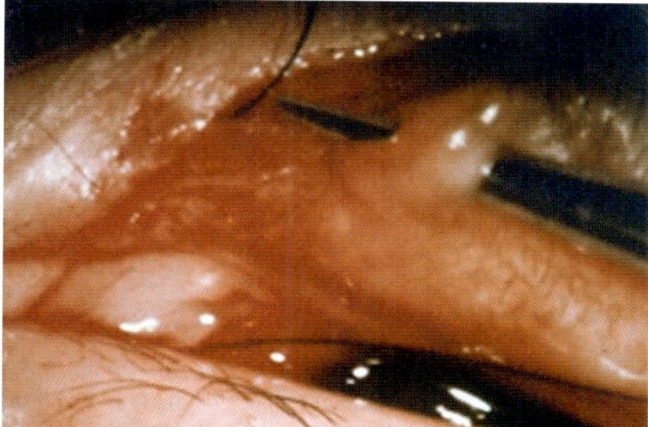

Fig. 5.3.6: The tip of punctum dilator emerges through the distal end of lacerated canaliculus

Figs 5.3.5a to c: (a) Mini-monoka silicone monocanalicular stent; (b) Bicanalicular self retaining stent: stent consists of two heads one each at two ends. Each head has two flexible flaps that fold inward during insertion through punctum; (c) Bicanalicular self-retaining stent in place: flaps open at lacrimal sac for fixation and fold outward upon stent removal

- Ritleng bicanalicular intubation system
- Bicanalicular self-retaining stent.

Intubation materials:
- *Probes:* 23 g, 11–18 cm long
- Tapered tips/olive tips (bulbous)
- *Silicone tubes:* 0.25/0.64 mm external diameter/ 30 cm long.

Bicanalicular Silicone Intubation Down the Nasolacrimal Duct

It is also known as BCSI with nasal fixation. Gibbs (1967) was the first one to describe a new probe for

intubation of lacrimal canaliculi with silicone rubber. The surgical site is scrubbed with diluted betadine. The problems frequently encountered during repair of canalicular lacerations include difficulty identifying proximal end of canaliculus, intubating the proximal injured system, retrieving stents in the nose in BCSI down the NLD technique, and repairing canalicular epithelium.

Surgical technique: Isolation of distal end of canaliculus.

Isolation of Proximal End of Canaliculus

Proximal end of canaliculus is easier to locate if laceration is close to the punctum. In lacerations close to sac, proximal end is deeper to medial palpebral ligament (MPL) (Fig. 5.3.6).

Methods to Identify Proximal End

- *Operative microscope:* The proximal end of canaliculus can be easily identified by typical appearance of the rolled/everted shiny white edges due to shiny epithelial lining under magnification. While looking for the proximal cut end the following steps help in finding the cut end.

  - Adequate retraction of wound edges particularly in patients with proximal cut end nearer to common canaliculus.

  - Achieve hemostasis with bipolar cautery. There should be no bleeding or oozing of blood that will obscure the cut end.

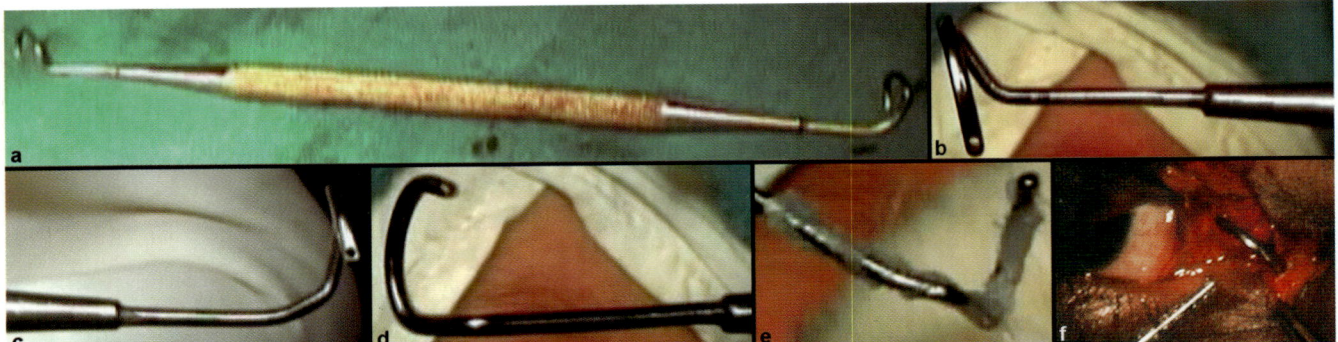

Figs 5.3.7a to f: (a) Modern pigtail probe in profile; (b) Smooth, blunt and round tipped pigtail probe with a French-eye at the tip; (c) Smooth, blunt and round tipped pigtail probe with a French-eye at the tip; (d) Smooth, blunt and round tipped pigtail; (e) Pigtail probe smeared with ointment probe with a French-eye at the tip; (f) Pigtail probe emerging from proximal end

– The application of adrenaline-soaked cottonbud at the site of torn canaliculus has proved very beneficial in author's experience. Local adrenaline serves dual purpose: 1. it stops bleeding, 2. it decreases soft-tissue edema and helps in identification.

- Passing a pigtail probe through the intact punctum and canaliculus, the tip of pigtail probe emerges from the cut end. This is a very good method but requires expertise and a smooth-tipped pigtail probe to avoid damage to uninvolved canaliculus. It should be used only by experienced lacrimal surgeons.

- Irrigation of saline through intact canaliculus after occluding the sac, otherwise the fluid reaches the sac and throat.

- Injection of air through intact canaliculus after pooling the saline in the lacerated area and occluding the sac. Air bubbles are seen emerging through the proximal cut end of the canaliculus. The air bubble test requires a closed system.

- Irrigation of various other fluids and dyes like fluorescein, methylene blue, steroids, sterile milk and viscoelastics have been advocated by different surgeons. However, the injection of dyes stains the tissues and makes the operation field look messy and may make the operative field obscure.

- A laser-directing method to search the nasal cut end of lacerated canaliculus has been recently described. It was a faster and more effective technique than conventional methods (Liang T, Zhao KX, Zhang LY, 2006).

- *Upper canalicular probing:* Recently, Cho et al (2008) have reported a simple and effective method of identifying the medial cut end of deep lower canalicular laceration by upper canalicular probing in 20 eyes. The lacrimal sac and canaliculus are lateralized after probing and facilitate locating the proximal cut end. This finding was demonstrated by dacryocystography (Figs 5.3.7 a to f).

Bicanalicular Silicone Intubation Down the NLD (Nasal Fixation): Surgical Technique

After isolation of distal and proximal lacerated edges, both the puncta are gently dilated with punctum dilator. One-snip punctoplasty may be done if required. The nasal pack is removed just before intubation. Intubation of injured canaliculus is performed first. Lacrimal probes with attached stent may be smeared with antibiotic ointment to facilitate its insertion and passage through the tracts. The probe with attached silicone tube is passed through the involved punctum at a right angle to the lid margin, inserted 1–2 mm. The probe is then passed horizontally while stretching the lateral aspect of the lid. The tip of the probe emerges from the distal torn edge of lacerated canaliculus. The probe is pulled through the cut end of distal canaliculus. The tip of this probe is now inserted in the cut edge of the proximal canaliculus and pushed gently in the canaliculus to cross the soft stop if any. Once the soft stop is passed, the probe is further advanced nasally, parallel to lid margin until the lacrimal sac was entered and the firm hard stop is encountered. The probe is rotated at 90° and directed inferiorly and posteriorly (in the direction of NLD). The presence of probe in the inferior meatus is confirmed by passing another probe and getting metal-on-metal sensation. The

OPERATIVE PHOTOGRAPHS OF SURGICAL TECHNIQUE OF BCSI DOWN THE NLD (NASAL FIXATION) (Figs 5.3.8–5.3.19)

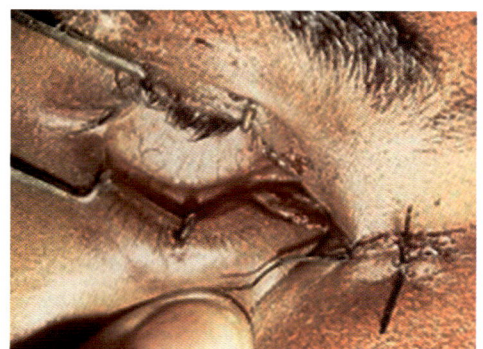

Fig. 5.3.8: Lower canalicular laceration right eye

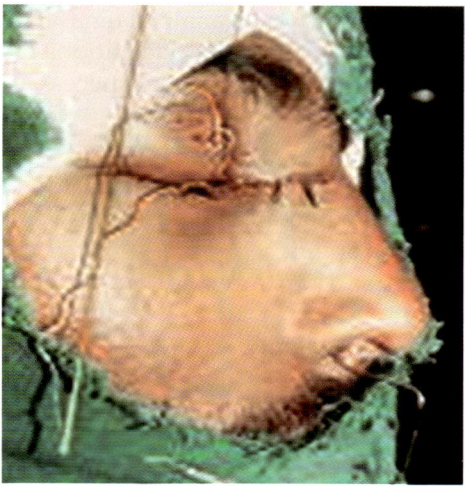

Fig. 5.3.9: Nasal BCSI for lower canalicular laceration

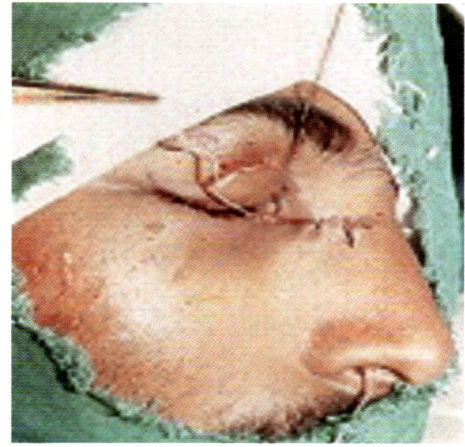

Fig. 5.3.10: Probe from upper punctum to the nose being pulled

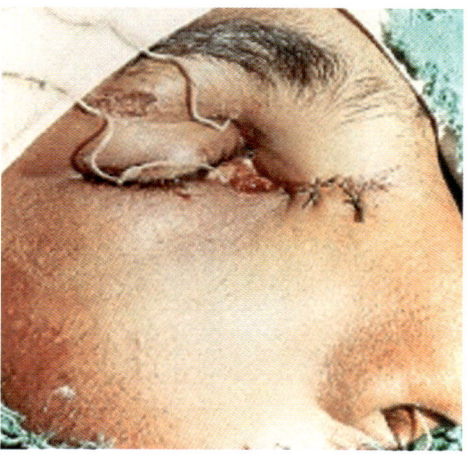

Fig. 5.3.11: Note the loop of silicone stent

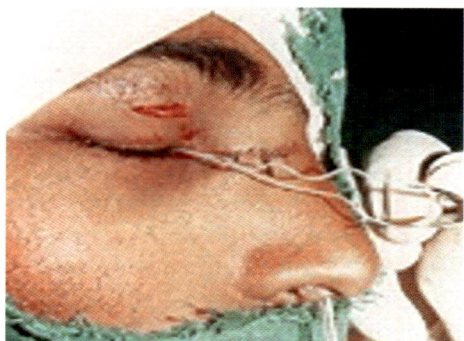

Fig. 5.3.12: Loop of silicone

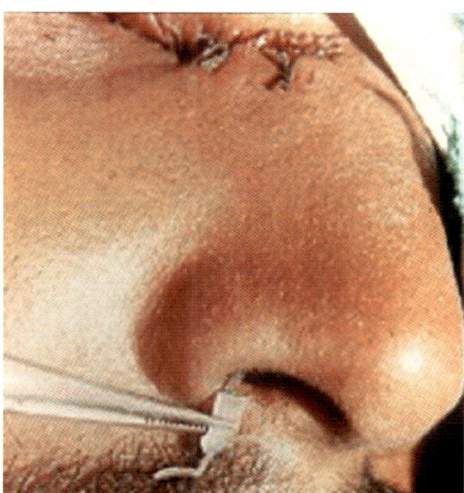

Fig. 5.3.13: Stent passed through a wide tube with multiple square knots

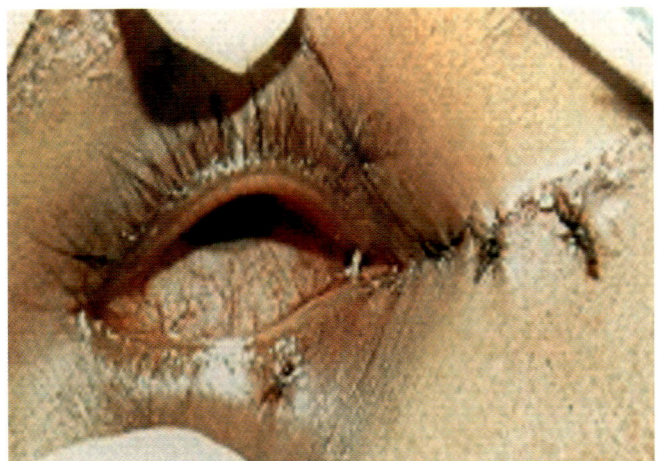

Fig. 5.3.14: Right eye BCSI down the NLD, wound closed in layers

probe in the inferior meatus is retrieved by grasping with small hemostat. Second probe was passed through the intact punctum and canaliculus and retrieved in the inferior meatus in the same manner. Two ends of silicone tube are secured with proper tension. The ends of the silicone tubing were passed through larger bore silicone tubing and then multiple square knots were tied. Additionally 6-0 prolene suture is used to secure the knots with outer wider silicone tubing. Excess length of the tube is cut and the knots left to retract in the nostril. Securing the nasal end of the stent with the ala nasi using 6-0 prolene in female patients was found to be very useful in author's hands.

Postoperatively the patients is put on frequent instillation of 0.3% moxifloxacin eye drops and 0.3% moxifloxacin eye ointment at night and oxytetrazoline 0.05% nasal decongestant drop in the ipsilateral nostril for 1 week. Postoperatively, all the patients are thoroughly examined for positioning of the stent: Its nasal and medial canthal ends and stent related complications.

Author's Results of BCSI Down the NLD
(Figs 5.3.15a and b)

- Forty-four patients, 1–50 years, 35 male, 9 female
- Forty monocanalicular lacerations, 24 lower, 16 upper
- Four bicanalicular lacerations
- Success rate—100%.

In a Japanese study of bicanalicular nasal intubation for the repair of 98 canalicular lacerations resulted in 80% anatomic and 85% functional success.

Advantages of BCSI Down the NLD

- Supports the medial canthal and lower eyelid tissues in proper anatomic position
- Prevents ectropion
- Avoids disadvantages of monocanalicular intubation
- *Success rate:* Excellent.

BCSI Down the NLD Disadvantages/Complications

- Difficult and challenging retrieval of probes in nose
- Out of reach for occasional lacrimal surgeon

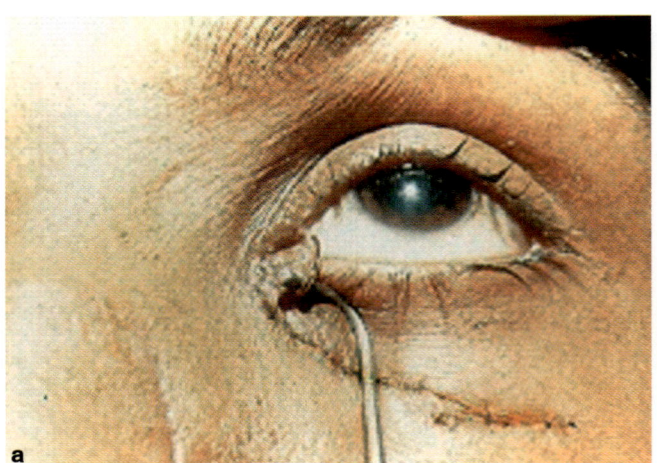
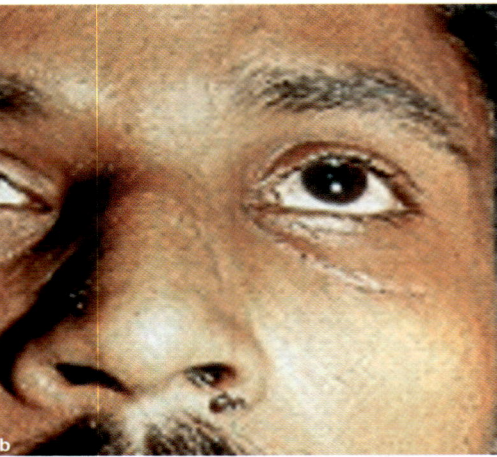

Figs 5.3.15a and b: Left eye lower canalicular laceration repaired by BCSI down the NLD. Note the silicone loop at medial canthus

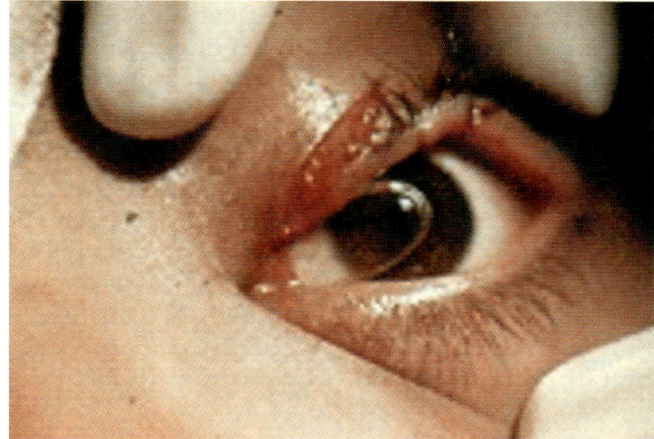

Fig. 5.3.16: Nasal BCSI before pericanalicular suturing

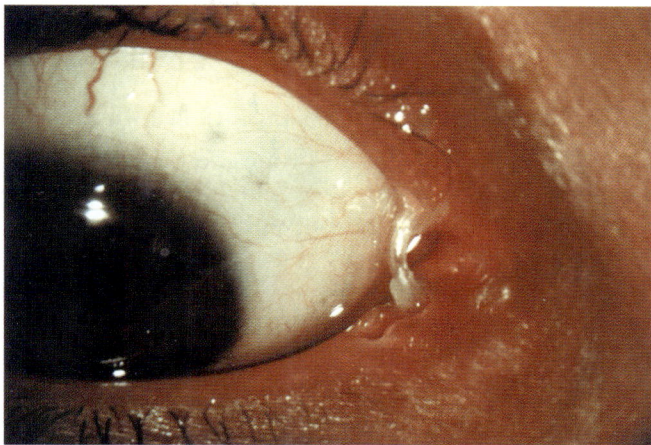

Fig. 5.3.18: Cheese—wiring of lower canaliculus

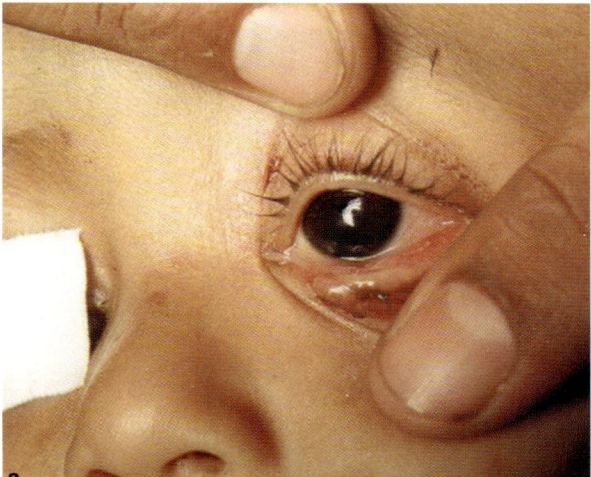

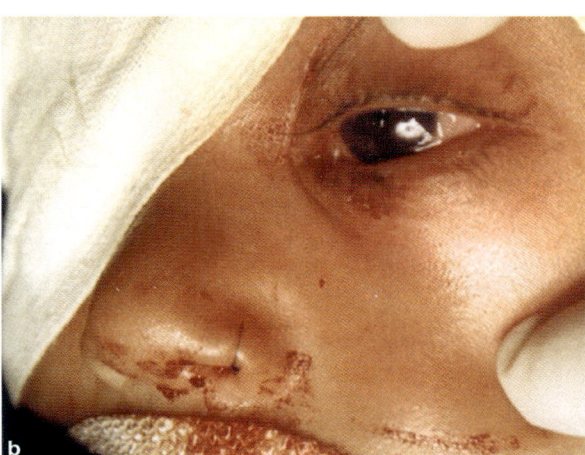

Figs 5.3.17a and b: Lower canalicular laceration left eye repaired by nasal BCSI

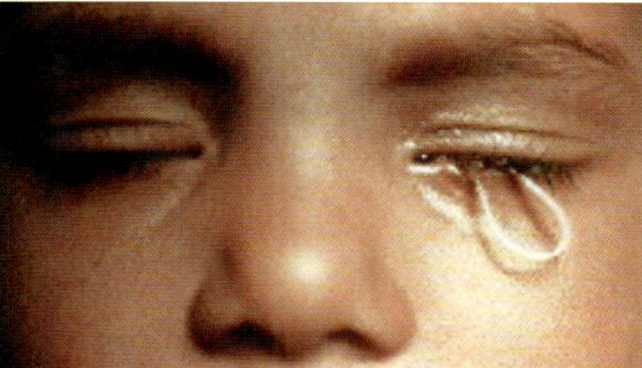

Fig. 5.3.19: Lateral prolapse of stent following BCSI down the NLD

- Special probes, grooved director/hooks with glued silicone tubing
- Brisk intraoperative bleeding
- Nasal packing required
- Narrow space in children
- Infracture of inferior turbinate
- Slippage of tube
- Cheese wiring of canaliculi.

The peripunctal or pericanalicular absorbable "anchor" suture may reduce the incidence of cheese-wiring by silicone bicanalicular stents after repair of canalicular lacerations or resections for stenosis (Benger and Nemet, 2008)

- Retrograde migration
- Lateral prolapse of stent-3
- Infection/dacryocystis/discharge
- Nasal discharge

- Conjunctivitis
- Postoperative care.

BCASI Using Pigtail Probe—Surgical Technique

Pigtail probe: Worst pigtail probe the original pigtail probe was designed by Worst in 1962. Worst probe was a spiral shaped probe with a miniature hook (sharp Crochet hook) in the tip. It was used for bicanalicular annular stent placement to repair canaliculus lacerations. The probe was used to help in location of the proximal cut edge of the lacerated canaliculus and insertion of the stent. The Crochet hook was a flaw in the design because it often caused false passage and injury to intact canaliculus. The hook caused severe injury to the lumen of the canaliculus while withdrawing the probe. It was also associated with high failure rate of 36–42%.

Modified pigtail probe: Beyer modified the probe in 1974. The modified probe is smooth, blunt and round-tipped probe with a French-eye at the tip. The hook at the tip was eliminated. This modern pigtail probe along with availability of fine, inert, soft, pliable, stable silicone stent have revived BCASI (Jordan and Nerad, 1990). Recently, pediatric-sized pigtail probes with an eyelet at the tip has been introduced (Forbes et al, 2008).

OPERATIVE PHOTOGRAPHS OF SURGICAL TECHNIQUE OF BICANALICULAR ANNULAR SILICONE INTUBATION (BCASI) USING PIGTAIL PROBE (Figs 5.3.20 to 5.3.33)

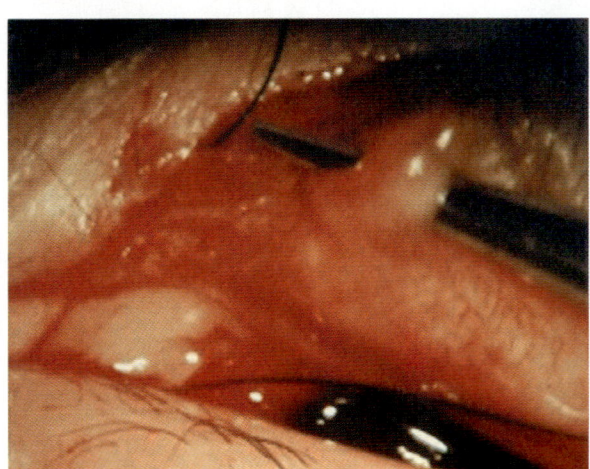

Fig. 5.3.20: Dilatation of lower punctum

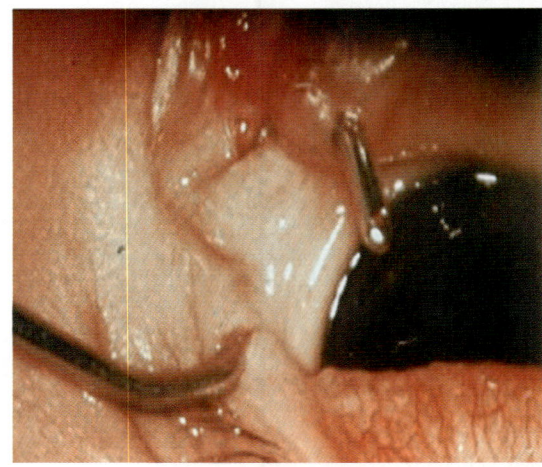

Fig. 5.3.22: Pigtail probe passed from upper to lower punctum

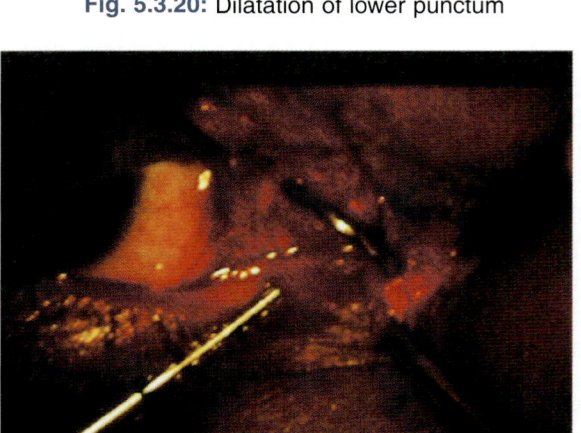

Fig. 5.3.21: Pigtail probe passed from lower canaliculus

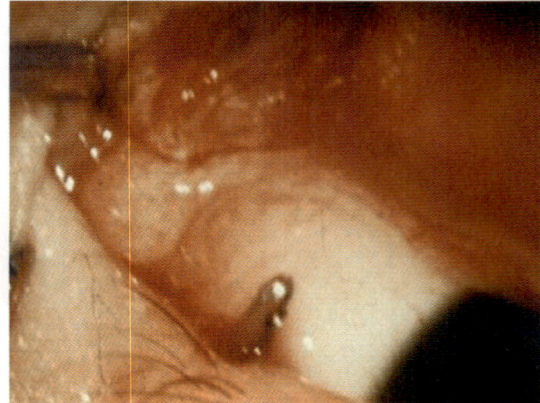

Fig. 5.3.23: Pigtail probe passed from the lacerated lower canaliculus to emerge from intact upper punctum

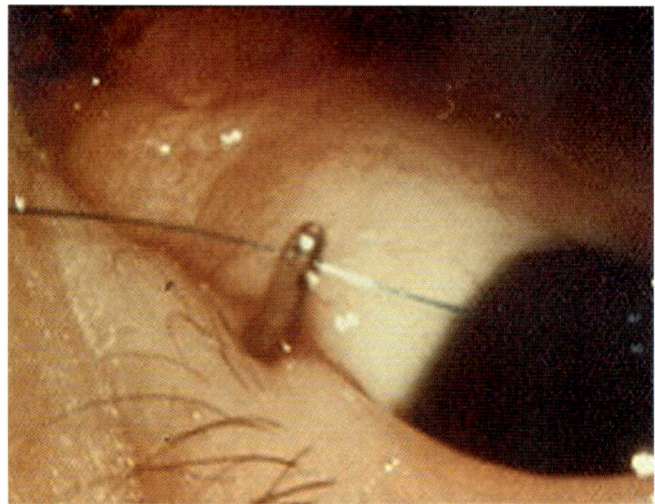

Fig. 5.3.24: 5/6-0 prolene suture threaded in the eye of the probe

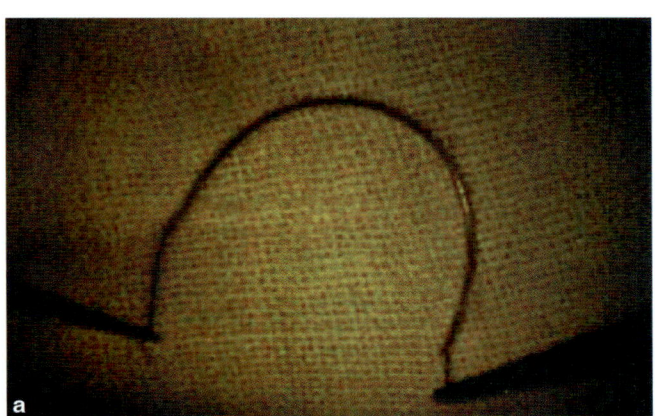

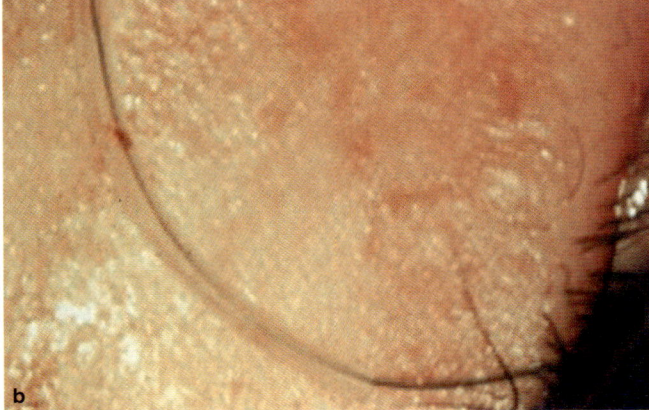

Figs 5.3.25a and b: 6-0 prolene suture is threaded inside the lumen of 2 cm long and 0.50 mm diameter sterile silicone tube

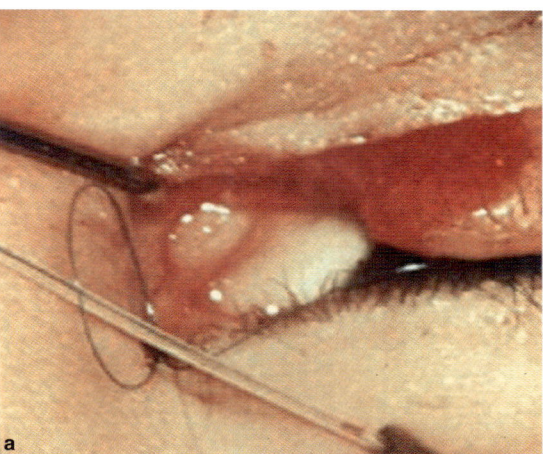

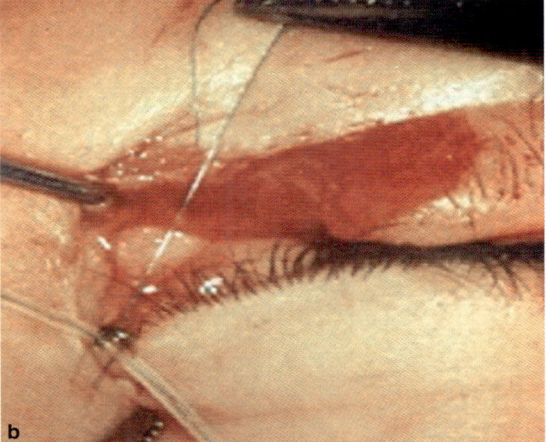

Figs 5.3.26a and b: The threaded tube passed through the punctum, intact canaliculus, common canaliculus, and proximal cut end

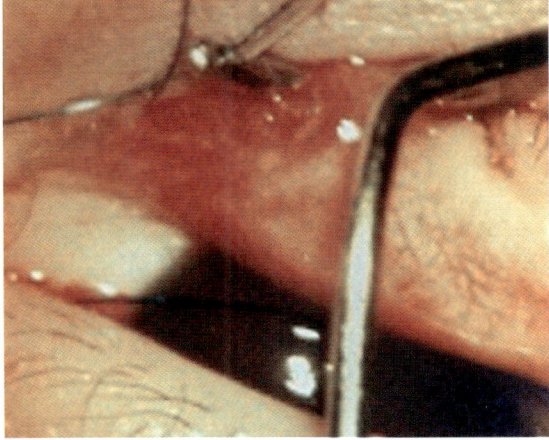

Fig. 5.3.27: The silicone tube being passed through the distal end of lacerated canaliculus

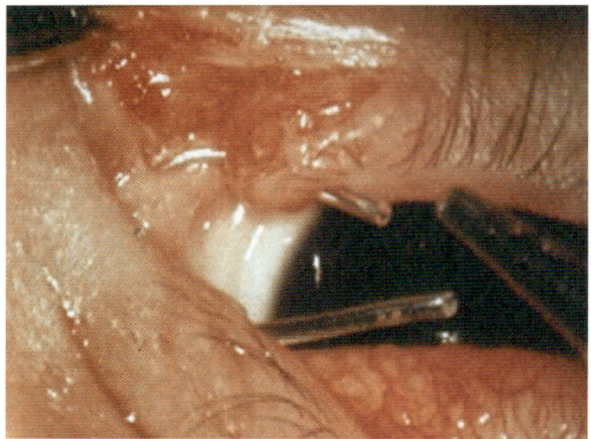

Fig. 5.3.28: Silicone stent from upper punctum to lower lacerated proximal and distal cut ends of canaliculus

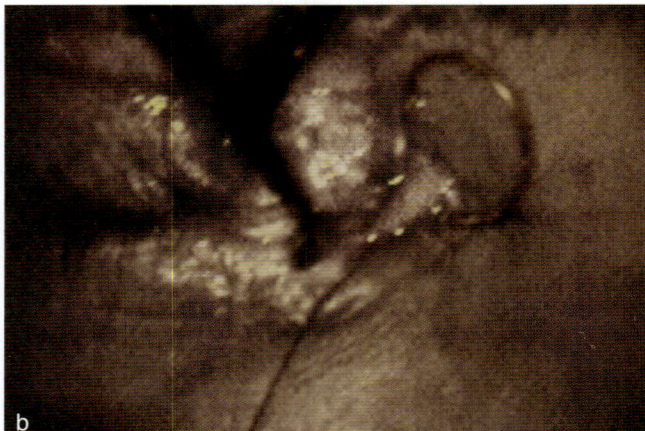

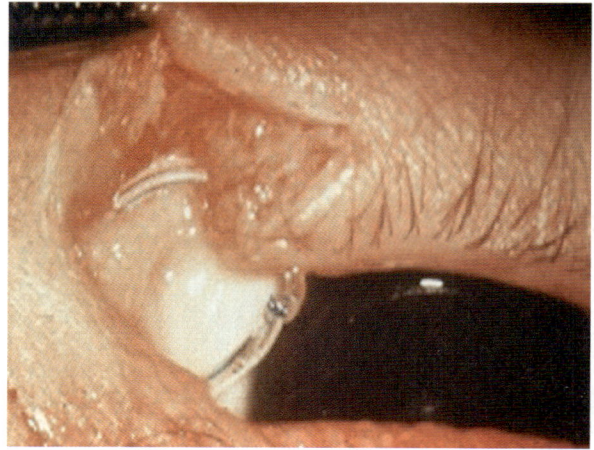

Fig. 5.3.29: Prolene suture tied. Stent bridging the punctum bridging the lacerated lower canaliculus

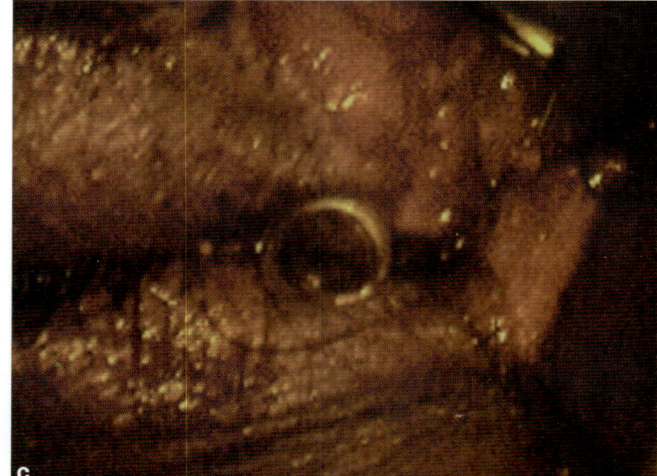

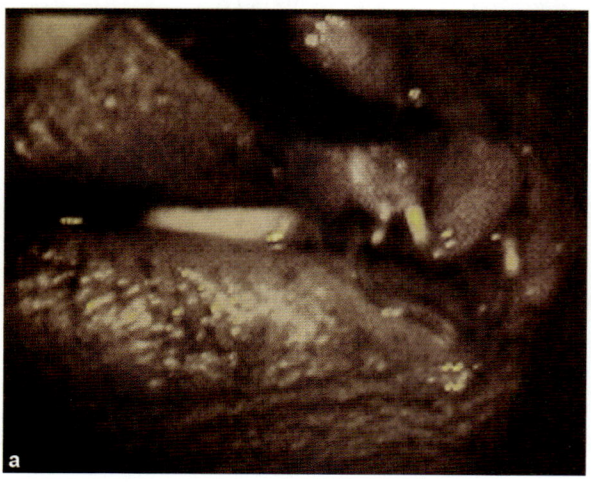

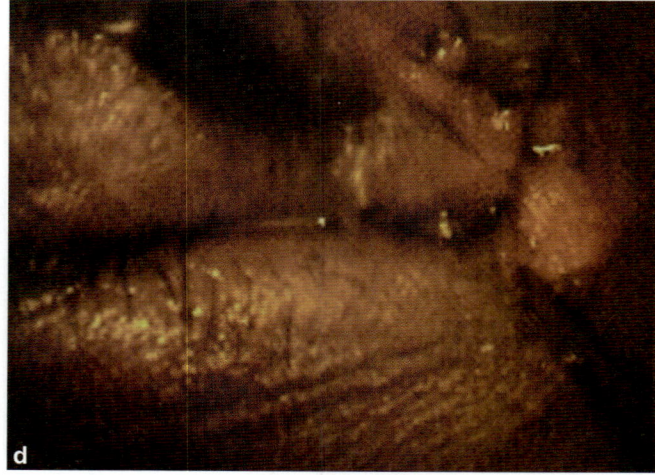

Figs 5.3.30a to d: Pericanalicular suturing using 7-0 vicryl

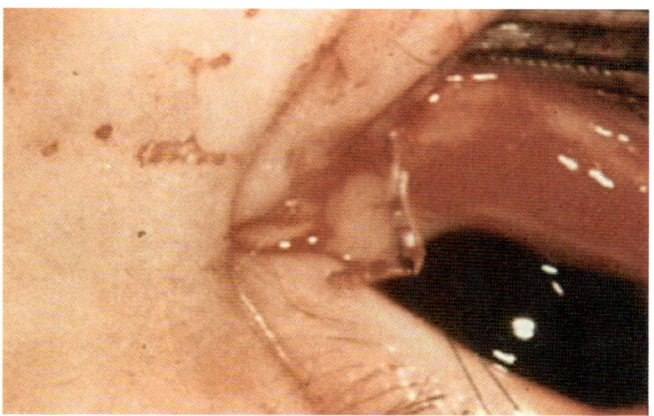

Fig. 5.3.31: 6-0 prolene suture tied, knot visible

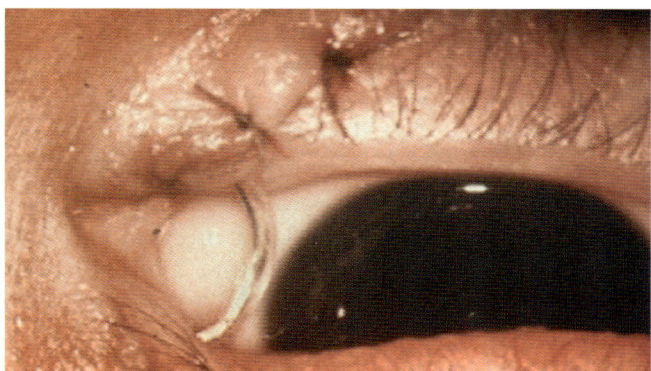

Fig. 5.3.32: Skin sutured and knot pulled in the canaliculus. BCASI—final appearance

Surgical Technique of Bicanalicular Annular Silicone Intubation Using Pigtail Probe

Both the puncta are dilated with punctum dilator. Pigtail probe is passed through the intact punctum and canaliculus and is gently and slowly negotiated through the common canaliculus, while the assistant pulls apart the medial parts of upper and lower lids to widen the angle between two canaliculi and facilitate the insertion of pigtail probe through the injured canaliculus. No force should be used while passing the probe. The probe emerges through proximal cut end (Figs 5.3.33 to 5.3.36).

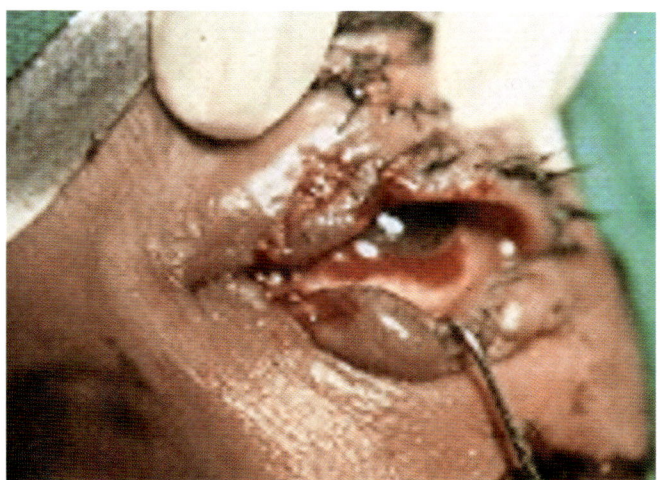

Fig. 5.3.33: Bicanalicular laceration left eye

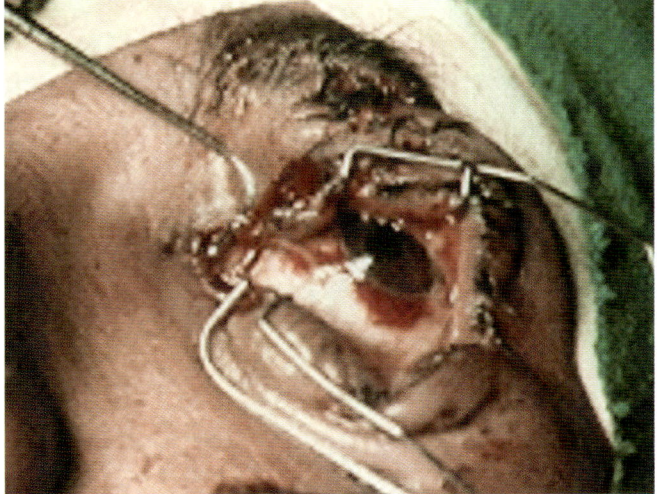

Fig. 5.3.34: BCASI for bicanalicular laceration left eye

The use of a pigtail probe is a simple technique that allows direct visualization of the proximal lumen of an injured canaliculus. Because of the risk of damaging the uninjured canaliculus or common canaliculus by creating a false passage or trauma to internal lining, some authors recommend this instrument as a last resort after failure to identify the injured canaliculus via direct visualization or irrigation. Many surgeons recommend the use of the pigtail probe be abandoned outright. Kennedy et al reviewed 222 canalicular laceration repairs and noted a higher incidence of postoperative epiphora in patients repaired with the pigtail probe (36.8% patients), and Saunders et al reported a 10% incidence of iatrogenic damage to the uninvolved ipsilateral canaliculus. Neither report specified if the worst probe (which has a hooked tip likely to induce trauma) or French-eyed probe (which has a smooth tip) was used.

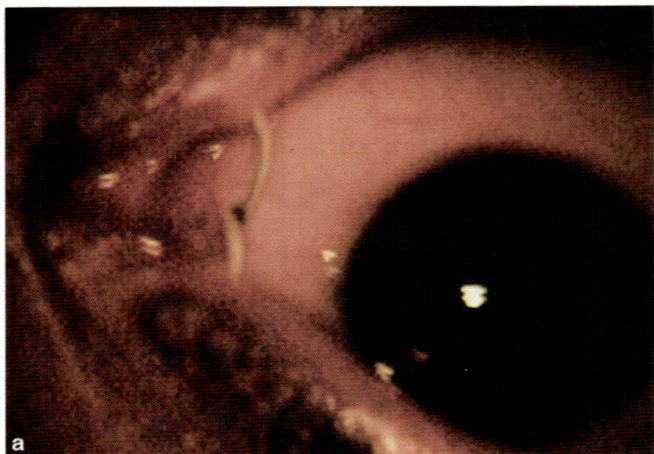

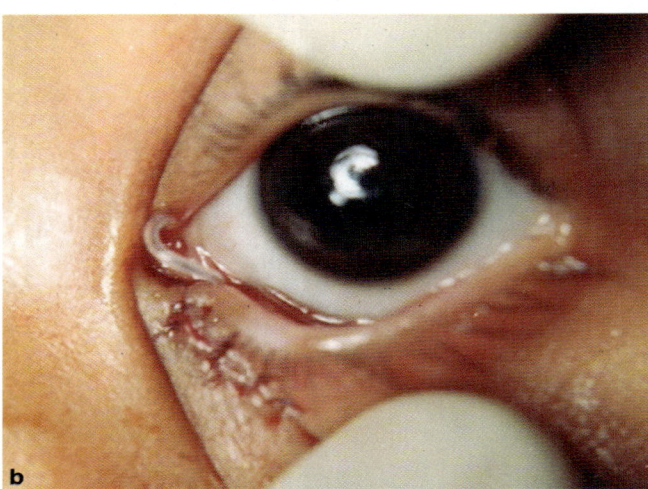

Figs 5.3.35a and b: BCASI—final appearance on the table

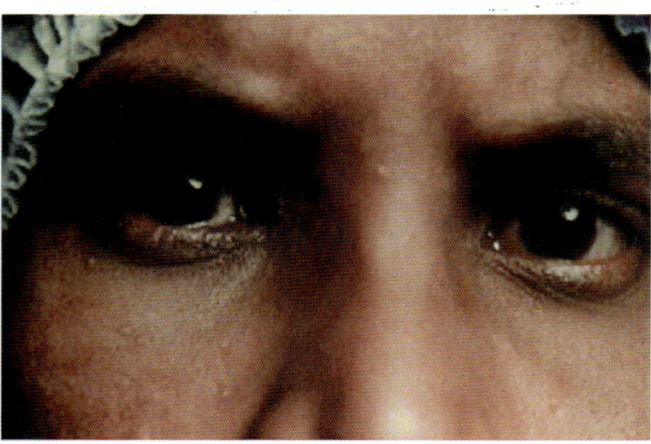

Fig. 5.3.36: Postoperative BCASI

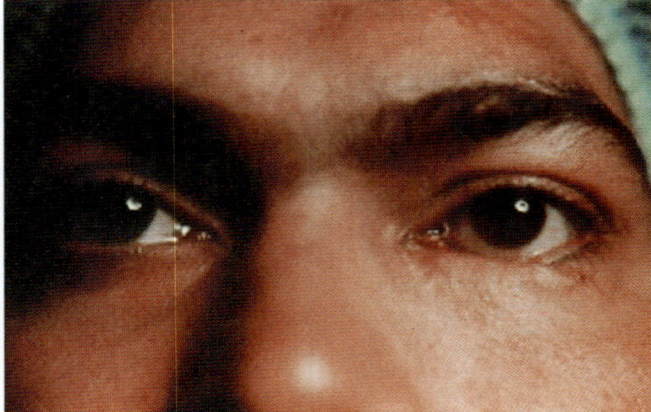

Fig. 5.3.37: Postoperative BCASI left eye

Postoperative Treatment

- Systemic antibiotics; 5–7 days
- Topical antibiotics; 2 weeks
- Follow-up once in 4 weeks
- Silicone stent left in place for 6–11 months
- Topical ketlur/diluted steroids if irritation

Results: BCASI-34 patients of monocanalicular laceration (18 lower, 16 upper), and 2 bicanalicular laceration, in the age group 2–50, years; 28 males, 6 females (Fig. 5.3.37)

- BCASI successfully performed in 32 cases
- BCASI abandoned in 4 cases
- No operative complications such as injury to intact canaliculus or false passage
- Postoperative complications
- Undue long loop: Two patients
- Punctal/canalicular cheese wiring: Nil
- Corneal abrasion, granuloma formation, loss of stent, infection: Nil
- Stent removal 6–11 months
- Follow-up period 6–24 months
- BCASI successful in 30 of 32 cases (93.7%)
- Criteria for success: Absence of epiphora, patent syringing after removal of stent.

Advantages of BCASI

- The procedure is simple, safe, effective
- Facilitates location of proximal cut end: Very important
- Mastered easily
- Intubation of sac, NLD and nasal fixation avoided

- No prolapse of stent as stent is in circle
- One study surveying 120 National Health Service-based consultants across UK regarding the management of of canalicular injury concluded that: 43% surgeons repaired a monocanalicular injury only if the lower canaliculus was involved, 40% always repaired a monocanalicular injury; 90% used magnification during surgery; 57% would never consider using the pigtail probe; 96% would use the bubble test and/or fluorescein dye to locate the severed medial canalicular end; the suture of choice was vicryl or dexon for (85%) and 71% surgeons would repair pericanalicular and canalicular tissues and 14.6%) respondents did not stent the canaliculus.

The round-tipped, eyed pigtail probe was used in a large series of 228 canalicular lacerations and was found to be safe and effective in silicone intubation of canalicular system with very high anatomic and functional success and without any incidence of damage to uninvolved canaliculus.

Monocanalicular Stenting

In this method, stenting of only injured canaliculus is performed. It is simple, safe and quicker technique than BCSI or BCASI. Various monocanalicular stents which have been used in the past are Vier's rod, Johnson's rod, Beyer's rod, polythene/silicone/teflon tubing.

Disadvantages of Monocanalicular Stenting

- Erosion through lid tissues
- Migration of stent
- Extrusion/spontaneous loss of stent
- Bulky lateral ends
- Conjunctival/corneal damage
- Does not provide support to medial, canthal and eyelid tissues in proper anatomic position
- Lower success rate: 50–94%.

Mauriello JA Jr, Abdelsalam A (1996) described a modified simple and effective method of monocanalicular silicone stent fixated to the peripunctal tissues by a 6-0 polypropylene suture as a practical alternative to bicanalicular intubation for canalicular lacerations. Dibble RF, Friedel SD (1990) reported a simplified method of monocanalicular silicone intubation which involved a monocanalicular

loop of tubing running from the punctum, through the lacerated canaliculus, and out the cutdown site over the lacrimal sac, provides a secure silicone tube stent.

Mini-Monoka Silicone Monocanalicular Stent

It consists of a modified punctual plug end which is attached to a silicone tube which is 40 mm long with 0.64 mm outer diameter. The stent is passed the dilated punctum and emerges through the cut end of canaliculus. The punctum plug is seated into the punctum. The nonpunctal end of the stent is inserted through the distal end of the canaliculus to the lacrimal sac thus the stent bridges canalicular laceration. The microsurgical pericanalicular anastomosis is performed in usual manner. Punctum plug remains fixed in the punctum. No sutures are required to fixate the stent to the lid.

Advantages

- Technically simple
- May be done under topical anesthesia
- No injury to uninvolved canaliculus
- No interpalpebral loop of the stent.

Drawbacks

- Punctual plug resting on the lid margin may irritate
- Does not aid in wound reapproximation
- Premature stent loss: 11–29% (Anastas et al 2001; Naik et al. 2008)
- Stent migration: 14%
- Canalicular patency: 79–90% (Anastas et al 2001; Naik et al 2008)

"One-stitch" canalicular repair: "One-stitch" canalicular repair using a single, fine, horizontal, mattress suture to reapproximate the overlying pericanalicular soft tissues combined with bicanalicular silicone intubation has proved to be highly successful in managing canalicular lacerations avoiding direct microsurgical reanastomosis of the canalicular epithelium.

Externalization of proximal end of lacerated canaliculus has been found successful in patients with tissue loss/infection/necrosis involving distal canaliculus and punctum, author has repaired such cases by BCASI or BCSI down the NLD so that the proximal end of canaliculus remains patent.

Conjunctival-Dacryocystorhinostomy (C-DCR)

An unrepaired canalicular laceration or failure after repair inevitably leads to extensive canalicular scarring with subsequent epiphora. A conjunctival: dacryocystorhinostomy with placement of a pyrex glass tube from carunculectomy site to the nose remains the treatment of choice. Complete microscopic resection of scarred canaliculus, anastomosis of normal canaliculus with bicanalicular annular silicone intubation may be tried before performing C-DCR.

Secondary repair of canalicular laceration: Recently Meltzer et al have described a new technique of secondary repair of traumatic laceration of lower canaliculus and punctum by lacrimal canalicular transplantation with composite eyelid graft from contralateral upper lid 3 mm lateral to the punctum and extended medially to include upper canaliculus. The patient was asymptomatic and was happy with the functional and cosmetic result. Syringing done at several visits was patent.

SUMMARY

Canalicular injuries remain the most common form of lacrimal trauma. Canalicular laceration must be suspected in any injury involving medial part of eyelid or medial canthal region. Passage of 00 lacrimal probe through the punctum confirms the diagnosis. As both upper and lower canaliculi play a role in tear drainage and modern techniques and instrumentation yield very high success rate after surgery, repair of all monocanalicular lacerations (upper or lower) is advocated. Basic principle of repair of such cases includes proper anatomical realignment of cut edges of canaliculus with insertion of silicone stent. Various surgical techniques to repair canalicular laceration are BCSI down the NLD/BCSI with nasal fixation, BCASI using modern pigtail probe and monocanalicular intubation. Each technique has its own merits and demerits. Controversy still exists about the best surgical technique. BCSI and BCASI, both are safe and effective. BCSI appears to be difficult and challenging. BCASI is not possible if both canaliculi open separately in the sac (10%). Pigtail probe should be rotated gently without any force. Mini-monoka silicone mono-canalicular stent is simple, safe, effective and does not threaten the uninvolved canaliculus. Silicone stenting and microsurgical pericanalicular anastomosis is essential and plays important role in all the techniques.

BIBLIOGRAPHY

1. Anastas CN, Potts MJ, Raiter J. Mini Monoka silicone monocanalicular lacrimal stents: subjective and objective outcomes. Orbit, 2001; 20 (3):189–200.
2. Benger RS, Nemet AY. Peripunctal "anchor" suture for securing the silicone bicanalicular stent in the repair of canalicular lacerations. Ophthal Plast Reconstr Surg. 2008; 24 (1):51–3.
3. Beyer CK. A modified lacrimal probe. Arch Ophthalmol 1974;92:157
4. Canavan YM, Archer DB. Long-term review of injuries to the lacrimal drainage apparatus. Trans Ophthalmol Soc UK. 1979;99(1):201–4. .
5. Cho SH, Hyun DW, Kang HJ, Ha MS. A simple new method for identifying the proximal cut end in lower canalicular laceration. Korean J Ophthalmol. 2008; 22(2):73–6.
6. Dibble RF, Friedel SD. A simplified method of monocanalicular silicone intubation. Ophthalmic Surg. 1990;21(2):134–5.
7. Dutton J. Atlas of Clinical and Surgical Orbital Anatomy. Philadelphia: WB Saunders; 1994:240.
8. Gonnering R. Periorbital animal bites. In: Linberg J, ed. Oculoplastic and Orbital Emergencies. Prentice Hall; 1990:215–228.
9. Gupta VP, Mittal S. Repair of canalicular laceration with bicanalicular silicone intubation down the NLD. Proceed. 57th AIOC (Cochin), 1999.
10. Gupta VP, Shrivastava S, Mittal S. Bicanalicular annular silicone intubation to repair canalicular lacerations. Proceed. 60th AIOC (Ahmedabad), 2002:503–504.
11. Gupta VP. Bicanalicular silicone intubation in lacrimal surgeries - A large series Proceed. 59th AIOC (Chennai), 2000:12–13.
12. Hawes M, Dortzbach R. Trauma of the lacrimal drainage system. In: Linberg J, ed. Lacrimal Surgery. New York: Churchill Livingstone; 1988:241–262.
13. Hawes MJ, Segrest DR. Effectiveness of bicanalicular silicone intubation in the repair of canalicular lacerations. Ophthal Plast Reconstr Surg. 1985;1(3):185–90.
14. Herzum H, Holle P, Hintschich C. Eyelid injuries: epidemiological aspects. Ophthalmologe. 2001;98(11): 1079–82.
15. Ho T, Lee V. National survey on the management of lacrimal canalicular injury in the United Kingdom. Clin Experiment Ophthalmol. 2006;34(1):39–43.
16. Jones LT, Marquis MM, Vincent NJ. Lacrimal functions. Am J Ophthalmol 1972;73:658.
17. Jordan DR, Gilberg S, Mawn LA. The round-tipped, eyed pigtail probe for canalicular intubation: a review of 228 patients. Ophthal Plast Reconstr Surg. 2008;24(3):176–80.
18. Jordan DR, Nerad JA, Tse DT. The pigtail prode, revisited. Ophthalmology. 1990;97:512–9.

19. Kennedy RH, May J, Dailey J, Flanagan JC. Canalicular laceration: An 11-year epidemiologic and clinical study. Ophthalmic Plastic and Reconstructive Surg. 1990;6:46–53.

20. Kersten RC, Kulwin DR. "One-stitch" canalicular repair. A simplified approach for repair of canalicular laceration. Ophthalmology. 1996;103(5):785–9.

21. Lemp MA, Weiler HH. How do tears exit? Invest Ophthalmol Vis SCI 1983;24:616.

22. Liang T, Zhao KX, Zhang LY. A clinical application of laser direction in anastomosis for inferior canalicular laceration. Chin J Traumatol. 2006;9(1):34–7.

23. Linberg J. Surgical anatomy of the lacrimal system. In: Linberg J, ed. Lacrimal Surgery. New York: Churchill Livingstone; 1988:1–18.

24. Linberg JV, Moore CA. Symptoms of monocanalicular obstruction. Ophthalmology. 1988;95:1077.

25. Loff HJ, Wobig JL, Dailey RA. The bubble test: an atraumatic method for canalicular laceration repair. Ophthal Plast Reconstr Surg. 1996;12(1):61–64.

26. Mauriello JA Jr, Abdelsalam A. Use of a modified monocanalicular silicone stent in 33 eyelids. Ophthalmic Surg Lasers. 1996;27(11):929–34.

27. McLeish WM, Bowman B, Andersaon RL. The pigtail probe protected by silicone intubation: A combined approach to canalicular reconstruction. Ophthalmic Surg. 1992;23:281–3.

28. Meltzer M A, Zatezalo C C, Zoltan S. Lacrimal Canalicular Transplantation With Composite Eyelid Graft. Ophthal Plast Reconstr Surg 2010; 26:1:23–25.

29. Morrison F D. An Aid to Repair of Lacerated Tear Ducts, Arch Ophthal 1964;72:341–342.

30. Naik MN, Kelapure A, Rath S, Honavar SG. Management of canalicular lacerations: epidemiological aspects and experience with Mini-Monoka monocanalicular stent. Am J Ophthalmol. 2008;145(2):375–380. Epub 2007 Dec 3.

31. Pecora JL. Pediatric pigtail probes. Ophthalmic Surg. 1980;11:249.

32. Reifler DM. Management of canalicular laceration. Surv Ophthalmol. 1991;36(2):113–32.

33. Saunders DH, Shannon GM, Flanagan JC. The effectiveness of the pigtail probe method of repairing canalicular lacerations. Ophthalmic Surg. 1978;9(3):33–40.

34. Saunders DH, Shannon GM, Flanagan JC. The effectiveness of the pigtail probe method of repairing canalicular lacerations. Ophthalmic Surg. 1978;9:33–40.

35. Savar A, Kirszrot J, Rubin PA. Canalicular involvement in dog bite related eyelid lacerations. Ophthal Plast Reconstr Surg. 2008;24(4):296–8.

36. Walter W. The use of the pigtail probe for silicone intubation of the injured canaliculus. Ophthalmic Surg. 1982;13:488–92.

37. Werb A. Panel discussion on the lacrimal system. In: Smith B, Converse JM, Wood-Smith, et al, eds. Plasic and Reconstructive Sutgery of the Eye and Adnexa: proceedings of the second international symposium. St. Louis: CV Mosby. 1967:182.

38. Worst JG. Method for reconstructing torn lacrimal canaliculus. Am J Ophthalmol. 1962; 53:520–522.

39. Wu SY, Ma L, Chen RJ, Tsai YJ, Chu YC. Analysis of bicanalicular nasal intubation in the repair of canalicular lacerations. Jpn J Ophthalmol. 2010;54(1):24–31.

5.4 TRAUMA AND OCULAR MUSCLE IMBALANCE

• Zia Chaudhuri • Rajat Chaudhary

INTRODUCTION

Traumatic strabismus may result from orbital or head injury which may be closed or open. These injuries usually get ignored during the initial part of management of trauma because the management is more concentrated on life-saving maneuvers. Thus, the presence of these complex injuries often delays the diagnosis and treatment of traumatic strabismus.[1] The main complaints with which patients with traumatic strabismus present with are ocular misalignment and diplopia. Loss of vision is an associated symptom, whose presence precludes the presence of diplopia.

Diplopia (i.e. double vision; a symptom) after extraocular muscle trauma following head injury is not uncommon, and it can be disabling. In addition to the distress diplopia generates, the cosmetic appearance due to ocular misalignment is usually unacceptable. Traumatic strabismus has three main causes:[2]

1. Direct injury to the muscles
2. Orbital injury
3. Neurological injury.

A careful workup including a complete eye examination and measurements of alignment, is used to evaluate the cause and suggest a treatment. In addition, imaging studies and forced ductions are sometimes required to assess the extent of muscle damage, any entrapment of the muscle and the associated neural trauma.

Treatment is closely related to the cause, and it varies from waiting for spontaneous recovery to prisms to surgery. The surgical decision process can be quite complex and should be based on an accurate knowledge of the etiology of the misalignment and on the principles of strabismus surgery.

ETIOLOGY OF TRAUMATIC STRABISMUS

Direct Trauma to Extraocular Muscles

Direct injury to the extraocular muscles can cause immediate diplopia with obvious misalignment of the eyes. Although uncommon, it is dramatic when it occurs.

When eyes with an anterior injury are explored surgically, most are found to have a superficial scleral laceration, with the muscle some 5–6 mm from its original insertion. The inferior rectus is the most commonly affected muscle, followed by the medial rectus, the lateral rectus, the superior rectus, the inferior oblique and the superior oblique.[3,4]

ORBITAL FRACTURE

An orbital fracture is one of the most common causes of traumatic diplopia. The classic blowout fracture of the floor of the orbit is the most common, followed by medial wall fractures. The roof of the orbit is uncommonly affected, and the lateral wall is protected by its strong bone structures. Approximately, one-third of patients with a blowout fracture have diplopia despite early repair of the fracture.[5,6]

Hypotropia from entrapment of the muscle or of orbital septae is the most common misalignment in cases of an orbital fracture (Fig. 5.4.1). The muscle itself may be trapped by the sharp edge of the fracture or may be herniated into a sinus (Fig. 5.4.2). Because the numerous connective tissue septae of the orbit are connected to the muscle sheaths, entrapment of the septae alone give a similar clinical result to muscle entrapment. Not infrequently, the orbital fracture repair itself causes entrapment of the muscle or incomplete release of an entrapped muscle. Forced duction testing generally shows a restriction of the entrapped muscle.

Hypertropia has also been described with posterior fractures.[5,6] The condition is thought to be caused by:

- One of the inferior rectus muscles being caught posteriorly on a sharp fracture step-off extraocular muscle trauma or
- A change in the angle of contact of the inferior rectus with the globe.

Patients with traumatic hypertropia have negative forced ductions, and 80% of the conditions are corrected with surgical elevation of the orbital contents to the posterior extent of the fracture.[6]

It is important to realize that nerve and muscle contusion can cause a temporary muscle dysfunction and that orbital swelling can also restrict ocular motility.[7]

Although a substantial number of patients with a blowout fracture experience spontaneous resolution of diplopia during the first 2–4 weeks after the injury,[5] large fractures should be operated on earlier before scarring makes repair more difficult.

NEUROLOGICAL INJURY

Cranial nerve palsies can occur in severe or mild head trauma, but palsy of the third cranial nerve is usually seen only in the setting of severe head injury. However, cranial nerve IV, with its long path, is susceptible to lesser trauma and may be paretic even when the patient had head trauma without loss of consciousness. These palsies are often transient and self-resolving. The correct mode of management is to keep the patient under observation till either the resolution of the palsy or the stabilization of the deviation. Patching of one eye to avoid diplopia, prisms or botulinum toxin injections may be tried as temporary measures to alleviate the diplopia. Surgery should not be attempted till the deviation is stable for a period of at least 6 months after the insult. Palsies of cranial nerve VI are relatively common. In the initial period after an injury to the sixth nerve, the alignment shows an obvious incomitance. With time there is a spread of comitance, however, as the antagonist shortens to match its chronically deviated position.[7]

Diplopia after relatively mild head trauma also may occur with a previously asymptomatic brain tumor.

DIFFERENTIAL DIAGNOSIS

Underlying strabismus and diplopia from other causes should be excluded. Long-standing strabismus should be considered in any case in which the ocular misalignment does not match the injury, but strabismus can confuse the examiner in the setting of a concussion. In addition to those with a known history of strabismus, patients with an absence of previous symptoms may have mild, congenital, fourth nerve palsies, phorias and Duane's syndrome. The stress of trauma or illness can cause some patients with phorias to breakdown into frank strabismus with diplopia, but these cases usually resolve in a few weeks. Careful measurements, old photographs, and occasionally forced ductions or examination under

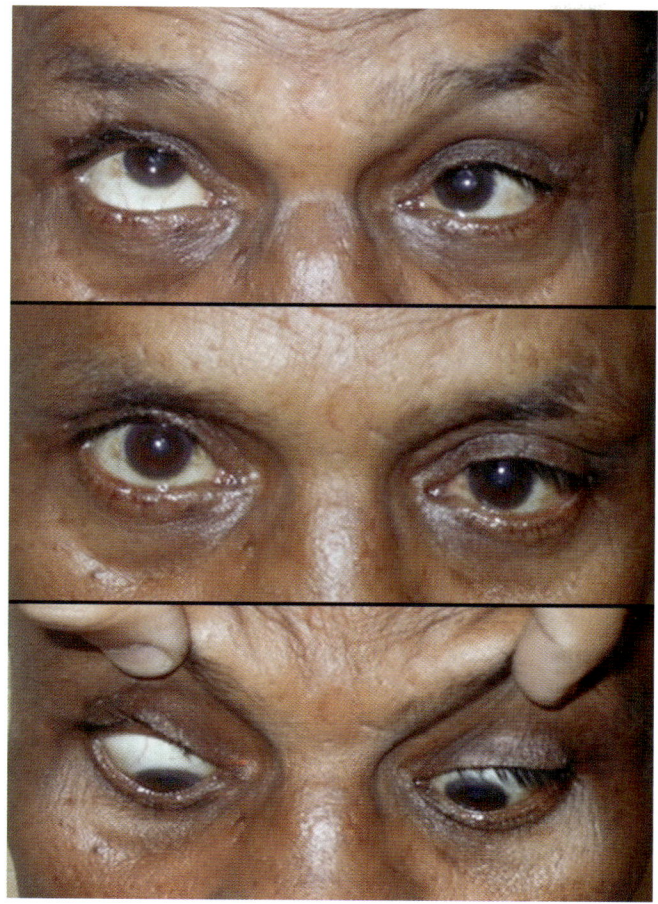

Fig. 5.4.1: Enophthalmos and restiction in up gaze and down gaze

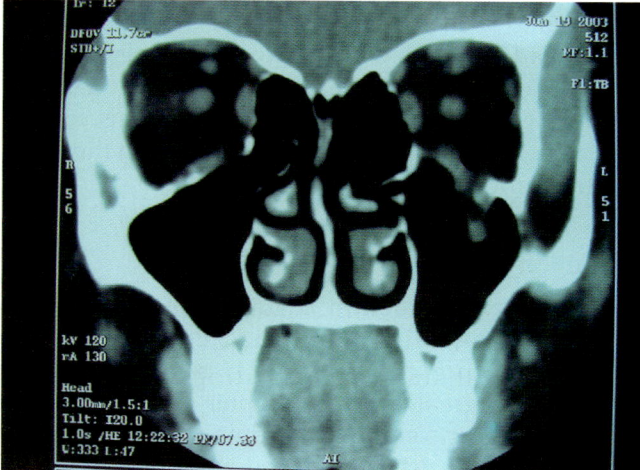

Fig. 5.4.2: MRI left eye blow out with hanging drop sign and displaced bony fragment in floor of orbit visible on MRI

anesthesia may be necessary to differentiate congenital fourth nerve palsies and Duane's syndrome from traumatic nerve injury.

Nonstrabismic diplopia is not uncommon in the setting of trauma and should be differentiated from diplopia-induced ocular misalignment. Usually, the diplopia is monocular because of cataract or regular or irregular astigmatism and is eliminated when the patient looks through a pinhole. In addition, a patient who has unilateral traumatic aphakia that is corrected by anisometropic spectacle lens may see two images due to aniseikonia. This problem is usually easily corrected with a contact lens.

EVALUATION

History

Past ocular history should include specific questions about childhood strabismus, previous muscle operations, and any family history of strabismus. A head posture from an unsuspected congenital superior oblique palsy or Duane's syndrome may be obvious from old photographs such as one appearing on a driver's license.

A patient with childhood strabismus usually has little or no diplopia. A patient with a resolving muscle contusion or a recovering nerve injury, on the other hand, may describe improving diplopia or an increasing diplopia-free field of gaze.

OCULAR EXAMINATION

Sensory Tests

When an asymmetrical visual acuity is uncorrectable by refraction and not caused by another obvious source, check for amblyopia with the crowding phenomenon. If the patient complains of diplopia but the eyes appear straight, occlude one eye to rule out monocular diplopia. The double Maddox's rod test is useful when palsy of the fourth cranial nerve is suspected. Bilateral traumatic fourth nerve palsies are common and usually have more than 10° of excyclotorsion between the eyes on this test.

Stereopsis and the worth four-dot test help to define the binocular status of the patient and can be used to demonstrate improvement after surgery.

Pupils

A careful pupil examination can reveal dilation from a third nerve injury. If a dilated pupil is observed, the pupil should be carefully examined with a slit lamp to rule out traumatic rupture of the iris sphincter or a tonic pupil.

Alignment

Alignment should be measured with the best spectacle correction. Traumatic misalignment can be complex, so measurements should be made in primary position, near-, up-, down-, left-, and right-gaze. In cases with a component of hypertropia or suspected fourth nerve palsies, the alignment should also be measured on head tilt to the left and to the right. In addition to standard prism testing, one of the most useful tests of alignment is the Lancaster red-green test. The Lancaster test gives a standard graphic plot of misalignment and can dramatically demonstrate torsional misalignment.

In cases of incomitant misalignment, the prism should be placed over the apparently paretic or restricted eye and the primary deviation measured. If the prism is placed over the apparently normal eye, the resulting measurement is called the secondary deviation and is larger than the primary deviation. Because muscle surgery is usually done on the eye with abnormal motility, the primary deviation is the most useful measurement to determine the extent of the muscle surgery to be performed.

Versions should be tested in all the cardinal positions of gaze.

A dilated fundus examination should be done to look for torsion. In straight eyes, the fovea will be observed to be in line with the lower third of the optic nerve head. Patients with fourth nerve palsy usually have observable excyclotorsion of 5–15°. Fundus photography can be used to document this torsion with a single photograph that includes both the fovea and the optic nerve.

Refraction

A cycloplegic refraction is important in cases of horizontal misalignment that could have an accommodative component. If an uncorrected hyperopia of greater than 1 diopter is discovered in the setting of concomitant esotropia, then putting this prescription in a trial frame (on another day, when the cycloplegia has worn off) may reduce or eliminate the misalignment.

CLINICAL TESTS

Forced ductions are often useful in the setting of traumatic strabismus and help to confirm a suspected diagnosis of rectus muscle restriction. In the setting of acute orbital injury, soft-tissue swelling by itself can cause restriction, so the results are most reliable 1 week after the injury. Most adults tolerate the procedure well with topical anesthesia alone, but occasionally it must be first done as part of the surgical repair of the misalignment. Caution and gentle technique should be used in patients older than 60 years of age, because the relatively friable conjunctiva of older adults may tear easily. A five-tooth Lester forceps tends to be gentler on the conjunctiva than a three-tooth standard forceps.

The eye is grasped at the limbus nearest the suspected restricted muscle and rotated in the direction of maximum deviation. It is important to avoid depression of the globe while rotating the eye, as this relaxes the muscle being tested. If the muscle is restricted, there usually is an apparent limitation in ocular rotation. Limitation is usually obvious when the restricted eye alone is rotated, but comparisons of the forced ductions of both eyes are sometimes necessary.

Some clinicians use a cotton-tipped applicator to rotate the eye, but this technique is useful only when the restriction is severe. The applicator must be applied with significant downward pressure, depressing the globe and relaxing the rectus muscle.

The results of clinical forced ductions should be confirmed at the time of surgery. Small amounts of restriction that were not revealed by clinical testing may become apparent. In addition, forced duction testing of the oblique muscles should be done under anesthesia. To test the superior oblique muscle, grasp the limbal conjunctiva nearest the medial rectus muscle. Depress and excyclotort the globe. This exaggerated forced duction puts the tendon on stretch and the examiner should feel the eye roll over the tight tendon. This test is useful to differentiate congenital from acquired unilateral fourth nerve palsy. In congenital cases, the superior oblique tendon is usually quite lax owing to a congenitally anomalous tendon. This test is also useful in diagnosing traumatic Brown's syndrome. The inferior oblique can be tested in a similar fashion, incyclotorting the globe.

Force generation testing is especially useful to differentiate paretic from restrictive misalignment and must be done while the patient is awake. The eye is grasped using the same technique as described for forced ductions, and the patient is instructed to look in the direction of maximum deviation.

Ancillary Tests

Binocular visual fields to determine the field of binocular single vision are especially useful in patients with blowout fractures, for whom the surgical goal may be to shift this field to the most useful areas: primary position and reading position (down-gaze).

Computed tomography scans with direct axial and coronal views are most useful in the management of orbital-fracture-associated strabismus but can also be used in some cases to evaluate lacerations of the muscle belly.

Magnetic resonance imaging provides high-resolution imaging of the muscles and is especially useful in evaluating cases of suspected laceration or loss of the muscle. In some cases, MRI has shown the correct etiology of post-traumatic strabismus prior to surgical exploration and repair. The use of fat-suppression MRI helps to reduce artifacts from the otherwise-bright orbital fat. Dynamic MRI (imaging the extraocular muscles during different gaze positions) can be used to differentiate a paretic muscle from a detached, functioning muscle.[8-10] Muscle bellies with normal contractility thicken when the patient attempts to gaze in the direction of action of that muscle.

MANAGEMENT

Preferred management options to treat the problems caused by extrocular muscle trauma include tincture of time, the use of spectacles and prisms, and occlusive filters in spectacles. In many cases, surgery should be considered only as a last resort.

Medical Options

Cranial nerve paresis often recovers spontaneously over a period of several months, and muscle contusions may recover in a few weeks. One long-term, prospective study[11] of traumatic sixth nerve palsy or paresis showed that spontaneous recovery is common. The prognosis was better if there was some sixth nerve function on the initial examination.

A few patients with concomitant esotropia and significant hyperopia benefit from spectacle correction. Before prescribing lenses, it is wise to evaluate the effect on alignment by putting the corrective lenses in a trial frame.

Prisms can help to treat diplopia caused by small amounts of concomitant tropias. In some cases they are the only treatment needed. They are easier to use if the patient already wears spectacles, as small quantities of prism can be obtained simply by displacing the optical center of the lenses. Most patients who did not previously wear spectacles will find those with prisms intolerable. Fresnel prisms are useful as a therapeutic trial and on a short-term basis. It is important to remember that prisms act in only one direction of gaze. This a should be explained to the patient properly.

Occasionally, a patient has a strabismus that cannot be adequately treated with surgery or prisms, or has incomitance such that the field of binocular single vision is nearly useless (e.g. complete third nerve palsies). These patients should be offered the option of cosmetically acceptable occlusive filters. In a few cases, the diplopia is only in one direction (e.g. down or laterally) and a partial occluder on the spectacle lens in the field of diplopia should be considered.

General Principles for Surgical Management

The choice of operation depends on the etiology, clinical measurements, forced duction and force generation findings and occasionally imaging results. Surgeons should bear in mind the following principles for surgical management of patients with extraocular muscle dysfunctions[12]

1. The patient should have realistic expectations. Although muscle surgery is generally successful, some patients will never have useful binocular single vision and should clearly understand this caveat before proceeding to surgery. They should also understand that reoperation may be required.

2. If orbital surgery is planned, do that first. Orbital surgery can relieve strabismus if there is an entrapped muscle.

3. It is wise to delay surgery up to 6 months in cases of traumatic nerve paresis. Spontaneous recovery generally begins by about 3 months, and the alignment is usually stable by 6 months.

4. Optimize the field of binocular single vision. One of the primary goals of surgery in non-concomitant cases is to increase the field of binocular single vision. This zone should be optimized for the individual consider the patient's occupation (e.g. professional drivers may need single vision in left gaze to avoid diplopia when looking out the driver's-side window) while deciding the surgical options.

5. Use adjustable suture surgery. Adjustment can be made up to 1 week after surgery if hyaluronic acid is placed between the muscle and the sclera.[13]

6. Reduce the risk of anterior segment ischemia. Blood supply to the anterior segment comes from three main sources: (1) ciliary vessels running through the rectus muscle, (2) the limbal conjunctiva and (3) the long posterior ciliary vessels at 3 o'clock and 9 o'clock. To prevent anterior segment ischemia avoid performing surgery on all four muscle on one eye, even if the operations are separated by time.[14]

7. Recess muscle that are tight on forced duction testing.

8. Operate on the muscle active in the field of greatest deviation. For example, in cases of long standing fourth nerve palsy, the antagonistic inferior oblique muscle is usually shortened, resulting in excyclotorsion and a deviation that is greatest in the action of the inferior oblique muscle. In these cases, the procedure of choice is to weaken the inferior oblique. This dictum must be tempered by the results of intraoperative forced ductions. For example, a tight superior rectus muscle will cause the greatest deviation to be in the field of action of the ipsilateral inferior rectus, but the procedure of choice is to weaken the tight superior rectus.

9. Cripple the yoke muscle in nonconcomitant strabismus using either recession of this muscle or a Faden procedure (posterior fixation suture). This intervention increases the field of of binocular single vision. For example a patient with a sixth nerve palsy will have a non-concomitant esotropia, with greatest deviation in the field of gaze of the paretic muscle. In this case, a transposition of the ipsilateral vertical recti to the lateral rectus combined with botulinum toxin injected into the ipsilateral medial rctus muscle will help straighten the eye, but a recession of the contralateral medial rectus will increase the field of binocular single vision.

10. Partial nerve palsies are often adequately corrected by recession of the antagonist and resection of the weak (but functional) muscle. In some cases, crippling the yoke muscle and injecting botulinum toxin into the antagonist gives best results. If the muscle is completely paralyzed, it is not worth resecting the same, as little effect will be obtained.

11. Transpositions of recti combined with injection of botulinum toxin into the antagonist are generally the best approach to complete isolated rectus muscle palsy (e.g. sixth nerve palsy).

MANAGEMENT OF LACERATED MUSCLES

The management of most lacerated muscles is similar to that of slipped or lost muscles.[15] If repaired early, a muscle that has been lacerated at its insertion is usually found 5–6 mm away from the original insertion. With time, the lacerated muscle and its antagonist shorten, making retrieval more difficult and requiring recession or botulinum toxin injection of the antagonist muscle.

When looking for the lacerated muscle, good illumination and exposure using malleable retractors are critical. Loupes and a strong overhead surgical light are usually sufficient, but a headlight or operating microscope may also be useful in some cases. The muscle is often found at its penetration through Tenon's capsule. If the patient has not received systemic atropine or a similar medication as part of anesthesia, then tugging on the muscle may help to differentiate it from the surrounding tissue by inducing the oculocardiac reflex.[15] If the muscle cannot be found after diligent efforts, it is not useful to open Tenon's capsule in a usually futile search for the stump: this procedure risks causing a fat adherence syndrome. Instead, the muscle should be declared lost and a transposition procedure performed to align the eyes.

REFERENCES

1. Subramanian PS, Birdsong RH. Surgical management of traumatic strabismus after combat-related injury. Mil Med. 2008;173(7):693–6.
2. Mines M, Thach A, Mallonee S, Hildebrand L, Shariat S. Ocular injuries sustained by survivors of the Oklahoma City bombing. Ophthalmology. 2000;107:837–43.
3. Harish AY, Ganesh SC, Narendran K. Traumatic superior oblique tendon rupture. J AAPOS. 2009;13(5):485–7.
4. Murray AD. Slipped and lost muscles and other tales of the unexpected. J AAPOS 1998;2:133–43.
5. Good WV, Hoyt CS, eds. Strabismus Management. Boston, Mass: Butterworth-Heinemann; 1996: Chap 20.
6. Seiff SR, Good WV. Hypertropia and the posterior blowout fracture: Mechanism and management. Ophthalmology. 1996;103:152–6.
7. von Noorden GK. Diagnosis of trauma-related strabismus. In: Freeman HM, ed. Ocular Trauma. New York, NY:Appleton-Century-Crofts; 1979: Chap 33.
8. Rubin SE. How to diagnose and manage paralytic strabismus Rev Ophthalmol. 1999;6(10):103–16.
9. Ward TP, Thach AB, Madigan WP, Berland JE. Magnetic resonance imaging in posttraumatic strabismus. J Pediatr Ophthalmol Strabismus. 1997;34:131–4.
10. Shin GS, Demer JL, Rosenbaum AL. High resolution, dynamic, magnetic resonance imaging in complicated strabismus. J Pediatr Ophthalmol Strabismus. 1996; 33:282–90.
11. Holmes JM, Droste PJ, Beck RW. The natural history of acute traumatic sixth nerve palsy or paresis. J AAPOS. 1998;2:265–8.
12. Wright KW, ed. Color Atlas of Ophthalmic Surgery: Strabismus. Philadelphia, Pa: JB Lippincott Company; 1991:241–3.
13. Granet DB, Hertle RW, Ziylan S. The use of hyaluronic acid during adjustable suture surgery. J Pediatr Ophthalmol Strabismus. 1994;31:287–9.
14. McKeown CA, Lambert HM, Shore JW. Preservation of the anterior ciliary vessels during extraocular muscle surgery. Ophthalmology. 1989;96:498–507.
15. Reineke RD. Treatment of ocular motility problems following trauma. In: Freeman HM, ed. Ocular Trauma. New York, NY: Appleton-Century-Crofts; 1979: Chap 34.

Anterior Segment Injuries

6.1 MECHANICAL TRAUMA
6.1.1 Mechanical Corneal Injuries

• G Mukherjee • Rajib Mukherjee

INTRODUCTION

Cornea is the most vulnerable ocular tissue to trauma due to its anatomical position as it is situated at the most anterior part of the eyeball, although it is adequately protected by bony orbital structures and strong blinking reflex of eyelids. There has been a marked increase in incidence of ocular injuries due to road traffic accidents, industrial development and agricultural revolution, gunshot and blast injuries due to worldwide terrorism and iatrogenic trauma following newer surgical intervention and procedures.

General incidence of corneal injuries reported is widely variable. WHO symposium (2004)[1] on corneal injury reported incidence varies from 1 to 5% in India.

Indian Council of Medical Research (ICMR) Study (1976–1979)[2] reported incidence of 1.2% ocular injuries while surveying over all blindness status in Indian population. National studies in (1986–1989)[3] and subsequently 1999, 2004 have also reported almost similar figures. A concomitant increase in corneal injuries were noted as one of leading cause of unilateral or bilateral blindness in last two decades. Primary ocular surface injuries involving conjunctiva, cornea and sclera reported as 80–85%, may or may not be associated with other intraocular or extraocular injuries.

Involvement of cornea as primary site of injury has been reported by authors[4,5] (Malik 55.8%, Koval 81.2%, Moreira 49.3%, Shukla and Verma 64%, Shukla 53%). Srinivasan et al (1997, 2003)[6] reported one of the most frequent cause of corneal infection is Ocular Trauma. WHO Collaborative Study (2006–2007)[7] also reported trauma is the most common cause of microbial keratitis (56.8%). The corneal blindness due to trauma is 28.6% and it is second to childhood keratitis 36.7% in children.

Since most of the time corneal injuries are associated with other ocular injuries like ocular surface injuries, intraocular and extraocular injuries, corneal injuries as a separate entity are not considerded. Trival corneal injuries as corneal abrasion, corneal foreign body (FB), etc. mostly are not taken into account and reported. So, all these factors makes it very difficult to know exact incidence of corneal injury as a separate entity.

TYPES OF CORNEAL INJURY

I. Mechanical injury
II. Non-mechanical injury
   a. Chemical injury—acid, alkali, etc.
   b. Radiational and thermal injury
   c. Electrical.
III. Iatrogenic
   • Birth trauma
   • Postsurgical trauma
   • Toxic keratopathy (drug-related).

Mechanical Injury

i. Blunt trauma
ii. Corneal abrasion
iii. Corneal FB
iv. Penetrating/open globe injury
   a. Clean cut wound
   b. Lacerated wound
   c. Corneal tissue loss.

This could be simple or uncomplicated and complicated.

- Uveal tissue trauma
- Lenticular trauma
- Vitreous disturbance
- Retinal injury
- Intraocular foreign body (IOFB)
- Damage to extraocular tissues
- Damage to bony orbital structures.

Approach to management depends on type of corneal injury.

Terminologies Related to Corneal Injuries

It is important to know and get used to various terminologies used in dealing ocular/corneal injury in order to maintain uniformity. It also helps to develop a good referral system and documentation. The new definitions are proposed by the American Ocular Trauma Society and these terminologies are accepted and followed by most traumatologist throughout the world.

- *Closed globe injury:* Where outer coat (cornea and selera) is intact and does not have a full thickness wound but there is damage to intraocular tissues, commonly seen with blunt trauma.

- *Open globe injury:* Involves full thickness wound of outer coat of globe.

- *Rupture of globe:* Where full thickness wound is caused by impact of trauma resulting in sudden markedly increased intraocular pressure (IOP) resulting rupture of weakest part of eyeball, usually due to blunt trauma.

- *Penetrating injury:* Single full thickness laceration of eyeball, usually caused by sharp objects.

- *Perforating injury:* Two full thickness laceration (entry and exit) of globe.

- *Intraocular FB:* Technically it is penetrating injury with retained IOFB (RIOFB). It should be put into separate category as management is totally different.

- *Contusion:* It is closed globe injury usually results from blunt trauma. Damage to ocular tissue takes place at the site of impact or at a distant site.

- *Laceration:* Could be full thickness or partial thickness of cornea, usually caused by a sharp object at the site of impact.

Documentation and Evaluation of Corneal Injury

Documentation and detail clinical assessment are absolute mandatory in all corneal injuries. This not only helps in proper management, prognostication rehabilitation but also in medicolegal point and compensation.

No time should be wasted in documentation, evaluation and collection of first hand information. Time lapse between the time of injury and the evaluation should be as little as possible as clinical picture changes very fast.

First Information

Following points must be noted in writing, as first hand information (at the place of trauma).

- Place and time of injury
- Causative agents leading to corneal trauma type and nature of object, e.g. metallic, nonmetallic, chemicals, vegetable matter, etc. Ocular infections are common with vegetable matter injury. Velocity of striking object at the time of impact to cornea. Blunt or sharp object.
- Note general condition of the patient. History of unconsciousness, convulsion, or any other associated injury to other part of body.
- Spectacle or any other protective devices using during trauma.
- History of ocular problem/visual acuity prior to injury.
- Any first-aid treatment given, if so details if available.

Assessment and Investigations

When the patient reports to ophthalmic surgeon or trauma center. It has three steps:

a. History
b. Examination
c. Investigations.

a. *History:* A careful history taking of the inciting events may suggest much about the nature and extent of cornea injury. This guides the examiner what to look for (e.g. corneal FB, abrasion, laceration, etc.) and workup in the right direction; for example, a suspected FB injury guides the examiner investigations needed.

A detail past history includes enquiry about pre-existing ophthalmic problems, e.g. amblyopia, previous ocular surgery or trauma. This will have direct bearing on visual outcome, prognosis and rehabilitation. This will also help in case of compensation.

b. *Examination:* It is better and safe to take written consent even before conducting examination and investigation. All finding must be documented, this is most important. Photographic documentation photo slit lamp is preferred in corneal injuries, if it is available. Otherwise a schematic representation of each corneal findings can be noted on corneal documentation chart (Mohan et al)[8] and it is adequate.

Complete ocular examination should be done. Starting with visual acuity of each eye if general condition permits. Projection of rays and perception of light (PR/PL) should be noted separately in each eye. Ocular surface including sclera and conjunctiva, should be examined on slit lamp in diffuse light and then proceed to examine each layer of Cornea, anterior chamber (AC), pupil, iris IOP and other intraocular tissues. One must look for any abnormal content in AC, e.g. blood, FB, etc. Ophthalmoscopic examination should be done if possible.

Word of caution while examining a traumatized eye

- Examination of traumatized eye should be carried out gently without jeopardizing an unstable globe. Forceful examination may lead to further damage. If the patient is not cooperative, due to pain or mentally traumatized it is better to sedate the patient and examine under local or general anesthesia. Children should examined under anesthesia.
- Magnetic resonance imaging (MRI) should never be done when a metallic foreign body is suspected.
- Detailed base line status of eyes prior to injury and after injury should be noted.

Special Investigations

a. *Ultrasonography (USG):* As primary investigative procedure both "A" and "B" scan are important. Lots of information can be collected through USG, e.g. IOFB, intraocular hemorrhage, retinal detachment, integrity of outer coat of eyeball, ruptured globe, condition of optic nerve, etc. It also helps in planning further management, e.g. anterior segment injury along with posterior segment

damage, a combined first time management gives better postoperative results. This test has lot of advantages and can be repeated several times if required, only disadvantage is it requires direct contact with the globe.

b. *Ultrasound biomicroscopy (UBM):* Extent of damage impregnated FB, lacerations can be better diagnosed.

c. *Anterior segment optical coherence tomography (OCT)* for anterior segment injury and both anterior and posterior segment OCT for combined injury is valuable in management.

d. *Radiography:* Plain X-ray of the eye and orbit must be taken, particularly when suspected injury to cornea is with a flying object.

e. *Computed tomography (CT) scan* is a superior radiographic investigation in localizing intra-ocular/orbital FB. It is also a valuable investigation in suspected intra-cameral FB (AC), FB in angle of AC, etc. It also helps in rulling out bony fractures of orbit and is superior to USG as it helps to know the size and location of FB without direct contact with globe.

f. *Corneal specular microscopy:* It gives valuable information about the status of corneal endothelium particular when damage to endothelium is suspected, e.g. blunt trauma, radiational, thermal injury, birth trauma, etc.

g. *Electrophysiological test:* Important to detect functional status of retina and optice nerve. This test has prognostic value. Electoretinography (ERG) can determine visual potential of injured eye. Only drawback is false result may be recorded in case of dense vitreous hemorrhage.

CORNEAL FOREIGN BODY

Injury to cornea with FB is the most common injury as seen by most ophthalmologist. WHO Study (2003) reported (56.8%) corneal FB injury the most important predisposing factor of infective keratitis. Damages to cornea with a FB depends on many factors, size and shape of the FB, nature of foreign body whether metallic, nonmetallic or a vegetable matter, single or multiple FB. Corneal injuries with metallic FBs are commonly seen amongst industrial worker where as injury with vegetable matter are seen amongst agriculture workers (Fig. 6.1.1.1.)

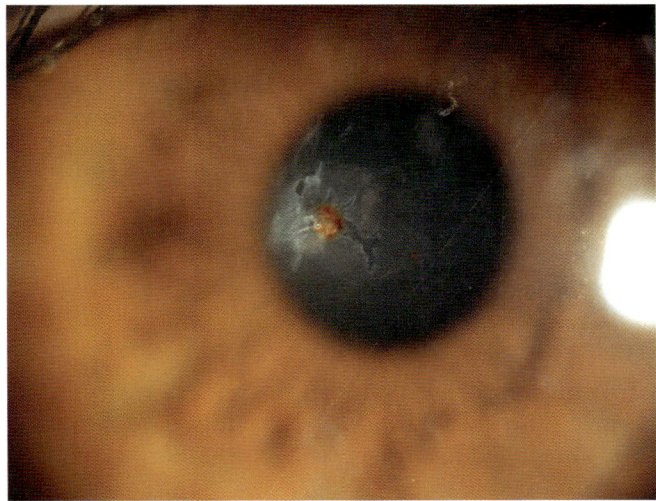

Fig. 6.1.1.1: FB iron

History

Detail history should be taken to know the nature of injury whether a flying FB from Laithe machine, chisel and hammer, etc. Type of FB should be noted. Flying FB from a machine strikes the eyeball with high velocity and results in deep penetration into the eyeball, may even result in double perforation.

Symptoms

Most common symptom is gritty feeling or FB sensation, watering, photophobia, red eye following history of trauma with flying objects.

Signs

Visual acuity should be noted at first instant. Sectorial conjunctival congestion near to corneal FB or generalized congestion. Lid edema if the patient reports late or another FB under the lid. Site and depth of FB, corneal edema, superficial punctate keratitis, rusting and infiltration around corneal foreign should be noted. Deep corneal FB may be associated with AC reaction. Corneal FB is detected or visualized best in slit lamp with indirect or retroillumination. Examination of cornea under magnification/slit lamp is mandatory. Look out for any other FB in conjunctiva, lids, canthus.

Iris hole or tear, localized lenticular opacity indicates IOFB. IOP should be noted. In self-sealed corneal wound, a RIOFB should be suspected and ruled out if there is history suggestive of FB injury. If possible a dilated pupil fundus examination should be done.

Plain X–ray eyeball and orbit, USG "B" scan CT scan (axial and coronal view 1 mm cuts), UBM should be done to exclude RIOFB.

Avoid MRI if history suggests a metallic FB.

Treatment

Superficial Foreign Body

Removal of corneal FB should be done under strict sterile conditions, under magnification and topical anesthesia, if patient is apprehensive peribulbar anesthesia should may be employed. Conjunctiva should be irrigated with povidone iodine before removal of FB is attempted. This protocol, should be strictly followed.

FB can be removed with a FB spud or with 20G needle. In case of multiple corneal FBs, a good irrigation of the ocular surface should first be done and removal should be attempted after that.

Corneal rust ring and infiltration should be scrapped thoroughly. Surface irrigation should be done with povidone iodine solution after removal of FB.

Patient should be advised frequent instillation of broad spectrum antibiotic drops and lubricants (artificial tear drops). Patient should be followed up within 24 hours. Patching of eye is required only with impacted FB.

Deep Intracorneal FB

It should be removed under peribulbar anesthesia and the same protocol should be followed as removal of superficial FB. Procedure should be carried out under operating microscope. Two needle technique should be used in deep FB to the avoid accidental displacement of FB in to AC. One needle should fix the FB and the other needle should displace the FB anteriorly.

Scrapped material should be submitted for microbiological investigation. This is mandatory in case patient presenting late. The patient with deep infiltration, AC reaction and nonhealing localized infective keratitis, should be suspected with intra-corneal FB, detailed investigation is warranted in such circumstances.

CORNEAL ABRASION

A breach in the corneal epithelial layer with intact Bowman's layer due to trauma is abrasion. Corneal abrasion could result from superficial corneal injury due to mechanical, chemical, toxic, radiational injuries. Epithelium mostly heals very fast without any problem. It is also commonly seen in contact lens wearer. Healing is delayed in diabetes mellitus, immunocompromised person, poor nutritional status, keratoconjunctivitis sicca, neuroparalytic, exposure keratopathy and primary basement membrane disorders. De-epithelialized area of cornea provides port of entry to microbial organisms resulting in infective keratitis in 60–65% cases of corneal abrasion. De-epithelialized cornea also provide instatility to tear film (Fig. 6.1.1.2).

Symptoms and Signs

Symptoms and signs of corneal abrasion depends on area of involvement and nature of causative agents, e.g. symptoms are severe in abrasion caused by chemical, toxic agents. Acute pain, red eye photophobia, FB sensation, profuse watering, distorted or hazy visual acuity are symptoms of abrasion.

Conjunctival congestion mostly circumciliary congestion, swollen eyelids, eptithelial surface defect could be detected along with altered corneal reflex and shine. Fluorescein staining demonstrates surface irregularity and demarcates area of involvement. Swelling of corneal stroma and few Descemet's membrane folds can be seen with large epithelial defect.

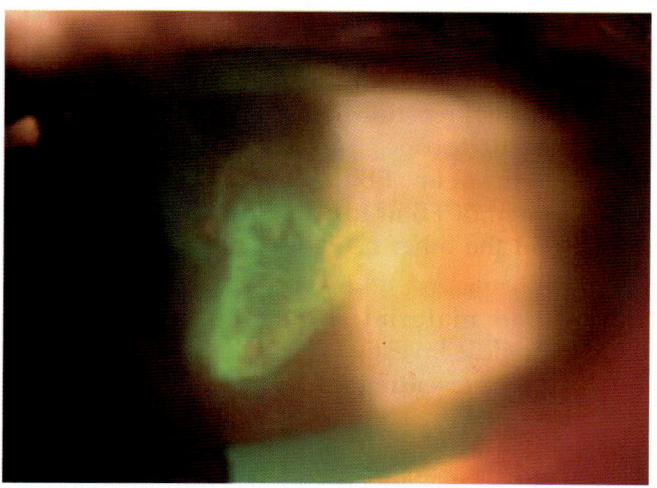

Fig. 6.1.1.2: Corneal abrasion

Corneal abrasion with low IOP can be seen in blunt trauma. Lid should be everted to look for any FB or displaced contact lens in contact lens wearer. Corneal abrasion with infiltration should be taken seriously and should follow protocol of management of infective keratitis.

Differential diagnosis of traumatic corneal abrasion.

a. Recurrent corneal erosion syndrome

b. Superficial herpetic keratitis.

Treatment

Cleaning of lid and thorough irrigation of ocular surface with sterile fluids and povidone lidine lotion should be used as antiseptic agent to sterilize cornea and conjunctiva.

Broad spectrum antibiotic drops and lubricating agent, e.g. tear substitutes with high viscocity, advised to instille frequently.

Patching of the eye practiced earlier days, not done presently unless patient having severe symptoms due to large abrasion. Bandage contact lens[10] or tape tarsorrhaphy is better choice. It helps frequent medication and examination. Ophthalmic ointments give comfort but may delay corneal epithelial healing. Steroid preparation are debrided to facilitate epithelial healing. The patient must be seen within 12–24 hours. and there after regularly till complete healing. Contact lens wearers should be instructed not to use contact lens till complete healing of epithelium occurs.

BLUNT TRAUMA CORNEA

The effect of blunt trauma on globe is variable from minor condition like corneal abrasion to destructive condition like rupture globe, orbital fracture. Magnitude of damage depends on the severity of force at the point of impact on the anterior part of the globe. Common causes of blunt trauma.

1. *Birth trauma:* Obstetrics forceps results in corneal edema, Descemet's tear, corneal abrasion (Fig. 6.1.1.3).

2. *Domestic:* Violence or accidental injury with fist of hand, elbow, etc. Color/water filled balloons during holi festivals cause damage to cornea (Fig. 6.1.1.4).

3. *Sports-related injury:* Golf ball, tennis ball, cricket ball, *Gulli-danda* injury and sports where physical/body contacts like boxing, wrestling cause blunt injury (Fig. 6.1.1.5).

4. *Industrial trauma* (Fig. 6.1.1.6).

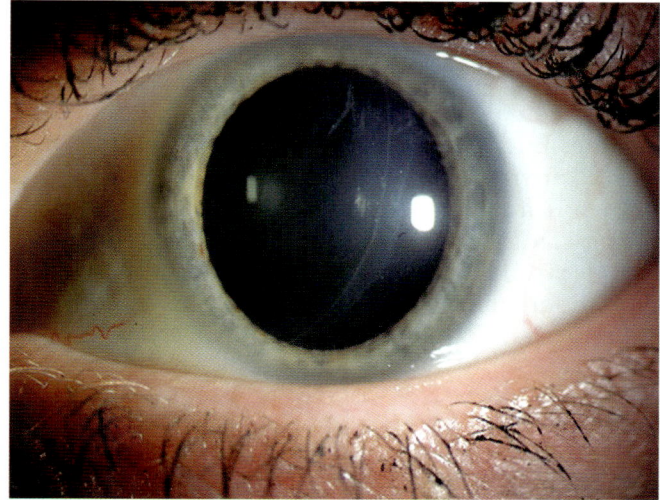

Fig. 6.1.1.3: Forceps birth trauma

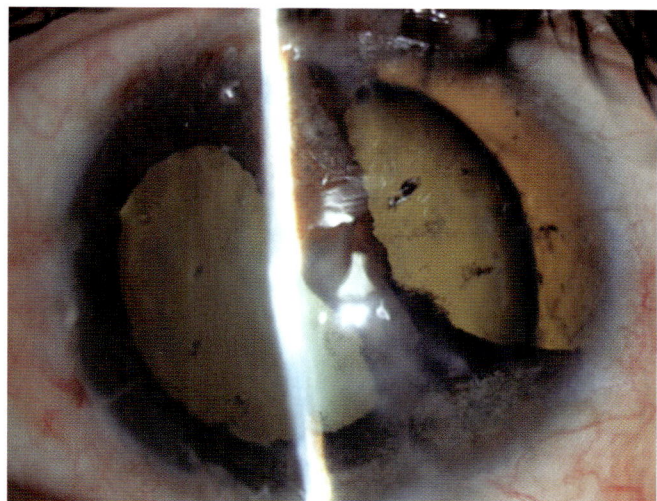

Fig. 6.1.1.5: Blunt trauma

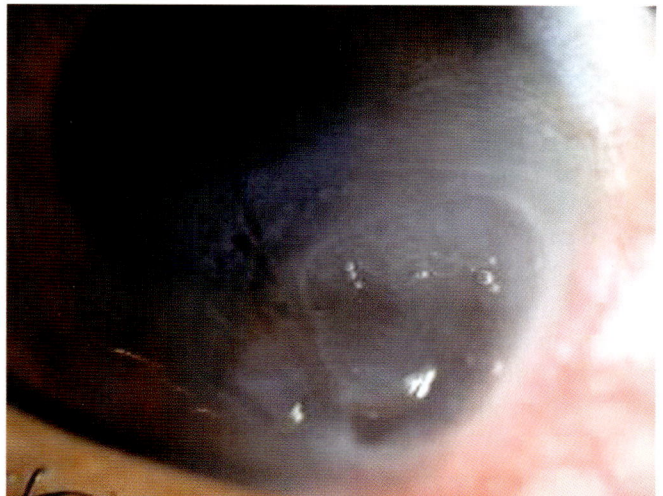

Fig. 6.1.1.4: Corneal burn-*agarbatti*

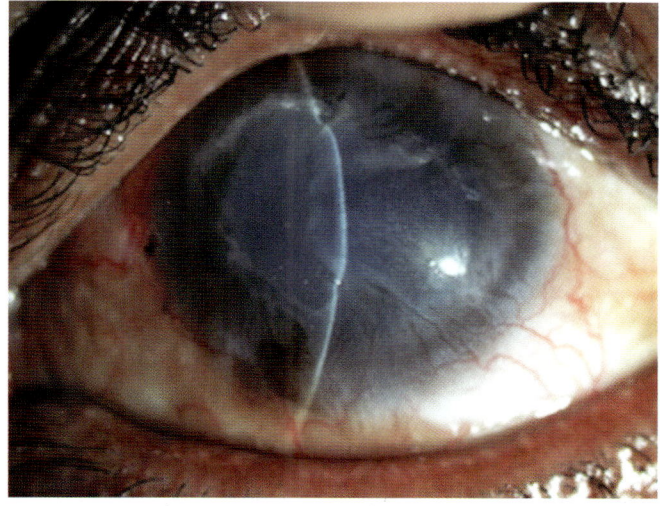

Fig. 6.1.1.6: Limbal cell loss chemical injury

Mechanism of Trauma

Partial (lamellar) or complete (total penetrating). laceration of cornea is mostly due to direct mechanical injury with any object. Damage to corneal cells can take place either due to direct contact (epithelial cell damage) or indirectly due to compression effect of eyeball (endothelial cell damage) or due to sudden rise in IOP. Endothelial cell layer and Descemet's layer may also be damaged due to hyphema or contact with intraocular tissues. Sudden anteroposterior compression with simultaneous expansion of equatorial region may result in damage to intraocular tissues, may even rupture of the globe at its weakest part. The primary impact of trauma is absorbed by cornea/corneosclera/iris lens diaphragm but secondary damage may take place at distant tissues in posterior pole.[9]

Clinical Manifestation of Blunt Trauma on Cornea

a. *Corneal abrasion:* Diagnosis and management same as other corneal abrasion.

b. *Acute corneal edema:* Traumatic decompensation of corneal endothelial cells with or without Descemet's membrane damage/rupture can cause edema. Specular microscopy should be done to know extent of endothelial cell damage. Status of Descemet's membrane can be detected with anterior segment OCT or UBM. Acute corneal edema could also be seen due to acute rise in IOP or in sever hyphema.

c. *Rupture of Descemet's membrane:* Conservative treatment should be done first if localized tear of Descemet's membrane occurs (Figs 6.1.1.7a and b). Air or injection of expensile gases (SF$_6$, C$_3$F$_8$) in AC may be helpful. Extensive damage may require corneal graft Descemet's stripping endothelial keratoplasty (DSEK) in future. Associated complication should be managed.

d. *Blood staining of cornea:* Blood staining of cornea can develop with or without raised IOP. Incidence reported is (2–11%).[11] Blood staining can also take place following hemorrhage from pre-existing deep intrastromal blood vessels. It appears as reddish-brown deep corneal opacity. With passage of time color changes. Recovery may take long time. Initial phase control of inflammation and IOP, are must. If irreversible damage has occurred then it may need corneal graft.

e. *Lamellar laceration cornea.*

f. *Rupture of cornea* may be seen associated with or without limbal or scleral rupture. This may also be associated with damage to intraocular tissues.

LACERATED INJURY

Lacerated injury of cornea is three times more common in males than in females. It is also common amongst younger age group. Corneal lacerations could either be partial or full thickness, and are potentially dangerous. It may lead to complete loss of vision and complication like sympathetic ophthalmia. Prompt diagnosis and meticulous management may save the eye visually and if not then at least cosmetically. Extent of damage caused depends on the size, sharpness of object and the speed at the time of impact to the cornea (Fig. 6.1.1.8).

Mode of Injury

Corneal lacerations are most commonly caused by direct trauma to cornea. In domestic setup, corneal laceration caused with sharp-pointed object, e.g. knife, needles, finger nails, screw driver, pen, pencils, bow and arrow, glass pieces, etc. Lacerated injuries in industries are mostly due to workers handling

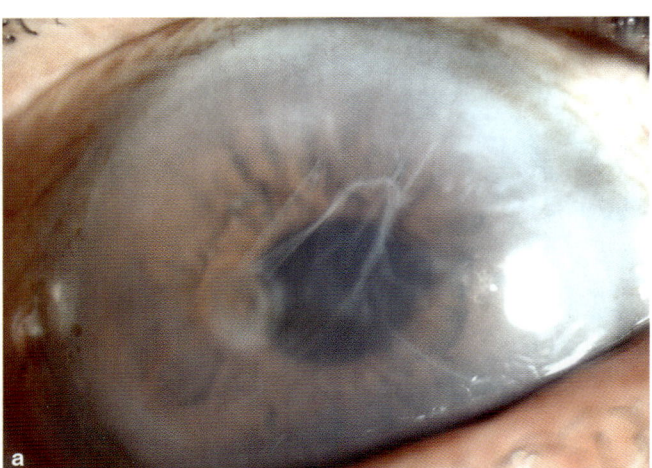

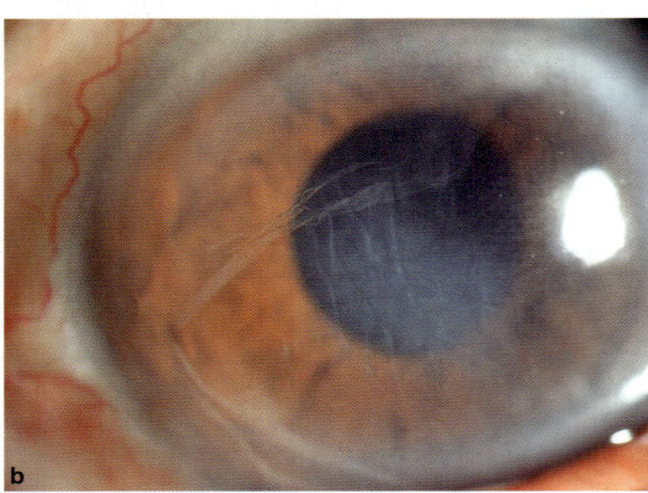

Figs 6.1.1.7a and b: DM detachment

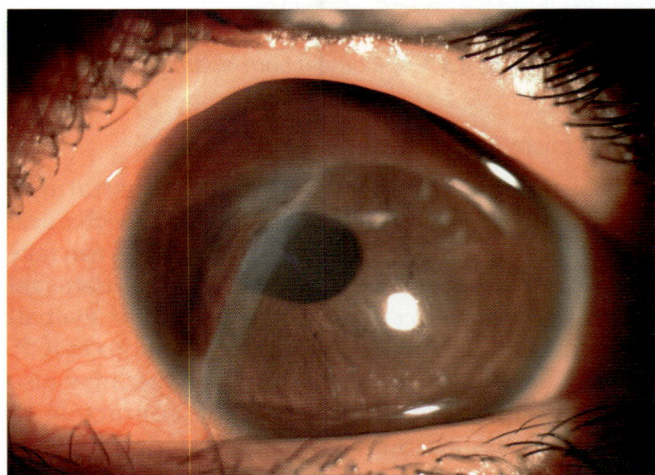

Fig. 6.1.1.8: Corneal laceration

machineries carelessly without using protective devices. Flying objects from machines lathe or from chisel hammer causes lacerated corneal injury. Gunshot, land mine blast injuries are common in war or terrorist attack. Lacerated injuries of cornea are also seen in automobile accidents and amongst agriculture workers.

Types of Corneal Laceration

Laceration of cornea could only be corneal or associated with limbal or scleral injuries. Corneal lacerations are commonly seen as:
- Partial thickness lamellar
- Full thickness
- Corneal tissue loss
- Complicated with prolapse of intraocular tissues
- Laceration with impacted FB.

Partial and full thickness corneal laceration could also be:
- Linear—regular or irregular
- Stellate shaped
- Zig-zag
- Corneal tissue loss.

All these lacerations could be either single or multiple.

Complications

a. *Infection:* Most dreaded complication.
   i. *Infective keratitis:* Mild superficial to sloughing corneal ulcer can develop depending on type of microbial agent. Most commonly seen in agricultural injury and road traffic accidents.
   ii. *Intraocular infections:* Easy penetration of microbial organism through open tract may lead to endophthalmitis, if not controlled lead to panophthalmitis and orbital cellulitis.
b. *Loss of AC:* Shallow or absent AC or persistent leakage of aqueous humor leads to peripheral anterior synechia and later may develop glaucoma. Persistent low IOP may lead to ciliary shock, choroidal effusion, choroidal detachment and macular edema.
c. *Lenticular change:* Lenticular changes are produced due to direct trauma along with corneal injury resulting localized opacity or rupture of anterior capsule and total cataracts. Lenticular changes can also develop following shallow AC, iris prolapse, etc. Subluxation or dislocation of traumatized lens are also seen.

d. Damage to intraocular tissues are variable from iris lens diaphragm to retinal detachment, anything can happen.

Management of Corneal Laceration

Management depends on type and magnitude of corneal laceration.

It may appear simple but may turn out to be complicated.
   i. Primary or secondary repair
   ii. Type and extent of damage
   iii. Complicated or uncomplicated.
      After noting down all relevant points trauma, detail examination should be carried out without wasting any time. Forcible retraction of eyelid must not be done as it may produce direct or indirect pressure on open globe and lead to expulsion of intraocular tissues. If the patient is apprehensive better to examine under local anesthesia as topical drops or with injection. Children must always be examined under anesthesia.
      - Visual acuity in both eyes should be noted at first instant it possible.
      - Examination of lids, conjunctiva with diffuse light.
      - Slit lamp examination of cornea in detail.
      First with diffuse illumination and then with optical slit examination.
      - Look for any FB.
      - Location zone of cornea extent and type of laceration.
      - Depth of laceration—better visualized with fine optical slit.
      - Damage prolapse of intraocular contents.
      - State of AC, pupil, iris, lens, etc.
   iv. IOP noted with almost care, digital or non-contact tonometry.
   v. Posterior-segment examination—if condition permits.
   vi. Seidel's test should be carried out in case of doubt about partial or full thickness corneal. Laceration, particularly when wound appears to be epithelized.
   vii. In all open globe injuries material should be taken for smear and culture sensitive (microbiology) test, this will help in postoperative management.
   viii. Other investigations should be carried out as situation demands.

Management strategy should be planned depending on magnitude of corneal laceration and or associated with other concomitant ocular damage. Surgeon should be prepared in every respect to face any eventualities during surgery.

Combined management by both anterior and posterior segment surgeons gives better result. Corneal laceration should be managed by an experienced surgeon to minimize complication and better results. If proper facilities and experienced surgeons not available, it is better to refer the case after giving first aid treatment. For example, a badly sutured corneal laceration may result in more damage to cornea than the primary trauma, e.g. gross astigmatism, thick bad corneal opacity, shallow AC and its subsequent complications.

Partial Thickness

Lamellar laceration: Management must be carried out under strict aseptic condition and under magnification.

- *Very small sized, superficial, regular linear wound:* Rule out any FB first, then clean the edges of the wound by good irrigation with sterile solution and wash with povidone iodine lotion. Patch the eye for 24 hours after application of broad spectrum antibiotic drops. Usually, heals without suture, bandage contact lens (BCL)[12] may be applied if the wound superficial but irregular or shelving. Advantage with BCL, allows frequent medication. BCL also has splinting effect to hold the wound against the movement of eyelids and thereby helps in faster healing. Along with application of broad spectrum antibiotic drops, short-acting cyclo-pelegic drops can be applied to prevent ciliary spasm, thus gives comfort to the patient. The patient should be examined frequently.
- Medium to large sized, irregular, half or more than half thickness, or stellate lacerated wound of cornea—need suturing.

Full Thickness Corneal Laceration

Management depends on the size of wound complicated or uncomplicated wound.

- Size of wound less than 3 mm, regular, shelved or flap like, edematous edges, simple toileting of wound, broad spectrum antibiotic drops and BCL may lead to healing of wound in 2–4 weeks time.

Edematous edges seals the wound water light supported by BCL. Suturing of such wound may result in more scarring and astigmatism. But, frequent observation is mandatory to look for wound leak and status of AC.

- Size of wound less them 3 mm, irregular but gapping of edges or tissue loss, AC shallow or flat. In such situation, cyanoacrylate tissue glue[13,14] should be applied along with BCL if inspite of application of glue and BCL. The AC does not remain stable or healing does not take place, suturing should be done. Advantage of application of glue is minimal anatomical and optical disturbance, especially if the wound is in or near the optical zone (central 5 mm). In children, application of glue and BCL may not be advisable as glue may get dislodged due to accidental rubbing of eye, under such circumstances it is safe of apply sutures.
- Size of laceration more than 3 mm ragged, regular or irregular, with or without tissue loss: suturing must be done as quickly as possible to prevent edema of edges of wound.

BASIC REQUIREMENT IN CORNEAL SUTURING
(Figs 6.1.1.9a to c)

- Absolute strict aseptic condition.
- Local/peribulbar block/general anesthesia (GA) as per case
- Under operating microscope
- Good surgical instruments atraumatic corneal forceps and 10-0 nylon suture with atraumatic needle
- Water tight closure of wound
- Good anatomical apposition particularly posterior layers of cornea
- Try to achieve asphericity, as possible minimal or no astigmatism
- Prevent uveal, lenticular or vitreous adhesion/incarceration to wound. It can be achieved with watertight closure and formation of AC with viscoelastics although during suturing.
- Eyeball should be stabilized with rectus sutures or application of Fleiringer rings, particularly in soft or collapsed globe.
- AC injections and manipulation should be done through the side port rather than corneal wound.
- Sutures should not be too-tight or loose, try to maintain anterior curvature of cornea. Intraopera-

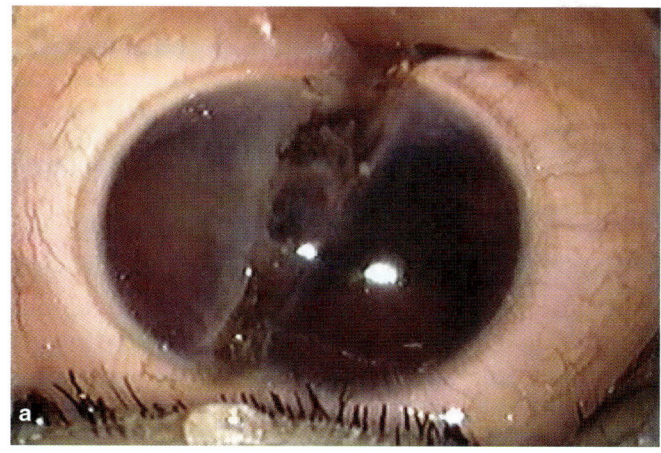

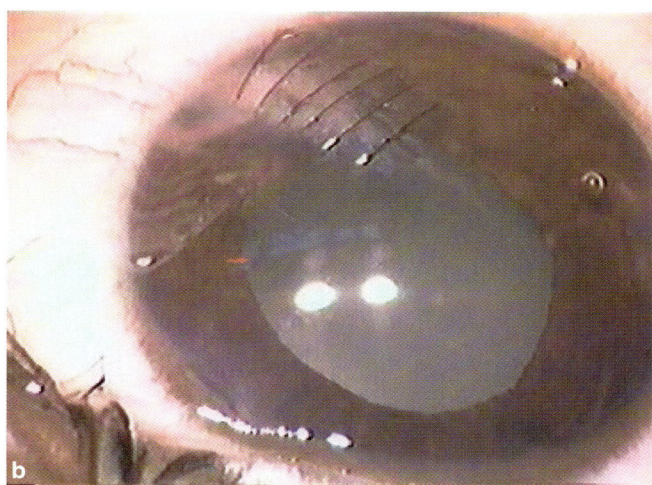

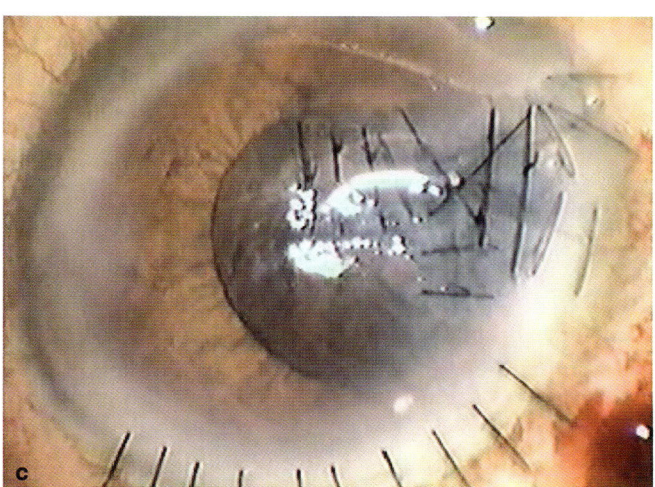

Figs 6.1.1.9a to c: Injury repair

tive keratoscope may be helpful. Depth of suture should be up to 90% in full thickness wounds.

- Limbal extension of corneal wound first apposition of limbus should be made, this will help further suturing rest of corneal wound.
- Any other associated injury like iris, lens, vitreous, etc. should taken care during corneal suturing.
- Iris prolapse should be thoroughly irrigated and then reposited. In vitreous prolapse, proper anterior vitrectomy with vitreotome or cutter should done rather than repeated cutting of vitreous with cellulose sponge.
- Wound edges should be held with atraumatic corneal forces, without any crushing effect of edges.
- Utmost care should be taken not to damage corneal endothelium, the most vital layer of cornea.

SUTURING TECHNIQUE

Corneal suturing can either be primary suture or secondary suture. Primary suture properly, applied gives better results. Sutures can be direct suture or indirect sutures continuous or interrupted. Suturing technique should follow keratorefractive principles.[15]

- Depth of sutures should be 90% of stroma. Through and through sutures can creat passage for microbial organism to AC.
- Equal and symmetrical sutures on either side of wound gives good apposition, unequal asymmetrical sutures causes over riding of edges.
- Corneal sutures should be 1.5–2.5 long depending on zone of corneal involvement. In peripheral zone, it should be longer and as we approach toward central optical zone it should be shorter.
- Attempt should be made to place all sutures equidistant from one and another.
- Anteriorly placed shallow sutures or tight sutures creates internal gaping (posterior layers), may lead to corneal edema, nonhealing and scarring.
- All suture knots should be cut small and buried away from visual axis. Exposed suture knots forms nidus for microorganisms, thick scar corneal neovascularization, top of that major discomfort to the patient.
- In irregular malaligned corneal laceration it is better to apply few temporary sutures first, then form AC. with viscoelastics and replace those temporary sutures with accurate regular sutures.

- Sutures in the visual axis should be avoided if possible or apply minimum number of shallow sutures, or some time apply indirect suture.
- Long deep slightly tight peripheral sutures and short shallow central sutures helps in maintaining normal corneal curvature and reduce astigmatism.

STELLATE LACERATIONS

Requires special approach.

- Indentify each portion of loose stellate corneal tissue, try to place them in normal place and see apposition. Pass few temporary sutures and form AC with viscoelastic substance through side port. Final suturing should be done according to each laceration.
- Linear cuts should be sutured first as described and then start suturing each tags individually, may require to place a few indirect suture to give support. Grossly lacerated wound with tissue loss may require purse string suture. BCL may be applied after suturing.
- Tectonic lamellar or penetrating grafts are indicated to replace disorganized mutilated corneal tissue or loss of tissue where suturing is not possible. Optical grafts are indicated in case of unsuccessful primary repair or failed teetonic grafts.

SUTURE REMOVAL

White the corneal healing is slow it may take 3–6 months for good sear through children may take letter less trail. There should be no hurry to remove stitches.

Following guidelines should be followed for suture removal:

a. Adequately healed corneal wound
b. Loose sutures
c. Exposed sutures causing symptom or collection of infiltrations around suture
d. Development of neovessels
e. Sign of suture infection
f. Gross astigmatism assessed by corneal topography
g. Children early suture removal.

Faulty placed sutures or sutures producing reaction should be removed early and should be replaced with a proper secondary suture.

There are many types of radiation energy that can cause damage to cornea. Cornea is rich in epithelial and endothelial cells (2,600–3,5000 cells per sq. mm) densely populated as compared to any other tissue in human body. Radiational energy mostly damage these vital cellular layers either directly or indirectly. Damage to these cells can also take place following direct effect of radiation on limbal cells and perilimbal capillaries.

Ionizing radiation of electromagnetic spectrum those cause damage to cornea are: ultraviolet (UV) light, infrared light, mircowaves, X–ray's, gamma rays, lasers, radio/television/rador signals and heat.[16]

Damage to cornea takes place by photocoagulation, photodisruption, and photochemical reaction. Photocoagulation causes cell destruction when the intraepithelial cell temperature is increased by 10°C or more. Photodisruption of cells are due to mechanical effect. Photochemical reaction to cornea is caused by radiation of short wavelength light and the tissue changes takes place due to chemical or enzymetic reaction. Radiation injury also causes impairment of DNA synthesis. Damage to corneal tissue depends on:

- Intensity of exposure
- Duration of exposure
- Type of radiation.

RADIATIONAL CORNEAL INJURY

Injury by physical agents are discussed in subsequent pages Ch 6.1.3.

REFERENCES

1. WHO–Collaboration with National Programme for Control of Blindess (NPCB) India "Symposium on Corneal injury and their management" 2004.
2. Indian Council of Medical Research (ICMR) – National blindness survey (1976–1979).
3. National Programme for Control of Blindness (NPCB) India 'Blindness Survey'. Ministry of Health and Family welfare. Govt. of India. (1986–1989), (1999) and (2004).
4. Shukla B, Nataranjan S. Book on 'Management of Oular Trauma', 1st edn 2005.
5. Shukla B. Epidemiology of Ocular Trauma, 1st edn 2002.
6. Srinivasan M, et al. Epidemiology and actioligical diagnosis of corneal ulcer in South India. Brit J Ophthal. 1997;81:965–971.
7. WHO Collaborative Study (2006–2007). Standard treatment guidelines, management of Corneal injury and infections.

8. Mohan M, Mukherjee G, Angra SK. Documentation of Corneal disorders. Indian J Ophthal. 1980;28:2.

9. Kirk Patrich, et al. No eye pad for corneal aberation, 1993; 7:468.

10. Broderick JD. Brit J Ophithal 1972;601;56:589.

11. Read J. Traumatic hypema: Surgical vs Meidcal management. Ann Ophthal 1975;7:659.

12. Leibowitz HM. Arch Ophthal 1972;88:602.

13. Hydiuk RA, Hall DS, Kinyoum JL. Ophthal Surgery 1974;5:50.

14. Weiss JL, William PJ, Lindstrom RL, Doughman DJ. Ophthalmology 1983;90:610.

15. Rowsey JJ, Itayer JC. Ophthalmic Surgery 1984;15:596.

16. Leibowitz HM, Waring George O. Book on "Corneal Disorders clinical diagnosis and management 1984.

6.1.2 Trauma to Crystalline Lens

• Jagat Ram • Neelam Verma

INTRODUCTION

Cataract formation is commonly observed as a result of direct injury to the crystalline lens by foreign object or due to blunt trauma to the globe.[1] Infrared energy (glass-blower's cataract), electric shock, and ionizing radiation are other rare causes of traumatic cataracts.[2,3] Lens dislocation and subluxation are found commonly in conjunction with traumatic cataract.[2,3] Other associated complications include glaucoma (phacolytic, phacomorphic, pupillary block, and angle-recession glaucoma) phacoanaphylactic uveitis; retinal detachment; choroidal rupture; hyphema; retrobulbar hemorrhage; traumatic optic neuropathy and globe rupture.[2] Traumatic cataract can present many medical and surgical challenges to the ophthalmologist. Careful examination and a management plan can simplify these difficult cases and provide the best possible outcome. In most cases, traumatic cataract interferes with the visual axis and needs removal.[4]

Trauma is the leading cause of monocular blindness in people younger than 45 years. Male to female ratio in cases of ocular trauma is 4:1. Childhood trauma of the eye and its adenexa represents approximately 4–20% of all eye injuries.[5] Incidence of traumatic cataract in children is reported as high as 29% of all childhood cataracts.[6] Majority of children suffer unilateral eye injury and boys are more often affected (over two-thirds) than girls.[7]

PATHOPHYSIOLOGY

Traumatic Cataract

Blunt trauma (Fig. 6.1.2.1) is responsible for coup and countercoup ocular injury. Coup and countercoup forces on the lens could cause rapid anterior-posterior shortening, leading to abrasion or rupture of the lens capsule with subsequent cataractogenesis. Direct anterior-posterior force also produces equatorial expansion of the lens, which can result in equatorial capsular rupture and zonular dehiscence. Equatorial capsular rupture can further stimulate cataract formation, although zonular dehiscence can lead to lens subluxation or complete dislocation, depending on the extent of zonular incompetence.[8,9] Blunt ocular

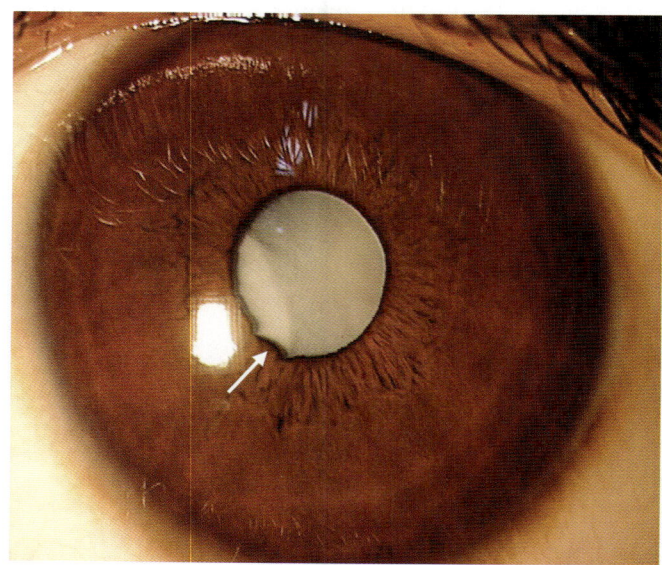

Fig. 6.1.2.1: Blunt trauma with a plastic object resulting in total lens opacification of crystalline lens. Note the sphincter tear (arrow)

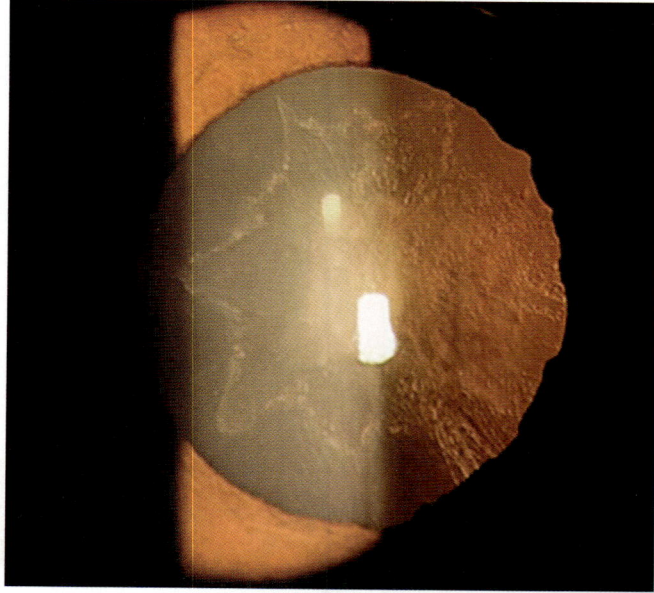

Fig. 6.1.2.2: Rosette cataract in an 8-year-old child with blunt trauma right eye

trauma typically leads to a stellate or rosette-shaped opacification (Fig. 6.1.2.2) that is axial in location that may remain stable or may progress.[10] In perforating trauma, direct contact of the lens capsule by the penetrating object leads to cortical opacification at the site of injury. If the capsular tear is large enough, the entire lens can rapidly opacify, (Figs 6.1.2.3 and 6.1.2.4) but a cataract caused by a small perforation may become sealed off and remain localized.[11]

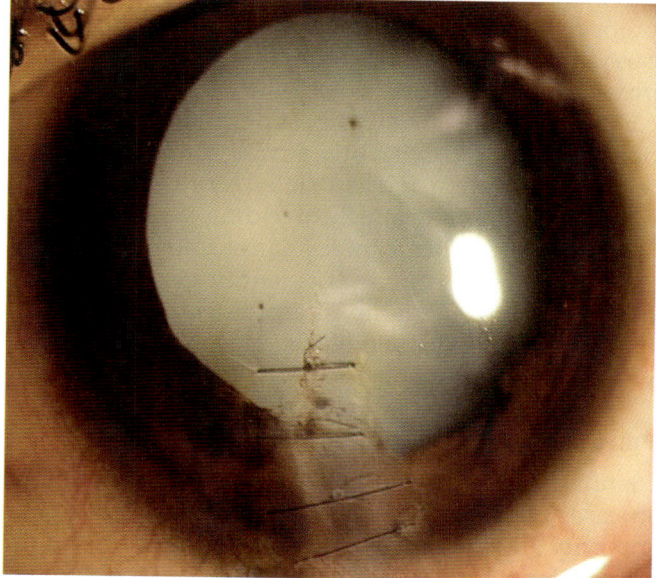

Fig. 6.1.2.3: Traumatic cataract in a 10-year-old boy with bow and arrow. Note the sutured corneal laceration sparing the central visual axis

The lenticular opacities following concussion comprises of:[12]

1. *Vossius's ring opacity:* The ring is typically about 1 mm in breadth and corresponds to the imprint of the pupillary border of the iris upon the capsule.

2. Localized opacities due to subcapsular changes; these opacities may be discrete, punctate and scattered (disseminated subepithelial opacities), film-like in distribution (cobweb opacities) or sufficiently numerous to develop into a zonular (lamellar) cataract. On the other hand, a diffuse subepithelial edema may give rise to a rosette-shaped opacity.

3. Diffuse cataractous changes (Fig. 6.1.2.5) may result, usually associated with a capsular tear and these may lead to total absorption of the lens in the young and its ultimate degeneration in the aged.

Two types of rosette-shaped opacities are generally recognized—those occurring very shortly after the injury and those appearing after sometime (late rosette).

I. Early Rosette Cataract

May appear in anterior or posterior subcapsular region and sometimes in both simultaneously. After concussion injury anterior opacities are more common; after a perforating injury the posterior rosette is perhaps more frequently seen. These may

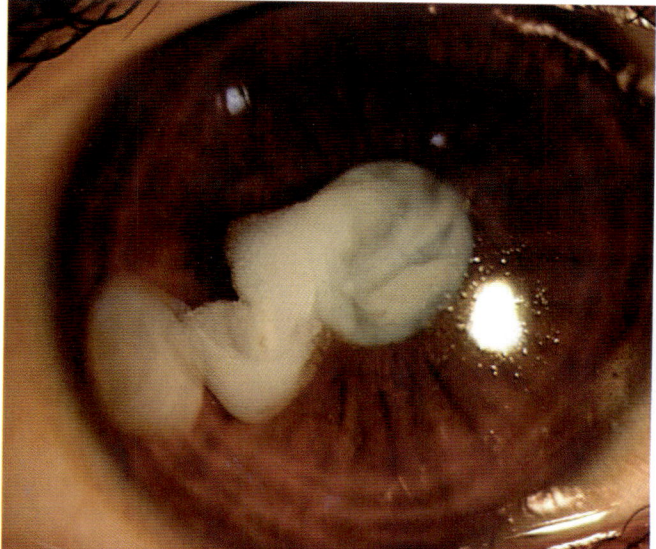

Fig. 6.1.2.4: Ruptured anterior capsule with flocculent lens matter in AC

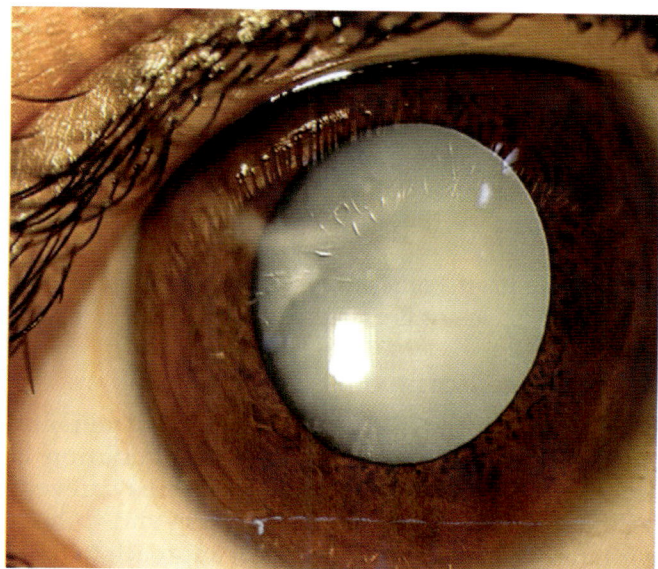

Fig. 6.1.2.5: Diffuse traumatic cataract following blunt trauma with a wooden object in a 10-year-old girl

be evident within few hours after injury or their appearance may be delayed for some weeks or months. The appearance of early rosette cataract is of feathery parallel rays running outward from the dark suture-lines. In this way a rosette-shaped figure is formed, determined by the arrangement of the sutures branching out from the axial region toward the equator.[12]

II. Late Rosette Cataract

Late rosette cataracts are seen some years after the trauma and are usually found lying deep in the cortex or in the adult nucleus, separated from the capsule by a clear zone of varying thickness. In such an opacity, the relationship of the sutures to the rays is the reverse of that found in the fresh cases, in this type the sutures run between the petals which are formed by the outcrop of rays from neighboring sutures.[12]

TRAUMATIC SUBLUXATION AND DISLOCATION OF LENS

Lens dislocation and subluxation are found commonly in conjunction with traumatic cataract. As a rule zonular tearing occurs most readily at its attachment to the lens; rupture at its ciliary insertion is rare. If subluxation is greater, the lens may slip from its axial position and its equatorial edge may appear as a crescent in the pupillary aperture, dividing it into a phakic and aphakic part (lateral subluxation). Such displacement may be combined with some rotator displacement so that the lens lies obliquely (axial subluxation); in both cases iridodonesis results and the AC becomes of unequal depth round its circumference. In complete traumatic luxation the lens may follow different routes into the AC, the vitreous, the interretinal space, the subscleral region, or outside the eye if the globe is ruptured so that it lies impacted in the rupture itself, comes to rest in the subconjunctival or Tenon's space or is extruded altogether.[12]

Preoperative Assessment

Before performing surgery to manage a traumatic cataract, a detailed preoperative examination is required to identify other pathology that may prevent optimal postoperative visual recovery and to help with the decision of which surgical approach to take. Open globe injuries and IOFBs must be ruled out before surgery.[13,14] A simple X-ray orbit helps to detect metallic retained intraocular or orbital FBs. Abnormal findings that predict a poor postoperative visual outcome include corneal disease, iridodialysis, a relative afferent pupillary defect, macular scarring, retinal detachment, and optic atrophy.[15] A B-scan USG is necessary if the posterior pole cannot be visualized. The physician should also examine patients for intraocular inflammation and increased IOP preoperatively and provide appropriate treatment. In carrying out a thorough lenticular examination, the physician should first determine the type (nuclear, cortical, subcapsular, etc.), location, and degree of lens opacification. Furthermore, a careful assessment for zonular disruption and associated lens subluxation or dislocation is important in deciding which surgical approach to take. Maximal pharmacologic pupillary dilation may be necessary to identify a subtle zonular dialysis. At the slit lamp, the physician should note the degree of zonular dialysis and phacodonesis, as well as the resting position of the lens.

Principles of Management

Planning surgical approach is of utmost importance in cases of traumatic cataract. Preoperative capsular integrity and zonular stability should be surmised. In cases of posterior dislocation without glaucoma, inflammation, or visual obstruction, surgery may be avoided. Indications for surgery include the following:

- Visually significant cataract
- Obstructed view of posterior pathology
- Lens-induced inflammation or glaucoma
- Capsular rupture with lens swelling
- Other trauma-induced ocular pathology necessitating surgery.

Standard phacoemulsification or phacoaspiration may be performed, continuous curvilinear capsulorhexis (CCC) is possible to complete in majority of eyes with traumatic cataract due to blunt trauma compared to those with sutured perforating (open globe) injury. If lens capsule is intact with sufficient zonular support, capsular bag fixation of posterior chamber IOL is achieved in majority and sulcus fixation in those where posterior capsule support is intact or adequate but capsular bag particularly anterior capsule cover is not adequate. Intracapsular cataract extraction is required in cases of anterior dislocation or extreme zonular instability. Anterior dislocation of the lens into the AC requires emergency surgery for its removal, as it can cause pupillary block glaucoma and also corneal decompensation. Pars plana lensectomy and vitrectomy may be best in cases of posterior capsular rupture, posterior dislocation, or extreme zonular instability.

Lens Implantation

Capsular fixation is the preferred placement if lens capsule and zonular support are intact (Figs 6.1.2.6 and 6.1.2.7).

- Polymethyl methacrylate (PMMA) capsular tension rings allow capsular fixation in cases of zonular dialysis less than 150°.[16]
- For more significant or progressive zonular dialysis, the Cionni-modified CTR (Morcher type) has been demonstrated to be a useful alternative to the conventional CTR. It can be sutured safely to the sclera without compromising the capsular bag, thus allowing the CTR and capsule to be held in place even in the presence of significant zonular incompetence.[17,18] Sulcus fixation is safe if posterior capsule is compromised but zonular support is maintained.
- Suture fixation is chosen if both capsular and zonular supports are insufficient and the angle is damaged minimally.
- Anterior chamber placement is an option in selective cases if no posterior support remains and iris or ciliary body trauma prevents suture fixation. However, AC intraocular lens (ACIOL) fixation it is best avoided in children.

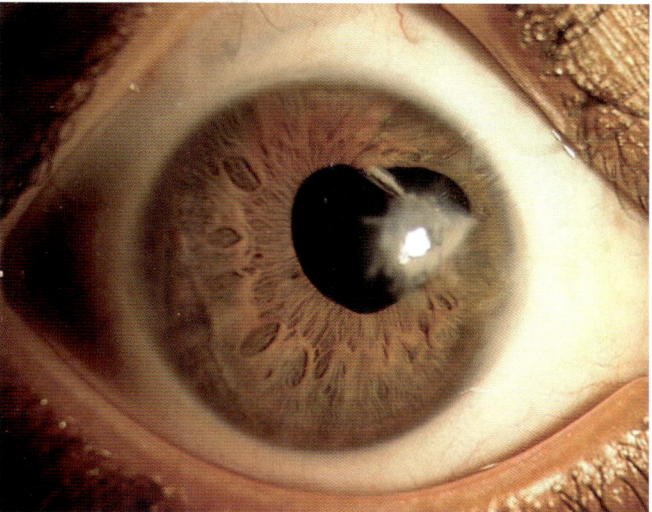

Fig. 6.1.2.7: Seven months postphacoaspiration with intracapsular square edge PMMA-IOL implantation. Note the corneal opacity sparing the visual axis. This child achieved a best-corrected visal acuity (BCVA) of 6/9

Timing of Surgery

All patients with penetrating eye injury need prompt primary repair (Figs 6.1.2.8 and 6.1.2.9). Cataract surgery is less often indicated at the time of primary intervention. The only situations for early/primary cataract removal are loose lens matter in the AC with uncontrollable inflammation and IOP control or corneal touch with decompensatory changes either

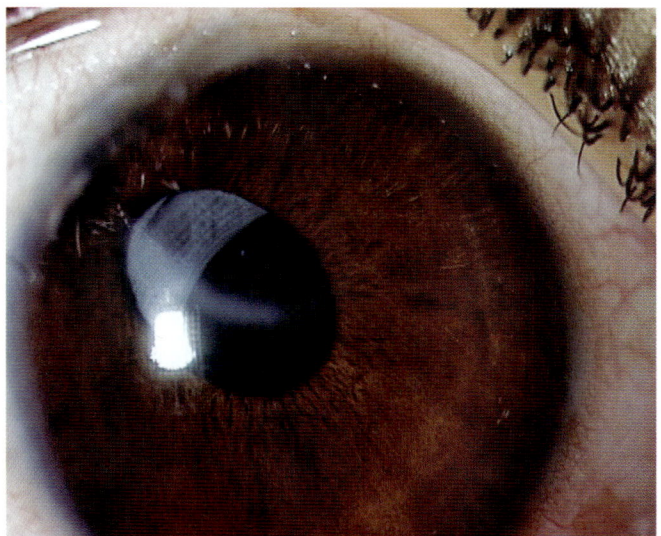

Fig. 6.1.2.6: Same eye as in Fig. 6.1.2.5 status 6 months post- cataract surgery and in the bag implantation of IOL

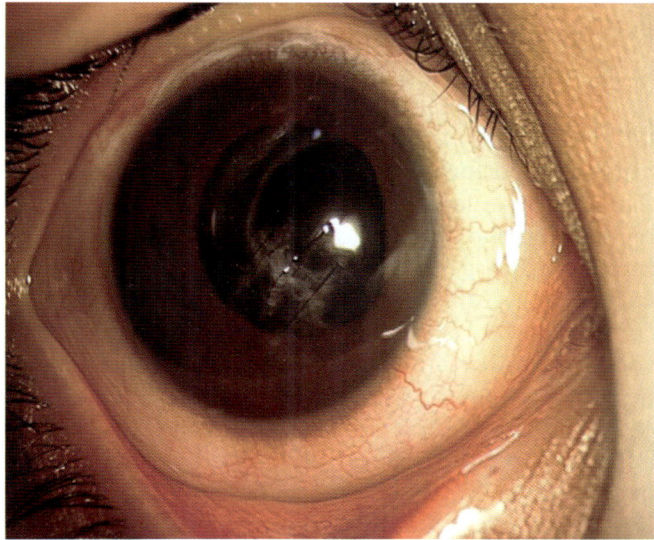

Fig. 6.1.2.8: Pseudophakia for traumatic cataract. Note the eccentric anterior capsulorhexis and repaired corneal laceration

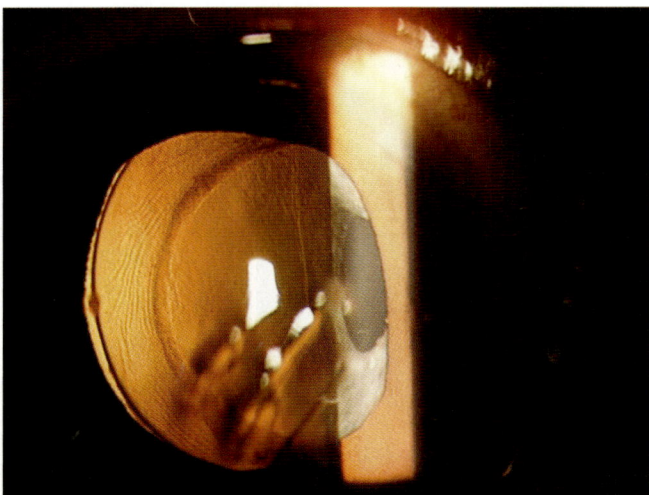

Fig. 6.1.2.9: Retroillumination photograph of the same figure as above showing in the bag implanted PMMA-IOL and a small defect of the posterior capsule

with lens matter or corneal touch by a subluxated lens. Except for the above mentioned circumstances, cataract surgery should be undertaken 3–6 weeks after trauma or primary repair to give adequate time for control of inflammation prior to cataract surgery.

Intraocular lens (IOL) power calculation is as for routine cases in adult patients but for the growing pediatric eye, poses several problems. The accumulating evidence on the myopic shift that occurs in pseudophakic children[19-21] have led to an almost unanimous agreement that the IOL power should aim for a certain amount of hypermetropia or emmetropia at time of surgery.

Surgical Steps

Surgery is performed under GA in pediatric patients. Anterior capsulorhexis formation is greatly facilitated by staining the anterior capsule with trypan blue or indocyanine green dye especially in traumatic cataracts where the red fundal glow is usually compromised. Use of superior viscoelastic agents like sodium hyaluronate (Healon GV or Provisc) are helpful in achieving CCC (Figs 6.1.2.8 and 6.1.2.9). The desirable size of CCC should be between 5.0 mm and 5.5 mm. In younger children posterior capsule opacification (PCO) is almost inevitable if posterior capsule management is not performed at the time of primary surgery. We have observed that anterior as well as posterior capsular thickening in several eyes

with traumatic cataract due to penetrating eye injury or blunt trauma and primary posterior capsulotomy is indicated in such cases for thickened posterior capsule. The PCO is amblyogenic and the purpose of surgery is defeated if long-term clear visual axis is not achieved. We perform primary posterior CCC (Figs 6.1.2.10 and 6.1.2.11) in children less than 8 years of age undergoing cataract surgery or in eyes with thickened posterior capsule. Technically, a posterior capsulotomy can be achieved in several ways. Primary posterior capsulorhexis (PCCC) makes a primary capsulotomy safe because of the smooth margin created at the opening resist peripheral extension of tears. Manual PCCC with the help of cystotome and forceps is preferable over other methods. Vitrector-assisted posterior capsulotomy is also done in selected situation. Use of high viscosity viscoelastic such as healon-GV → or viscoat → helps to achieve PCCC. The desirable size of posterior rhexis is 3–3.5 mm. Most of the surgeons prefer to perform primary PCCC and anterior vitrectomy to decrease the incidence of PCO. Anterior vitreous acts as a scaffold and helps in lens epithelial cell (LEC) migration and proliferation. The vitrectomy may be performed using limbal or pars plana route. In children, the aim is to remove only

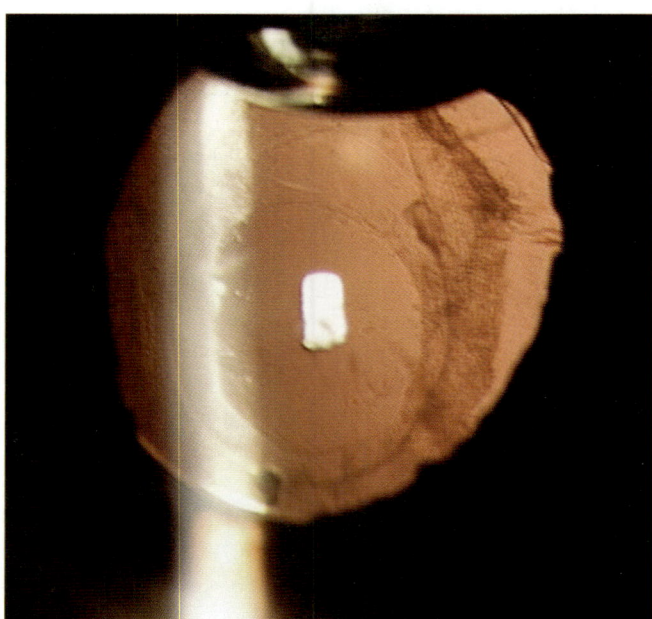

Fig. 6.1.2.10: First postoperative day photograph of an 8-year-old child with traumatic cataract. A square edge PMMA-IOL has been implanted in the capsular bag and a primary posterior capsulotomy with anterior vitrectomy has been performed

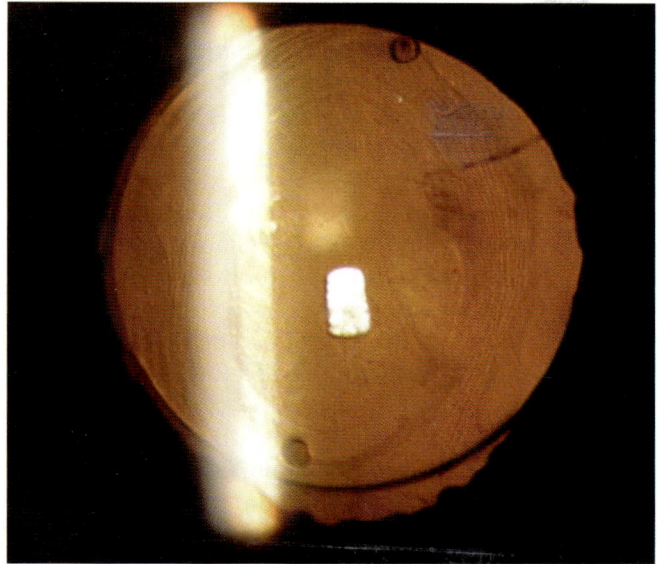

Fig. 6.1.2.11: Same eye as in Fig. 6.1.2.10 status 6 months after surgery

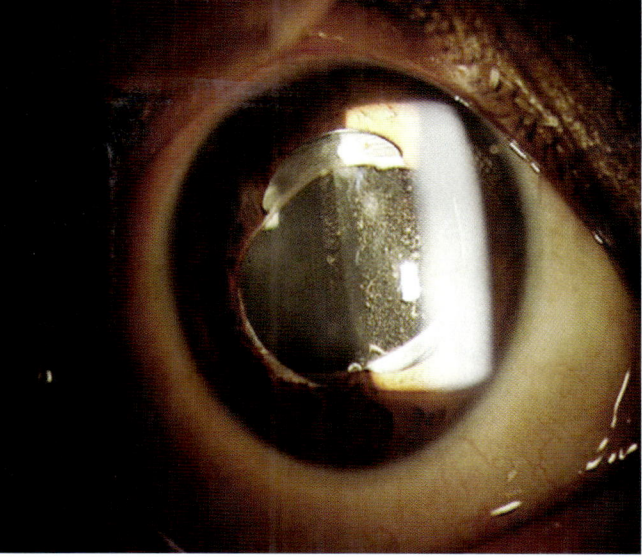

Fig. 6.1.2.12: In the bag implantation of square edge PMMA-IOL following blunt trauma with in a child of years with pigment deposits on the IOL surface

central anterior vitreous in the posterior capsulotomy opening it may be achieved using limbal route. Two ports vitrectomy is ideal. It is performed from the side ports incision on the clear cornea.

IOL Implantation

Capsular bag implantation of IOL (Fig. 6.1.2.12) is best choice to reduce the contact of IOL with uveal tissue and to achieve IOL centration. This may not be possible in cases where there is a dehiscence of the anterior capsule due to the injury and a CCC cannot be fashioned. In such cases, the IOL optic may be captured into the PCCC although the maneuver is technically very demanding and should be attempted only by the very experienced surgeon. Optic capture of IOL is equally effective in reducing PCO and achieving IOL centration.

Postoperative Care

Postoperatively, these eyes tend to show more tissue reaction. We use intensive topical steroids (as frequently as 8–10 times a day). The topical steroids are tapered over a period of 6 weeks. Topical antibiotics are instilled three times a day for 10–14 days. Cyclopentolate eye drops 1% or homatropine 2% three times or atropine eye ointment should be used for about 4 weeks to prevent posterior synechiae

formation in pediatric patients. The risk of postoperative complications is higher due to the greater inflammatory response and early detection and management of complications is must.

Amblyopia is one of the most important vision-threatening complications in children undergoing cataract surgery. The aphakic or pseudophakic child must be provided with suitable optical correction after surgery. Postoperative occlusion of the normal eye in cases of unilateral traumatic cataract is done to achieve binocular vision and stereopsis.

Postoperative Complications

Fibrinous uveitis (Fig. 6.1.2.13) is a common postoperative complication due to increased tissue reactivity especially in children that may lead to posterior central synechiae, pupillary block glaucoma and lenticular membrane formation.[22] Fibrinous uveitis following cataract surgery with posterior chamber intraocular lens (PCIOL) has also been reported in various studies. Brar et al[23] noticed fibrinous uveitis in 40.9% of eyes in the blunt trauma group compared to 61% eyes in the penetrating group.

Increased uveal contact in eyes with sulcus fixation of IOL leads to a persistent low grade uveitis that predispose to synechiae formation and subsequent pupillary capture (Fig. 6.1.2.14). There is no doubt that

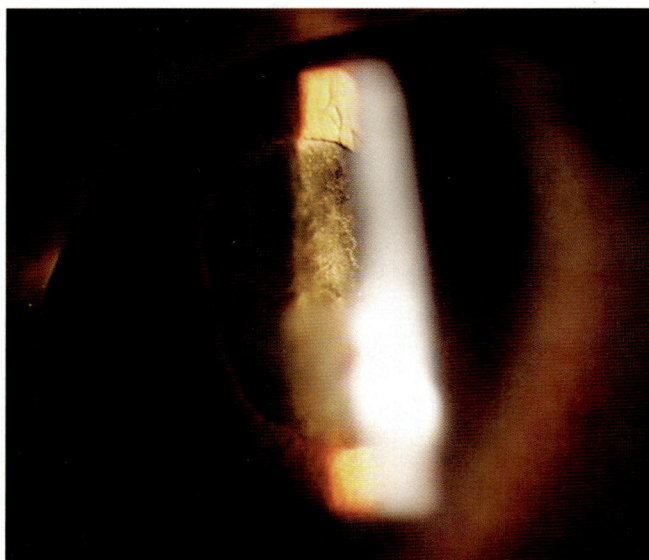

Fig. 6.1.2.13: Severe fibrinous reaction in an 11-year-old boy on the second postoperative day. A much greater tissue reaction is expected in children with traumatic cataracts

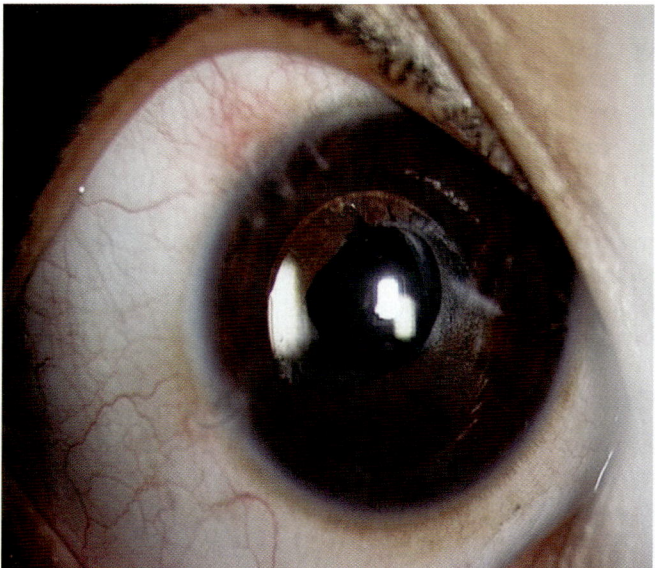

Fig. 6.1.2.14: Partial pupillary capture of a square edge PMMA-IOL in a child with perforating trauma with wooden piece. Note the clear visual axis 8 months following cataract surgery

in-the-bag fixation of IOL and less associated post-operative uveitis are important factors in decreasing this complication. Pupillary capture can occur despite angulated (10°) haptics. In a study by Pandey et al,[24] higher incidence of pupillary capture was noted in

sulcus fixated IOLs (40%) compared to capsular bag fixated lenses in pediatric traumatic cataracts. It is suggested that use of a larger optic size IOL in capsular bag-fixated lenses or a capsulorhexis smaller than the IOL optic would help to reduce the incidence of pupillary capture.

The incidence of glaucoma following pediatric surgery varies from 3 to 32%.[25] Glaucoma occurring soon after surgery is usually due to pupillary block or peripheral anterior synechiae formation while open-angle glaucoma may occur late, which emphasizes the need for the life long follow-up of these cases.

The most common and vision impairing complication is posterior capsular opacification (Figs 6.1.2.15 and 6.1.2.16), particularly after pediatric cataract surgery. The incidence of PCO varies from 21 to 100%.[26] Some authors have suggested that the incidence of PCO may be greater in patients with traumatic cataracts.[30,35] View record in Scopus cited by in Scopus (62)[27] younger the child, the higher the incidence and earlier the onset of PCO. Maintenance of a clear visual axis remains a high priority when planning management of the posterior capsule in the amblyogenic age group.[28] To restore a clear visual axis, yttrium aluminium garnet (YAG) laser (Fig. 6.1.2.17) or surgical capsulotomy must be undertaken in these

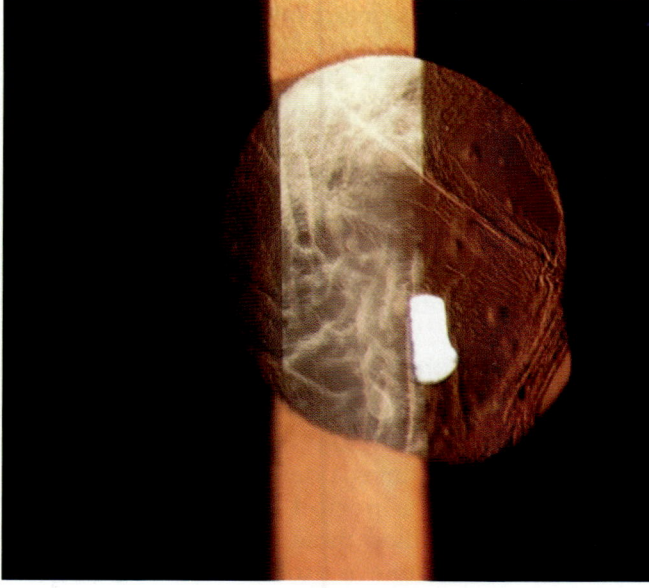

Fig. 6.1.2.15: Visually significant fibrous type of PCO in a 9-year-old child

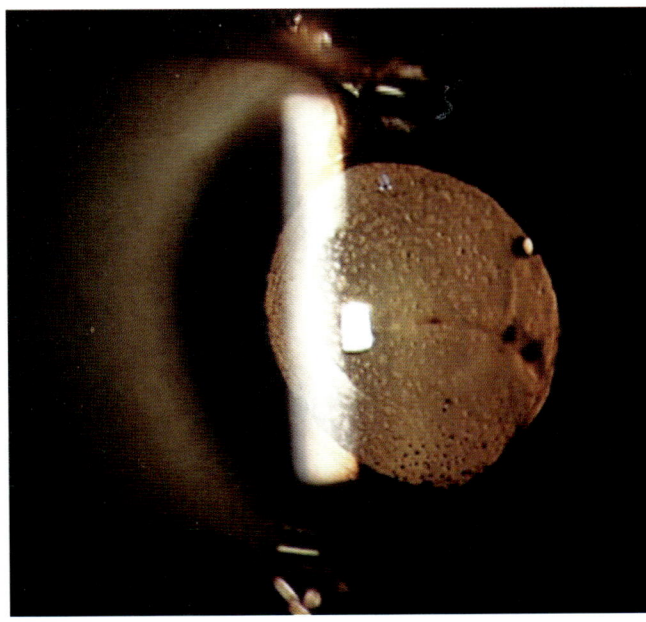

Fig. 6.1.2.16: Fibrotic PCO following capsular bag implantation of square edge PMMA IOL. No primary posterior capsulotomy has been performed

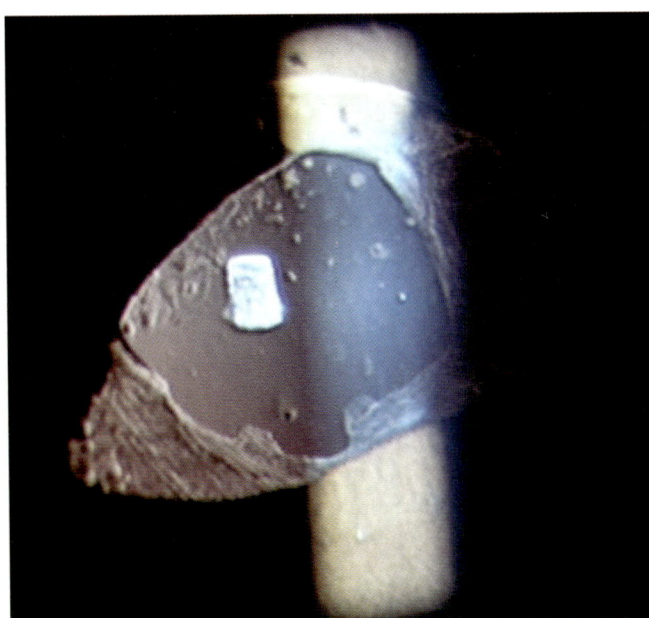

Fig. 6.1.2.17: Eye after Nd:YAG capsulotomy with clear visual axis

children to prevent poor visual acuity and amblyopia.[29] Various surgical techniques, such as primary capsulotomy, primary capsulotomy with

anterior vitrectomy, optic capture, epilenticular IOL implantation, have been employed to maintain a clear visual axis. Although various options to prevent PCO have been suggested, none is foolproof. Most of the surgeons believe that primary management of the posterior capsule and anterior vitreous is important during cataract removal in young children. Ram et al[30] and Vasavada et al[31] have reported significantly less chances of visual axis opacification in eyes undergoing PCCC with vitrectomy. Fenton et al.[32] reported that 15.6% of children with PCCC and no vitrectomy required neodymium-doped: yttrium aluminium garnet (Nd:YAG) capsulotomy for PCO. Hemo, et al[33] supported posterior capsulotomy as a part of the management of traumatic cataract, particularly in young children, combined with anterior vitrectomy before IOL implantation because of their tendency to fibrinous inflammation. Buckley et al[34] successfully avoided any secondary intervention for PCO by performing a standard endocapsular technique followed by a pars plana anterior vitrectomy and posterior capsulotomy in 20 children and Gimbel et al[35] has advocated a posterior capsulorhexis at the time of surgery.

CONCLUSION

In summary, a traumatic cataract is common after any form of injury to the eye. A thorough preoperative ocular examination is essential to properly assess the eye with a traumatic cataract. The surgical approach, potential use of capsular tension devices, and choice of IOL are all dictated by the inherent integrity of the zonules, lens capsule, and other associated anterior segment structures. Excluding other intrinsic causes of visual dysfunction, an eye with a traumatic cataract is amenable to treatment and has an excellent potential for significant postoperative visual improvement.

REFERENCES

1. Moisseiev J, Segev F, Harizman N, et al. Primary cataract extraction and intraocular lens implantation in penetrating ocular trauma. Ophthalmology 2001;108: 1099–103.
2. Shingleton B J, Hersh PS, Kenyon KR, et al. Lens injuries. Eye Trauma. 1991;126–34.
3. Schwab IR. Anterior Segment Trauma. AAO Basic and Clinical Science Course Section 8. 1997;285–6.
4. Macewen CJ. Eye injuries: A prospective survey of 5671 cases. Br J Ophthalmol. 1989; 73:888–94.

5. Lambert SR, Drack AV. Infantile cataracts. Surv Ophthalmol 1996;40:427–58.

6. Eckstein M, Vijayalakshmi P, Killedar M, et al. Aetiology of childhood cataract in South India. Br J Ophthalmol 1996;80:628–32.

7. Tomazzoli L, Renzi G, Mansoldo C. Eye injuries in childhood: a retrospective investigation of 88 cases from 1988 to 2000. Eur J Ophthalmol 2003;13:710–3.

8. Wolter JR. Coup-contrecoup mechanism of ocular injuries. Am J Ophthalmol. 1963;56:785–96.

9. Weidenthal DT, Schepens CL. Peripheral fundus changes associated with ocular contusion. Am J Ophthalmol. 1966;62:465–477.

10. Johns KJ, Feder RS, Bowes Hamill M, et al. Lens and Cataract. *AAO* Basic and Clinical Science Course Series. San Francisco: The Foundation for the American Academy of Ophthalmology; 2001;50–54:213–6.

11. Shock JP, Adams D. Long-term visual acuity results after penetrating and perforating ocular injuries. Am J Ophthalmol 1985;100:714–8.

12. Duke-Elder S, MacFaul PA. Injuries. System of Ophthalmology. Henry Kimpton Publishers. London, 1972. 26, 30–34, 42–44, 125.

13. Kwitko MR, Kwitko GM. Management of traumatic cataract. Curr Opin Ophthalmol. 1990;1:25–7.

14. Irvine JA, Smith RE. Lens Injuries in trauma. In: Shingleton B, Hersh PS, Kenyon KR, eds. Eye Trauma. St. Louis: CV Mosby; 1991:126–35.

15. Greven CM, Collins AS, Slusher MM, Grey Weaver R. Visual results, prognostic indicators, and posterior segment findings following surgery for cataract/lens subluxation-dislocation secondary to ocular contusion injuries. Retina. 2002;22:575–80.

16. Jacob S, Agarwal A, Agarwal A, et al. Efficacy of a capsular tension ring for phacoemulsification in eyes with zonular dialysis. J Cataract Refract Surg. 2003;29:315–21.

17. Ahmed IK, Crandall AS. Ab externo scleral fixation of the Cionni modified capsular tension ring. J Cataract Refract Surg. 2001;27:977–81.

18. Moreno-Montanes J, Sainz C, Maldonado MJ. Intra-operative and postoperative complications of Cionni endocapsular ring implantation. J Cataract Refract Surg. 2003;29:492–7

19. Awner S, Buckley EG, DeVaro JM, Seaber JH. Unilateral pseudophakia in children under 4 years. J Pediatr Ophthalmol Strabismus. 1996;33:230–6.

20. Vanathi M, Tandon R, Titiyal JS, Vajpayee RB. Case series of 12 children with progressive axial myopia following unilateral cataract extraction. J AAPOS. 2002;6:228–32

21. Jaworowska-Cieslinska I, Kaluzny J. Refractive changes in children with pseudophakia Klin Oczna. 2004;106:760–4.

22. Koeing SB, Ruttum MS, Lewandowski MF, Schultz RO. Pseudophakia for traumatic cataracts in children. Ophthalmology 1993;100:1218–24.

23. Brar GS, Ram J, Pandav SS, et al. Postoperative complications and visual results in uniocular pediatric traumatic cataract. Ophthalmic Surg Lasers 2001;32:233–8.

24. Pandey SK, Ram J, Werner L, et al. Visual results and postoperative complications of capsular bag and ciliary sulcus fixation of posterior chamber intraocular lenses in children with traumatic cataracts. J Cataract Refract Surg 1999;25:1576–84.

25. Brady KM, Atkinson CS, Kilyy LA, Hiles DA. Glaucoma after cataract extraction and posterior chamber lens implantation in children. J Cataract Refract Surg 1997;23:669–74.

26. Menezo JL, Taboada JF, Ferrer E. Complications of intra-ocular lenses in children. Trans Ophthalmol Soc UK 1985; 104:546–52.

27. Reddy AK, Ray R, Yen KG. Surgical intervention for traumatic cataracts in children: Epidemiology, complications, and outcomes. J AAPOS 2009;13:170–4.

28. Vasavada AR, Bharti RN. Pediatric cataract surgery. Curr Opin Ophthalmol 2006;17:54–61.

29. Brady KM, Atkinson CS, Kilty LA, Hiles DA. Cataract surgery and intraocular lens implantation in children. Am J Ophthalmol 1995;120:1–9.

30. Ram J, Brar GS, Kaushik S, Gupta A, Gupta A. Role of posterior capsulotomy with vitrectomy and intraocular lens design and material in reducing posterior capsule opacification after pediatric cataract surgery. Journal Cataract Refract Surgery 2003;29:1579–84

31. Vasavada A, Trivedi RH, Singh R. Necessity of vitrectomy when optic capture is performed in children older than 5 years. J Cataract Refract Surg 2001; 27:1185–93.

32. Fenton S, O'Keefe M. Primary posterior capsulorhexis without anterior vitrectomy in pediatric cataract surgery, longer term outcome. J Cataract Refract Surg 1999; 25:763–767.

33. Hemo Y, BenEzra D. Traumatic cataracts in young children. Correction of aphakia by intraocular lens implantation. Ophthalmic Paediatr Genet 1987; 8:203–7.

34. Buckley EG, Klombers LA, Seaber JH, et al. Management of the posterior capsule during pediatric intraocular lens implantation. Am J Ophthalmol 1993;115:722–8.

35. Gimbel HV, DeBroff BM. Posterior capsulorhexis with optic capture: maintaining a clear visual axis after pediatric cataract surgery. J Cataract Refract Surg 1994; 20:658–64.

6.1.3 Glaucoma due to Ocular Trauma

• **Barun Kumar Nayak** • **Sunil Kumar Jain**

INTRODUCTION

Ocular trauma is a leading cause of ocular morbidity with early and late-onset complications that may affect the final visual outcome. It has been reported to be one of the most important causes of unilateral vision loss in developing countries.[1,2] The injured eye may demonstrate obvious signs of damage or the clinical signs of trauma may be largely inapparent.

Trauma-related glaucoma is a potentially devastating complication that may present acutely or develop later on in an individual's lifetime. Thorough evaluation of the anterior segment as well as careful follow-up is necessary to detect the predilection for glaucoma and to initiate management.

PREVALENCE AND INCIDENCE OF OCULAR TRAUMA

Ocular trauma is not uncommon and frequently results in hospitalization. In a survey of hospital discharge data between 1984 and 1987, the average annual rate of principal diagnosis of ocular trauma was 13.2 per 100,000.[3] Of these patients 40% were diagnosed with primary contusion of the eyeball, adnexa or orbital fracture. Most ocular trauma patients are young, typically less than 30 years of age.[4-6] Children represent 27–48% of the total number of patients with ocular trauma.[5,6] Males are more likely to sustain an ocular injury than females: the male to female ratio ranges from 3.4:1 to 13.2:1.[5,7] The circumstances that lead to ocular trauma vary considerably and are influenced by numerous factors. Geographic, socioeconomic, and cultural influences factor into the etiology of ocular trauma. Patients from lower socioeconomic groups have a higher incidence and severity of ocular trauma. Sporting and domestic accidents accounted for almost two-thirds of the injuries, with the remaining known causes divided between industrial accidents and malicious acts. Among the sport-related ocular contusion, ball games are the most common cause. Another cause of ocular trauma with a relatively recent increase in prevalence is airbag injury related to motor vehicle accidents.[8]

INDIAN DATA

There are very few studies that have looked at ocular trauma from a population based perspective in India.[9-11] In the rural setting[9,10] a total 4.5–10.6% persons gave a history of ocular trauma in either eye, including 0.4–1% persons reporting trauma in both eyes. Blunt injuries were the major cause for trauma reported in this population. Men were more likely to have an eye injury than women. Ocular trauma was significantly more frequent among laborers when compared with other occupational groups. Injury with vegetable matter such as a thorn, branch of a tree, plant secretion, etc. was the major cause of trauma reported in this population. The majority of the eye injuries occurred at the workplace, followed by home. The majority of those affected did not wear any eye protection at the time of trauma. In the urban population,[11] the majority of the trauma resulting in blindness occurs during childhood and young adulthood, and slightly more than half occurs while playing.

GLAUCOMA

Following an ocular injury, the IOP may be found initially to be high or low. Several mechanisms exist to explain a low intraocular pressure (Table 6.1.3.1). Low IOP may result from aqueous hyposecretion due to ciliary contusion and inflammation, increased uveoscleral/vortex outflow due to cyclodialysis cleft, tears through trabecular meshwork into Schlemm's canal, or loss of integrity of the globe due to sclera or corneal perforation.

Low IOP can often convert to high IOP as a result of treatment, normal healing processes and the long-lasting effect of the injury itself on trabecular meshwork outflow.

Table 6.1.3.1: Low intraocular pressure after trauma

IOP after trauma may be low:
- Aqueous hyposecretion due to ciliary contusion
- Increased uveoscleral/vortex outflow due to cyclodialysis cleft
- Full thickness corneal or sclera laceration

Table 6.1.3.2: Immediate and delayed causes of traumatic glaucoma

Immediate	Delayed
• Contusion	• Angle recession
• Trabecular disruption	• Peripheral anterior synechiae
• Hyphema	• Lens induced
• Massive choroidal hemorrhage	• Ghost cells
• Chemical (alkali)	• Closure of cyclodialysis cleft
	• Fibrous/epithelial downgrowth
	• Retained IOFB
	• Rhegmatogenous retinal detachment

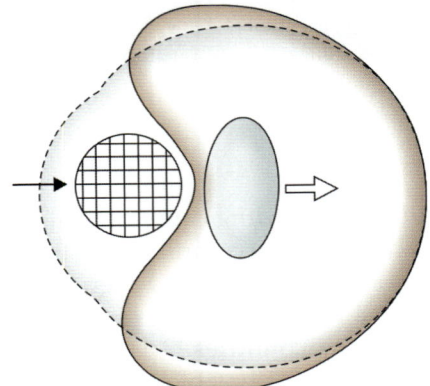

Fig. 6.1.3.1: Diagrammatic representation of compensatory expansion of globe in the equatorial direction

Elevated IOP has multiple causes, but they all tend to reflect a reduced facility of outflow of aqueous through the trabecular meshwork. It is useful to categorize the types of glaucoma associated with trauma as either immediate onset or delayed onset (Table 6.1.3.2). The type of trauma is also important to consider and is conventionally divided into blunt and penetrating trauma. A broader classification would include chemicals, electromagnetic radiation, and surgery as additional causes of trauma that might induce glaucoma.

Traumatic glaucoma can be also be classified as either open-angle or closed angle.

In the open-angle variety, the obstruction to aqueous outflow can be pretrabecular (e.g. epithelial down growth), trabecular (hyphema and ghost cell glaucoma) or post-trabecular (elevated episcleral venous pressure following carotid cavernous fistula).

Angle closure happens following adherence of peripheral iris to the trabecular meshwork or peripheral cornea.

Injuries to the anterior segment, which cause glaucoma most commonly, follow blunt injury. The impact from the blunt injury results in a sudden compressive deformation of the eye. The cornea and sclera are displaced posteriorly and there is a compensatory expansion of the globe in the equatorial direction[12] (Fig. 6.1.3.1).

Early Onset Glaucoma after Eye Injury

Contusion with Intraocular Inflammation

Occasionally, IOP elevation in the setting of blunt trauma is noted in the absence of any obvious intraocular damage. The angle is typically open and there is no evidence of angle recession, trabecular disruption, or hyphema. Inflammation in the form of cells and flare in the AC may be present. The presumed mechanism of this IOP rise is acute inflammation of the trabecular meshwork with a corresponding reduction in the facility of outflow. This pressurerize is typically self-limited, and improvement may be hastened by a short course of topical anti-inflammatory agents.

Trabecular Disruption

Herschler has shown that gonioscopy early after blunt injury may demonstrate trauma-related changes in the trabecular zone.[13] A full thickness tear in trabecular meshwork may occur and a trabecular flap may be created at the point of rupture. Inflammation is invariably associated with this type of injury. IOP may or may not be elevated, depending on the amount of aqueous production. Indeed, IOP may actually be subnormal in the early peritraumatic period, due to direct access of aqueous to Schlemm's canal, bypassing the trabecular meshwork. Small clot may be noted in the area of the trabecular meshwork tears due to bleeding from the Schlemm's canal.

Traumatic Hyphema

Significant bleeding in the AC associated with blunt ocular trauma increases the chance for elevation of IOP. The IOP may be elevated due to all the factors noted under contusion injury and trabecular meshwork damage as well as red blood cell obstruction of the outflow pathway.

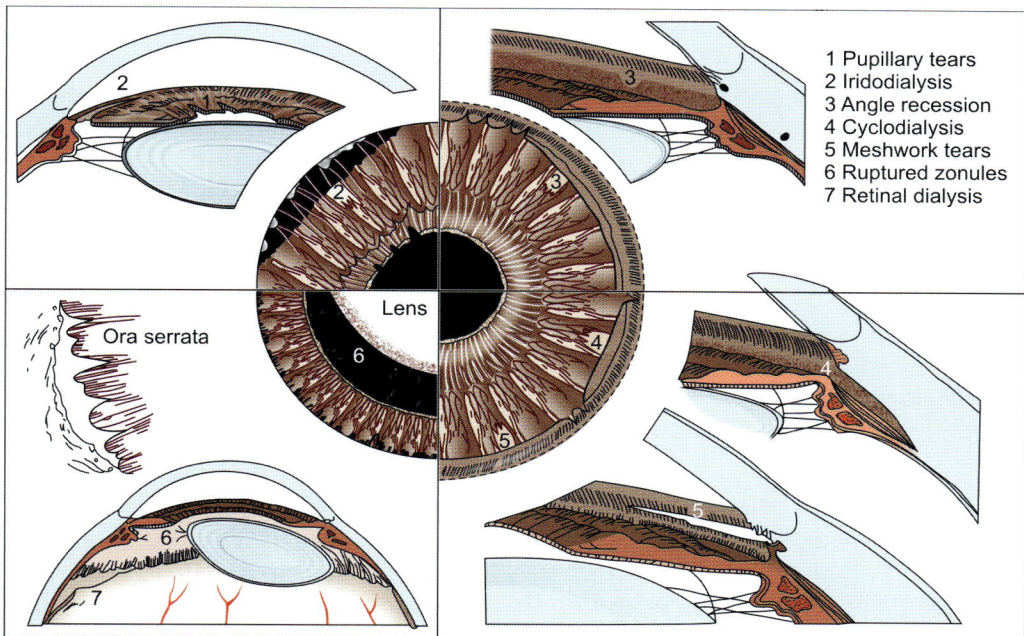

1 Pupillary tears
2 Iridodialysis
3 Angle recession
4 Cyclodialysis
5 Meshwork tears
6 Ruptured zonules
7 Retinal dialysis

Fig. 6.1.3.2: Campbell's seven rings or circles of tissue, anterior to the equator of the globe that suddenly expand with blunt impact

Campbell[14] has graphically described seven rings, or circles of tissue, anterior to the equator of the globe that suddenly expand with blunt impact. Because the internal fluids of the eye cannot compress, the forces are transmitted to the seven rings of tissue. This often results in splitting or tearing of tissues which may manifest as radial sphincter tears, iridodialysis, angle recession, cyclodialysis, trabecular meshwork tears, zonule separation, or peripheral retinal dialysis (Fig. 6.1.3.2).

Moderate elevation up to 10 mm Hg above baseline may occur in as many as 30% of patients with traumatic hyphema.[15] Because the vast majority of these patients have healthy optic nerves, they can tolerate an elevation of IOP for a moderate period of time. The elevation tends to be self-limited and clears as the blood cells are normally processed through the aqueous drainage channels. A given patient's susceptibility to IOP elevation in the setting of trauma is highly variable. Read and Goldberg[15] found that the IOP levels to 35 mm Hg or more that persist beyond 5–7 days may be associated with an increased risk of glaucomatous optic atrophy, particularly in presence of sickle cell disease, but not restricted to that group. Higher pressures for a shorter period may be even more poorly tolerated.

In patients with normal hemoglobin, the greatest concern for serious elevation of IOP is in those hyphema patients who suffer rebleeding. The incidence of rebleeding is highly variable depending on type of injury and the patient population. If rebleeding occurs, it tends to occur in the first 2–5 days after the injury. Although the majority of patients who lose vision in the setting of traumatic hyphema do so secondary to macular problems rather than secondary to glaucoma, every effort should be made to minimize the risk for sudden elevation of IOP. Treatment is directed toward minimizing the risk of rebleed.

Medical treatment for glaucoma in the setting of traumatic hyphema involves aqueous suppressants as the first line of defense (Table 6.1.3.3). Cycloplegics agents and topical steroids are often used to reduce the associated iritis and minimize outflow pathway edema.

Surgical treatment is indicated for those patients who do not respond satisfactorily to medical therapy. A host of procedures have been described to handle hyphema. Washing out the circulating red blood cells from the AC may be all that is required. If that does not lower IOP to an acceptable level, the washout can be repeated or additional techniques employed as

Table 6.1.3.3: Management of hyphema associated with glaucoma

First line of therapy: Medical management
- Aqueous suppressants
- Topical steroids
- Cycloplegic agents

    If medical management is ineffective, with concern for glaucomatous optic nerve damage and/or corneal staining, then surgical therapy is indicated.
- Anterior chamber washout
- Expression of blood clot
- Delivery of clot with cryoprobe
- Automated hyphemectomy with vitrectomy cutter
- Trabeculectomy

noted in the Table 6.1.3.3. Paracentesis and AC washout seems to be the simplest procedure, and this may be coupled with a bimanual irrigation system. The entire clot needs to be removed, as circulating red blood cells obstruct the outflow pathways.

Sickle cell hemoglobinopathy and traumatic hyphema: one of the groups at highest risk for optic nerve damage in the setting of traumatic hyphema are those patients with sickle cell hemoglobinopathy.[16] These patients are susceptible to even marginal IOP elevation and are also predisposed to profound IOP spikes. The sensitivity of the optic nerve to marginal IOP elevation is presumably related to restricted blood flow to the optic nerve in sickle cell disease. A high increase of IOP that may occur in these patients seems to be related to the restricted egress of rigid sickled red blood cells through the trabecular meshwork outflow pathways. A vicious cycle develops in that the sickle cells cannot clear from the AC and there is a stagnation of cells. A relatively acidotic pH develops in the AC, leading to further sickling. The accumulating sickled red cells have no greater chance of clearing through the trabecular outflow pathway and the cycle feeds on itself. Our traditional means of treating glaucoma in this setting may actually contribute to an exacerbation of the sickling process. Use of carbonic anhydrase inhibitor and the associated metabolic acidosis that results may increase sickling. If a systemic carbonic anhydrase inhibitor is required in this condition, methazolamide may be the preferred choice as it causes less systemic acidosis. Miotics may increase inflammation. Topical aqueous suppressants are the treatment of choice. Mention systemic steroids for reducing rebleed and other agents like.

Chemical Trauma

Alkaline agents have the capability of penetrating ocular tissues and may lead to glaucoma. This is uncommon with acid burns. A number of researches have studied the nature of the IOP rise following alkali exposure.[17] A "dicrotic" pressure rise has been noted with an immediate IOP rise up to the level of 40–50 mm Hg within the first 10 minutes of the injury. The pressure tends to return to normal after a short time and then gradually rises to high levels at the end of the first hour or two. It is believed that the shrinkage of the outer collagen coats of the eye may cause the initial IOP spike. Prostaglandin release has been implicated as the major factor in the second hypertensive phase. Weeks to months later, the IOP may be elevated due to angle closure as a result of peripheral anterior synechiae formation. If there is severe damage to the ciliary body, decreased aqueous production may produce early hypotony. Patients with severe alkali burns may not recover from this hypotonous phase.

Because of the corneal changes that may arise from a chemical injury, IOP elevation may be overlooked. Treatment for the IOP elevation, if necessary, is focused on aqueous suppressant therapy, both topically and systemically. Miotics are generally avoided because of the intense inflammation that is associated with chemical burns. Topical steroids, if even of cornea is abraded totally steroids may be indicated for initial 10 days.

Acidic chemicals cause coagulation of tissue proteins, which limits the penetration, resulting in more superficial injuries, unless the acid concentration is high or there is prolonged exposure. The IOP has been shown to become elevated after acid burns in rabbits. A spike in IOP occurs acutely, lasting up to 3 hours. Similar to alkali burns, the shrinkage of corneal and scleral tissues is thought to cause the initial rise in IOP. A sustained elevated IOP is thought to be mediated by prostaglandin release. Treatment of any resultant glaucoma is similar to alkali burns.

Late Onset Glaucoma after Eye Injury

Angle Recession

A tear in the ciliary body results in angle recession. The typical tear occurs between the circular and the longitudinal muscle in the ciliary body. There is a resulting posterior displacement of the iris root, which results in the clinical appearance of irregular broadening of the ciliary body band. Collins was the first to give pathologic description of angle recession in 1892.[18] Wolff and Zimmerman presented a classic correlation between traumatic glaucoma and angle recession in 1962.[19]

Angle recession is common following blunt ocular trauma. In patients with traumatic hyphema, angle recession occurs in 71–100% of eyes.[20-23] Despite this high incidence of angle recession, glaucoma is uncommon, occurring in approximately 7–9% of eyes.[20,22,24] Alper[25] believed that the risk of glaucoma developing was highest if more than 240° of angle appeared recessed.

Elevated IOP may occur months or decades following the initial injury. Blanton[20] observed a bimodal pattern with glaucoma occurring either within first year or after 10 years. The earlier onset group often had less angle recession, and the IOP rise was transient in some patients.

The diagnosis of angle recession is made by careful gonioscopic examination (Figs 6.1.3.3a and b). The ciliary body band tends to be broader in certain zones and there may be baring of ciliary processes. The sclera spur may appear abnormally white. Differences between the eyes may be remarkably subtle. The most useful technique for documenting angle recession is to compare quadrants between the injured eye and the noninvolved eye of a given patient.

The treatment of angle recession glaucoma follows the pattern used for primary open-angle glaucoma. Inadequate control with topical and oral therapy may lead one to consider laser trabeculoplasty. Argon laser trabeculoplasty is rarely effective and may also be associated with a higher incidence of acute IOP elevation. Filtration surgery is often required.

The mechanism of glaucoma in angle recession depends on the timing of the IOP elevation after injury. Early IOP increase is due to trabecular inflammation and the presence of circulating blood and inflammatory products. This often resolves within weeks to months, and the patient may enter a "honeymoon period", with normalization of IOP. The ophthalmologist must be aware that this period of normal IOP can be short lived; such eyes deserve close follow-up, at least every 6 months.

Late angle recession glaucoma is secondary to the formation of a "glass membrane" over the trabecular meshwork, thought to be an extension of Descemet's

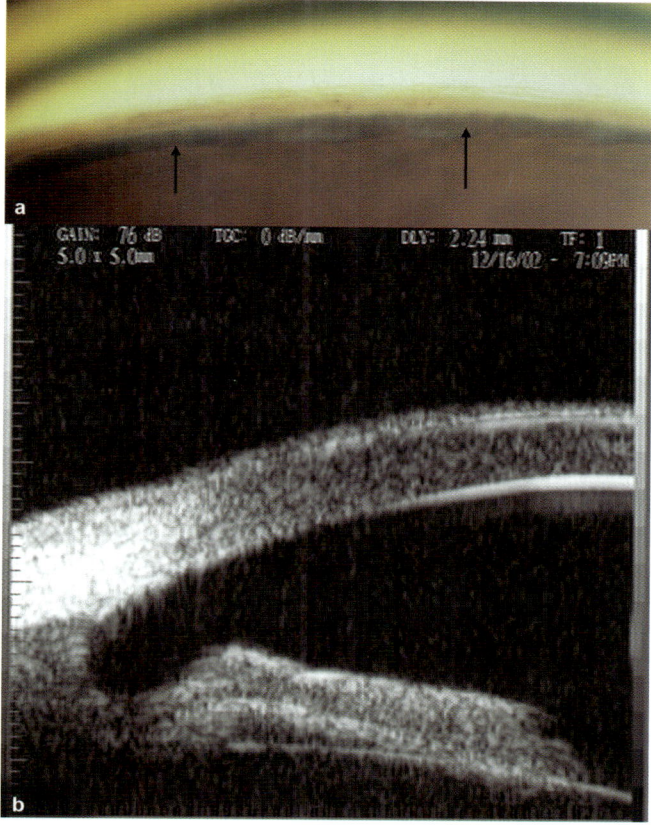

Figs 6.1.3.3a and b: (a) Goniophotograph showing angle recession; (b) UBM demonstrating angle recession

membrane. This explains the poor response to conventional medical and laser treatment in angle recession glaucoma.

Ghost Cell Glaucoma

Ghost cell glaucoma can occur when injury to the globe causes disruption of the anterior hyaloids face and is associated with blood accumulation in the vitreous Fig. 6.1.3.4. However, disruption of the hyaloid face is not a prerequisite for the development of ghost cell glaucoma.

Ghost cell glaucoma was initially described by Campbell et al.[26] They showed that following vitreous hemorrhage, fresh red blood cells degenerated into ghost cells in the vitreous usually within 1 or 2 weeks, resulting in a secondary elevation of IOP. This occurs when red blood cells, usually in the vitreous, but occasionally in long-standing hyphema, convert to less pliable, rigid, khaki colored ghost cells that do not pass

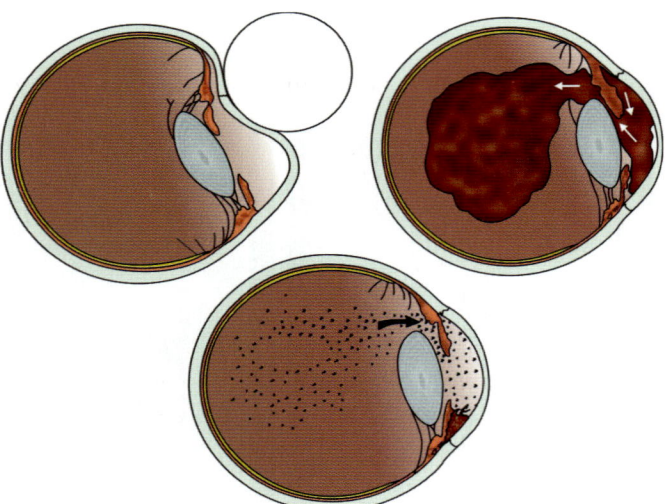

Fig. 6.1.3.4: Schematic demonstrates the effects of blunt injury, equatorial globe expansion, hyphema and vitreous hemorrhage, disruption of the anterior hyaloid face, passage of rigid khaki colored ghost cells into the AC and blockage of trabecular meshwork

easily through the trabecular meshwork. The cells obstruct aqueous outflow with a resulting rise in IOP. The khaki ghost cells can often be identified at the slit lamp and may occasionally layer in the inferior angle recess as a "pseudohypopyon". The glaucoma occurred anywhere from 2 weeks to 3 months following the trauma but was most common 1 month after the injury. AC aspirates demonstrate cells with a characteristic shrunken appearance by phase contrast microscopy. Heinz bodies represent denatured hemoglobin present in the cytoplasm of some ghost cells.

The treatment of ghost cell glaucoma includes conventional medical therapy, with surgery as necessary. Most patients can be controlled with topical aqueous suppressants, including β-adrenergic antagonists, carbonic anhydrase inhibitors, and α_2-agonists. In some situations, the use of oral carbonic anhydrase inhibitors and intravenous hyperosmotic agents may become necessary. Refractory cases may require surgical intervention. AC washout may temporarily control IOP. If the reservoir of khaki ghost cells is large enough, there may be recurrent elevation of IOP despite AC washout. A pars plana vitrectomy may be necessary to ensure complete removal of all blood components trapped in the vitreous. If IOP is still uncontrolled, filtration surgery may be required. Ghost cell glaucoma in aplakia desereves mention.

Lens-induced Glaucoma

Lens-induced glaucoma is a varied group of secondary glaucomas that has the lens as a factor in the cause of IOP elevation. The angle in this category of glaucoma may be open or closed. The four major categories include: (1) lens dislocation, (2) lens swelling, (3) phacolytic glaucoma and (4) lens particle glaucoma. Each type may arise with trauma to the globe (Fig. 6.1.3.5 and Table 6.1.3.4).

Lens Dislocation or Subluxation

Dislocation or subluxation of the crystalline lens most commonly occurs with blunt trauma. Disruption of the zonules allows the lens to move anteriorly or posteriorly. Depending on the position of the lens and the vitreous status, pupillary block may occur (Fig. 6.1.3.6). Pupillary block may lead to angle closure with a precipitous increase in IOP. Creeping angle closure may develop in a more sub-acute or chronic form, leading to late onset development of glaucoma. Rarely, complete dislocation of the lens may allow vitreous to come forward to fill the AC and lead to vitreous block glaucoma.

Treatment of lens induced glaucoma depends on the type of glaucoma. Careful examination is critical to determine the presence or absence of pupillary block. If pupillary block is present, a laser iridotomy

Table 6.1.3.4: Insights into mechanisms of lens induced glaucoma	
• Phacomorphic	Lens swelling—mass effect leading to direct mechanical angle closure or pupillary block glaucoma
• Phacotropic	Lens dislocation/subluxation—pupillary block with secondary angle closure, direct mechanical angle closure or vitreous block glaucoma
• Phacolytic/phacoparticle	Lens particle/high molecular weight proteins obstructing trabecular meshwork with an open angle
• Phacotoxic	Inflammatory material obstructing trabecular meshwork with an open angle

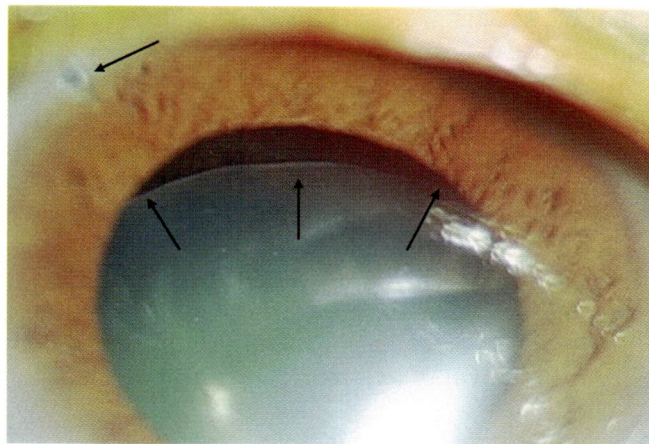

Fig. 6.1.3.5: Lens-induced glaucoma

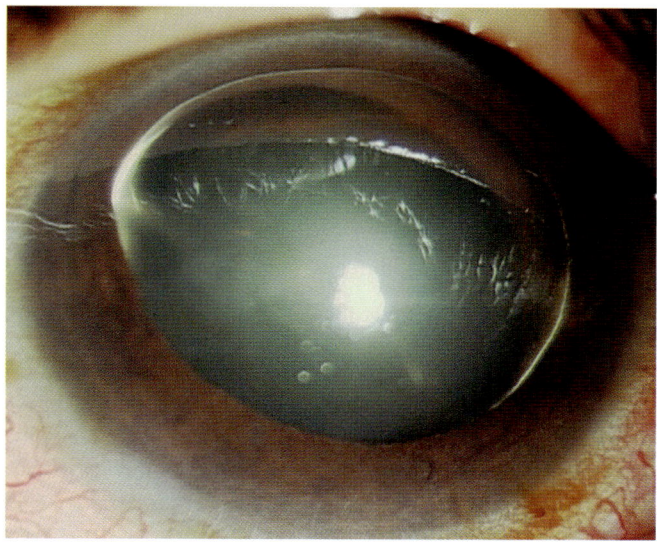

Fig. 6.1.3.6: Anterior subluxation of lens post-trauma

or surgical iridectomy is indicated. Lensectomy may be required for visual reasons and for recurrent episodes of pupillary block. The technique of lensectomy will depend on the degree of subluxation. Surgical removal may involve a planned intracapsular or extracapsular lens extraction or phacoemulsification or pars plana lensectomy with vitrectomy depending on the amount of subluxation and density of the lens nucleus.

Lens Swelling

Blunt or penetrating trauma may alter lens fibers or capsule sufficiently to result in lens swelling. The lens may hydrate and become a mature cataract with development of phacomorphic glaucoma (Fig. 6.1.3.7). Pupillary block may occur or the lens may swell enough to directly close angle structures. A previous history of trauma and asymmetry of AC depth on clinical examination are vital in establishing the reason for this type of glaucoma. Cataract surgery is required for visual rehabilitation and correction of the glaucoma.

Phacolytic Glaucoma

Phacolytic glaucoma is seen in the setting of a mature or a hypermature cataract. Open-angle glaucoma occurs as a result of leakage of high molecular weight proteins through an intact lens capsule. There is a rapid onset of pain and redness in the eye. IOP may become extremely high. Corneal epithelial edema is usually present. Patches of white material, probably macrophages are also seen on the anterior capsule (Fig. 6.1.3.8). Inflammatory precipitates such as keratic precipitate (KP) may or may not be present on the corneal endothelium. Cellular reaction in the AC in some cases is slight, but more often is moderate, and in rare instances is accompanied by hypopyon.

Cataract extraction is the definitive treatment. Prior to cataract surgery, medical therapy should be used to reduce the IOP and inflammation. Surgery may be delayed for several days in cases with severe uveitis to allow for intensive topical steroid therapy. Patients should be evaluated daily. Suppression of uveitis and control of IOP before surgery are beneficial, although not always possible. Exracapsular cataract surgery has been used successfully for phacolytic glaucoma. The IOP usually returns to normal within a few days after cataract surgery.

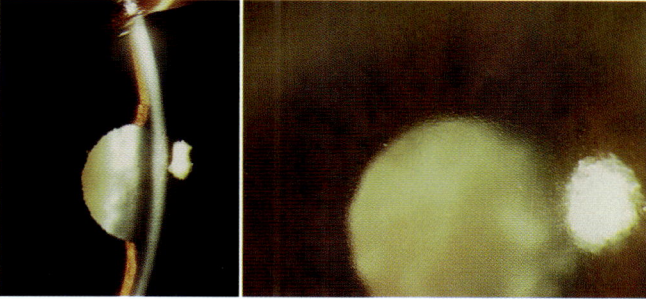

Fig. 6.1.3.7: Lens swelling/intumescent cataract resulting in shallowing/intumescent cataract resulting in shallowing of the AC and epithelial edema due to rise in IOP

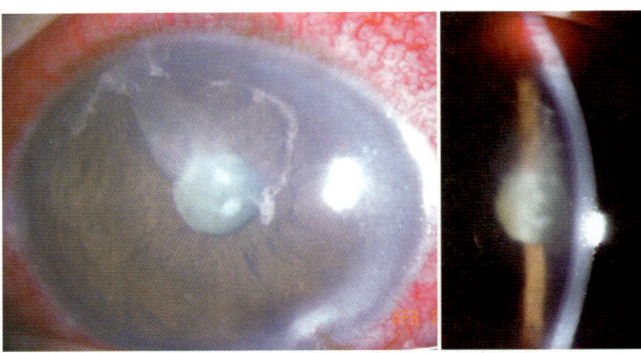

Fig. 6.1.3.8: Phacolytic glaucoma: presence of severe AC inflammation in form of coagulum, dense flare and cells. Also the anterior capsule shows white patches indicating macrophages

Lens Particle Glaucoma

Frank disruption of the lens due to penetrating trauma, and rarely blunt trauma,[27] may lead to fragments of lens material in the AC (Fig. 6.1.3.9). This will be obvious at the time of initial injury or rarely have a delayed onset[27] and will require surgical decision making based on other associated findings. Most of these are associated with corneoscleral lacerations that require primary repair. Lens particle glaucoma is a limited response that consists mainly of bloated macrophages and lens debris and is not the severe granulomatous uveitis seen in lens induced uveitis. The severity of glaucoma is proportional to the amount of free cortical material in the aqueous humor. The lens protein is the major component that causes obstruction of outflow facility in lens particle glaucoma such as in phacolytic glaucoma.

If treatment is delayed, peripheral anterior synechiae and posterior synechiae can form. Medical therapy is useful for eyes with minimal to moderate amounts of free cortical material. Treatment with aqueous suppressants, cycloplegics, and topical steroids often suffice until residual lens material is absorbed. Intensive topical steroid therapy can delay the absorption of lens protein and should be avoided. Surgical removal of lens debris is recommended.

Peripheral Anterior Synechiae

Ocular injury often results in inflammation and blood in the AC peripheral anterior synechiae may from due to prolonged iridocorneal apposition and pupillary block. Peripheral anterior synechiae (PAS) may form. Hyphema that persist for an extended period of time in the setting of significant inflammation are the most common cause of PAS formation in setting of blunt trauma. Penetrating trauma commonly results in PAS formation, particularly if the laceration crosses the limbus.

Late Closure of a Cyclodialysis Cleft

A separation of ciliary body from the sclera spur results in a cyclodialysis cleft. This may occur following blunt trauma or after surgical intervention. This may result in temporary or permanent hypotony. Goldmann has postulated that a reduction in the normal flow of aqueous across the trabecular meshwork results in reduced permeability of the meshwork to aqueous outflow. This may account for the marked, acute IOP elevation that occurs following closure of cyclodialysis clefts.

Delayed closure of a cyclodialysis cleft can be a difficult diagnosis to make. The IOP increase tends to be severe and is associated with significant pain. A previous history of trauma should raise the suspicion of the examiner. Treatment involves use of aqueous suppressants, oral or intravenous hyperosmotics as well as alpha agonists. When closure of a cleft is suspected treatment with miotics and phenylephrine may be effective in reopening the cleft and in lowering the pressure. A repeat gonioscopy then often provides the diagnosis.

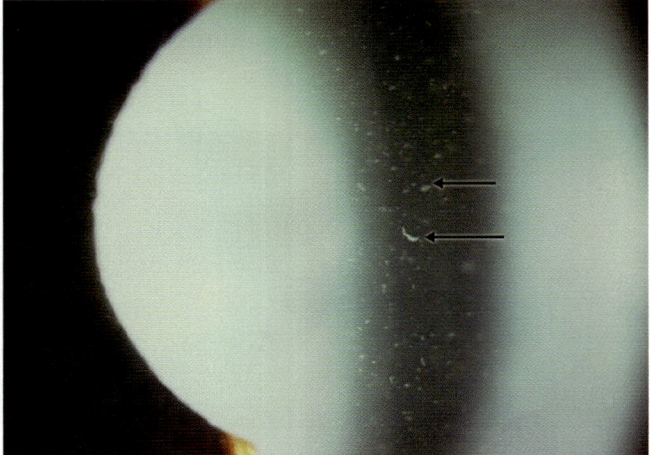

Fig. 6.1.3.9: Free floating lens particles in the AC causing glaucoma

Epithelial Downgrowth

Lacerating trauma to the eye may lead to a fistula that develops from the external surface of the eye to the AC. This provides a conduit for epithelium to enter the anterior segment. This is an uncommon problem in the setting of microsurgical repair, but must be searched for in eyes that develop glaucoma at a time remote from the initial lacerating injury. The characteristic slit lamp appearance of a scalloped endothelial membrane is diagnostic for epithelial downgrowth. Argon laser applications to the involved iris make a white spot. These two findings confirm the diagnosis, although histopathologic confirmation via iris biopsy may be required in certain cases. Treatment involves excision of all involved iris and explanation of the intraocular lens, if present. Cryotherapy is applied to the involved ciliary body and cornea. Visual prognosis is guarded in these cases. Tube shunt procedures may be effective.

Retained Intraocular Foreign Body

Penetrating ocular trauma should always raise a high suspicion for a retained IOFB. All patients with penetrating injuries should undergo radiographic imaging to evaluate for any potential metallic FBs.

The IOP after a penetrating ocular injury is usually low because of the open wound, but after surgical repair glaucoma may develop because of intraocular changes induced by the penetrating injury. During the early postinjury period the IOP may be elevated secondary to hyphema, inflammation, or angle closure due to lenticular trauma. As these conditions subside, chronic changes may develop as a result of the inflammation. Cyclitic membranes may form in the AC, pulling the lens-iris diaphragm forward with secondary angle closure or obstructing the pupil with subsequent iris bombe. Peripheral anterior synechiae may also develop, leading to angle closure due to chronic inflammation or a prolonged shallow/flat AC.

Prompt administration of topical anti-inflammatory agents and cycloplegics may prevent synechiae formation and decrease the strong inflammatory response. Additionally, reformation of the AC early on is important to prevent peripheral anterior synechiae.

Patients with a retained IOFB may develop elevated IOP through all the same mechanisms as described earlier for simple penetrating trauma, but may also develop glaucoma due to the late sequela of retained metallic FBs. Iron released from a retained metallic FB is toxic to the trabecular meshwork, leading to a decreased outflow and elevated IOP (siderosis). Copper may be oxidized within the eye, causing similar trabecular changes as with iron, but with less frequency (chalcosis).

Patients may present immediately with a clear history and evidence of an IOFB, or they may appear months or years after the initial event in a more subtle fashion with unilateral cataract, chronic inflammation, glaucoma, or reduced retinal function. Ocular examination is directed at looking for evidence of penetration such as discrete area of iris transillumination, a small lenticular rupture or a corneal or sclera wound.

Rhegmatogenous Retinal Detachment

It is most commonly associated with ocular hypotension due to decrease in aqueous production. However, 5–10% of the patients may develop elevated IOP (Schwartz syndrome). The mechanism for increased IOP is most likely due to direct photoreceptor obstruction of aqueous outflow in the anterior segment.[28] Schwartz's syndrome can be difficult to diagnose, and commonly occurs in the setting of a shallow, peripheral retinal detachment with the appearance of an AC inflammatory reaction. It is not unusual for Schwartz's syndrome to be misdiagnosed as inflammatory glaucoma. Repair of the retina detachment most commonly results in a prompt and permanent return of IOP to normal, assuming there are no associated problems in the anterior segment that might exacerbate a tendency toward glaucoma.

REFERENCES

1. Thylefors B. Epidemiological patterns of ocular trauma. Aust N Z J Ophthalmol 1992;20:95-8.
2. Negrel AD, Thylefors B. The global impact of eye injuries. Ophthalmic Epidemiol 1998;5:143-69.
3. Klopfer J, Tielsch JM, Vitale S, et al. Ocular trauma in the United States. Eye injuries resulting in hospitalization, 1984–1987. Arch Ophthalmol 1992; 110:838-42.
4. Blomdahl S, Norell S: Perforating eye injury in the Stockholm population. An epidemiological study. Acta Ophthalmol 1983; 62:378-390.
5. Canavan YM, Archer DB. Anterior segment consequences of blunt ocular injury. Br J Ophthalmol 1982; 66:549-55.

6. MacEwen CJ. Eye injuries: a prospective survey of 5671 cases. Br J Ophthalmol 1989;73:888-94.

7. Moreira CA, Debert-Ribeiro M, Belfort R: Epidemiological study of eye injuries in Brazilian children. Arch Ophthalmol 1988;106:781-8.

8. Lesher MP, Durrie DA, Stiles MC: Corneal edema, hyphema, and angle recession after air bag inflation. Arch Ophthalmol 1993;111:1320–22.

9. Nirmalan PK, Katz J, Tielsch JM, et al. Ocular trauma in a rural south Indian population: the Aravind Comprehensive Eye Survey. Ophthalmology. 2004;111(9): 1778–81.

10. Krishnaiah S, Nirmalan PK, Shamanna BR, et al. Ocular trauma in a rural population of southern India: the Andhra Pradesh Eye Disease Study. Ophthalmology. 2006;113(7):1159–64.

11. Dandona L, Dandona R, Srinivas M, et al. Ocular trauma in an urban population in southern India: The Andhra Pradesh Eye Disease Study. Clin Experiment Ophthalmol 2000;28:350-6.

12. Thompson JT. Traumatic retinal tears and detachments. In: Shingleton BJ, Hersh PS, Kenyon KR, Eye Trauma. St. Louis, Mosby Year Book, Inc., 1991;196.

13. Herschler J, eds. Trabecular damage due to blunt anterior segment injury andits relationship to traumatic glaucoma. Trans Am Acad Ophthalmol Otolaryngol 1972;83:229.

14. B Campbell DG. Traumatic glaucoma. In: Edited by Shingleton BJ, Hersh PS, Kenyon KR eds Eye Trauma. St. Louis, Mosby Year Book, Inc., 1991;117–125.

15. Read J, Goldberg MF: Comparison of medical treatment for traumatic hyphema. Trans Am Acad Ophthalmol Otolaryngol 1974;78:799.

16. Goldberg MF. The diagnosis and treatment of sickled erythrocytes in human hyphemas. Trans Am Acad Ophthalmol Otolaryngol 1978;76:481.

17. Paterson CA, Pfister RR. Intraocular pressure changes after alkali burns. Arch Ophthalmol 1974;91:211.

18. Collins ET. On the pathologic examination of three eyes lost from concussion. Trans Ophthalmol Soc UK 1992;12:180.

19. Wolff SM, Zimmerman LE. Chronic secondary glaucoma associated with retrodisplacement of iris root and deepening of the anterior chamber angle secondary to contusion. Am J Ophthalmol 1962;84:547.

20. Blanton FM. Anterior chamber angle recession and secondary glaucoma. A study of the after effects of traumatic hyphemas. Arch Ophthalmol 1964;72:39.

21. Tonjum AM. Intraocular pressure and facility of outflow late after ocular contusion. Acta Ophthalmol 46:886, 1968.

22. Monney D. Angle recession and secondary glaucoma. Br J Ophthalmol 1973;57:608.

23. Canavan YM, Archer DB. Anterior segment consequences of blunt ocular injury. Br J Ophthalmol 1982;66:549.

24. Kaufman JH, Tolpin DW. Glaucoma after traumatic angle recession. A ten year prospective study. Am J Ophthalmol 1974;78:648.

25. Alper MG. Contusion angle deformity and glaucoma. Gonioscoic observations and clinical course. Arch Ophthalmol 1963;69:455.

26. Campbell DG, Simmons RJ and Grant WM: Ghost cells as a cause of glaucoma. Am J Ophthalmol 1973;97:2141.

27. Jain SS, Rao P, Nayak P, et al. Posterior capsular dehiscence following blunt injury causing delayed onset lens particle glaucoma. Indian J Ophthalmol 2004;52:325.

28. Matsuo N, Takabatake M, Ureno H, et al. Photorecptor outer segment in the aqueous humor in rhegmatogenous retinal detachment. Am J Ophthalmol 1986;101:673.

6.2 CHEMICAL TRAUMA

• Ritu Arora • Shailley Jain

INTRODUCTION

Chemical burns are an ocular emergency which requires immediate management. The rapid dilution of the corrosive chemical by an irrigating fluid, even water, may be the single most important factor in determining the final outcome of the injured eye.

Chemical injuries may occur in an industrial or agricultural setting, at home, in criminal assaults, in chemical warfare and occasionally in medical setting (for example in treatment of conjunctival papilloma with silver nitrate applicator sticks).[1] The agent may be in solid, liquid or gaseous form. Other factors influencing the injury may be present such as pressurized ammonia, flakes of sodium hydroxide (NaOH) and lime (which are retained in fornices and provide a continuous reservoir causing severe injury), thermal injury as in magnesium hydroxide which is present in fireworks, sulphuric acid causing thermal injury with high velocity penetration of foreign body following automobile battery explosions. Automobile airbags occasionally release sodium hydroxide as part of the chemically driven rapid inflation process causing mild alkali injury. Industrial accidents are more frequent with labor and construction, chemical plants and machine factories.

Epidemiology

In series from western literature, most victims are young males with injuries being most common in industrial accidents.[2] Other common causes are exposure at home with cleaning agents and those associated with criminal assaults. Alkali injuries are far more frequent than acid injuries which can be attributed to their presence in household cleaning agents and building materials. Morgan[3] reviewed 221 chemical injuries in 180 patients presenting to the Croydon Eye Unit, UK between January 1, 1985 and February 28, 1986. Most patients were between 16 years of age and 25 years of age, 75.6% were male while 24.4% were female. Alkali injuries were twice as common as acid injuries. 89.4% injuries were accidental while 10.6% resulted from chemical assault. Among the accidental cases, 63% occurred at work, 33% at home and 3% at school. In another series by Kuckelkorn[2] at the Eye Center Serving Aachen, Germany, 236 chemically injured eyes of 171 patients were seen between September 1990 and August 1991. 70% were adult males, 23% were adult females while 7% were children. Most patients were between 16 years at age and 45 years of age. 61% injuries were industrial accidents, 37% occurred at home and in 2% the cause was unknown. In another series by Kuckelkorn,[2] in 42 patients with severe chemical injuries which required admission to the RWTH Aachen, Germany, between 1985 and 1992 only six patients could be rehabilitated visually. Most patients were between 20 years of age and 40 years of age. 73.8% injuries were industrial accidents while the rest occurred at home. A population-based study of chemical eye injury in the chemical industry from Manchester Royal Eye Hospital,[4] University of Manchester, UK reported 60 eye injuries (45.1% of all eye injuries) due to chemicals (eye injury incidence 11.4 per 1,000 employees per year) in a population of 62,839 workers studied for 1 month (approximately 10 million man-hours). Six patients (10%) required hospital attention. No sight-threatening injuries occurred. Most of these injuries were avoidable. Eye protectors were not a requirement in some situations where injury occurred (one-third of injuries), were not used where specified in some cases, and in others failed to prevent injury even when worn.

In a series from Postgraduate Institute of Medical Education and Research (PGIMER), Chandigarh,[5] clinical and demographic profile of 145 chemical eye injuries in 102 patients was analyzed. Forty-three patients (42.1%) suffered bilateral injuries. Acids and alkalis together were responsible for 80% of the chemical injuries. Young people working in laboratories and factories constituted two-thirds of the patients. Fifty-two eyes (35.9%) suffered severe (grade III/IV) injuries. Injuries caused by assault were more severe and proportionately lost more eyes. Visual outcome correlated with severity of injury at initial presentation.

CHEMICALS AND PATHOPHYSIOLOGY OF OCULAR TRAUMA

General Reactions of Chemicals and their Outcome[2,6-8]

The nature and extent of the injury caused by the action of a chemical upon the eye depends on several factors which determine the type and severity of damage in each particular case, these factors being:

1. Intimacy and duration of contact with ocular tissues
2. Physical properties of the chemical which determine its penetrability
3. Chemical reactivity with the tissue components, the extent and reversibility of which determines the degree of permanent damage.

Alkalis (bases) are agents with a pH in the higher than normal physiological range. In contrast to acids, alkaline agents rapidly penetrate the cornea, reacting with the cellular lipids to form soaps. They essentially dissolve the cell membranes and continue destroying tissues much longer than acids, permanently damaging ocular tissues and entering the AC in as short a time as 5 seconds. Alkalis also dehydrate cells and destroy enzymatic and structural proteins. The most severe effects occur in the pH range 11.0–11.5. Penetration rates differ by the type of base; ammonium hydroxide is one of the fastest penetrating bases, followed by NaOH, potassium hydroxide (KOH) and calcium hydroxide. The hydroxyl ion (OH^-) saponifies the fatty acid components of the cell membranes resulting in cell disruption and death, while the cation is responsible for the penetration of the specific alkali.

Acids (substances with lower than normal pH values) precipitate tissue proteins, creating a barrier to further ocular penetration. The corneal epithelium offers some protection against weaker acids. Very weak acids may cause only temporary loss of the corneal epithelium with minimal damage to the deeper structures. In the case of acids, the H^+ ion causes damage due to pH alteration, while the anion produces protein precipitation and denaturation in the corneal epithelium and superficial stroma.

Damage may occur to proximal and distal bulbar conjunctiva, palpebral conjunctiva and anterior orbital tissues in addition to the corneal and intraocular injury. Necrosis of bulbar conjunctival tissue is associated with infiltration of leukocytes, which is a source of continued ocular surface inflammation and associated release of increased levels of N-acetyl-glucosaminidase and cathepsin D into the preocular tear film. There is a loss of vascularization at the limbus due to ischemic necrosis of the conjunctiva and this reduces the availability of vascularly derived collagenase inhibitors, which may contribute partially to subsequent corneal ulceration and perforation. There also occurs hydration of collagen fibrils causing their thickening and shortening. This distortion of the trabecular meshwork along with release of prostaglandins may result in acute rise in IOP immediately after the injury.

Acids vs Alkalis: Biochemical Changes[2,6-8]

Alkalies

1. *pH changes:* Cations react with carboxyl group of stromal collagen and glycosaminoglycans resulting in thickening and shortening of trabecular meshwork and loss of stromal clarity. Distortion of trabecular meshwork and release of prostaglandins are responsible for the elevation in IOP, which is often seen immediately following alkali injuries. The alkali makes the collagen more susceptible to enzymatic degradation by the hydrolysis of the protective interfibrillary glycosaminoglycans by the hydroxyl ions. Depending on the degree of penetration, there may be damage to corneal and conjunctival epithelium, basement membrane, stromal keratocytes, stromal nerve endings, endothelium, and lens epithelium, resulting into vascularization of the conjunctiva, episclera, iris and ciliary body ultimately.

   Depending upon the amount of penetration, there is a change in the aqueous pH, which returns to normal within 30 minutes to 3 hours if the external pH is restored.

2. *Collagen synthesis defects:* Damage to the ciliary body epithelium results in decreased secretion of ascorbate and a reduction in its AC concentration, potentially compromising subsequent corneal keratocyte collagen synthesis and stromal repair. Irreversible intraocular damage with hypotony and phthisis bulbi may follow prolonged aqueous pH values of 11.5 or greater.

3. *Ulceration and proteolysis:* Alkali burns commonly cause stromal ulceration which is secondary to the initial effects of the chemical on the tissues, usually

occurring approximately 2–3 weeks after the burn as a result of accelerated proteolytic processes coupled with inadequate collagen synthesis.

After chemical injury, polymorphonuclear (PMN) cells are attracted to the region of tissue damage, infiltrating the stroma. Corneal stromal fibroblasts, corneal epithelium and PMN release collagenases. The peak of collagenase activity does not occur till 14–21 days after the burn.

Free radicals may also play a role in the tissue destruction and ulceration. A relative deficiency of superoxide dismutase could occur in association with epithelial loss and with the decrease in this superoxide scavenger, tissue destruction would be potentiated.

Acids

The H$^+$ ion causes damage due to pH alteration, while the anion produces protein precipitation and denaturation in the corneal epithelium and superficial stroma. It is this coagulation of proteins that produces the characteristic ground glass appearance of the epithelium. This functions as a barrier to further penetration and limits further intraocular injury. Also, tissue proteins in turn have a buffering effect on the acid. With the exception of hydrofluoric acid and sulphurous acid, acids penetrate much less than alkalies. If stromal penetration occurs, alterations similar to alkali burns may occur.

Causative agents and pathophysiology

In general, chemicals can be classified as:
1. Acids or alkalies or toxins
2. Inorganic or organic.

ALKALI INJURIES[2,6,8]

Most common alkalies causing ocular burns are ammonia, lye, KOH, magnesium hydroxide and lime. Most serious alkali injuries are associated with ammonia and lye: both penetrate immediately into the eye, potentially producing serious damage to the anterior segment. Magnesium hydroxide can produce a devastating injury because of a combined thermal injury. Most common alkali producing ocular injury is lime, which does not inflict as much damage as the more rapidly penetrating alkalies as it forms calcium soaps that precipitate and hinder further penetration. Lime particles retained in the superior fornix provide a continuous reservoir of alkali after injury and increase the severity of the injury (Table 6.2.1).

Table 6.2.1: Common alkalies causing chemical injuries

Compound	Sources/uses
Lime	Chuna packets, plaster, mortar, cement, whitewash
Ammonia	Fertilizers, refrigerants, cleaning solutions
Lye	Drain cleaners
Potassium hydroxide	Caustic potash
Magnesium hydroxide	Sparklers
Hydrogen peroxide	Household item as milk preservative

Common Alkalies Causing Ocular Injury

1. Ammonia (NH$_3$)

It is a colorless gas and a component of fertilizers, refrigerants, cleaning agents (7% solution), and manufacture of other chemicals. Ammonia fumes stimulate the eye to secrete tears, which tends to dilute the chemical, reducing its potential for major ocular damage unless there is a direct blast of the gas onto the ocular surface. However, on prolonged exposure it dissolves in water and tears to form ammonium hydroxide fumes, which does cause major ocular damage. As it is highly lipid soluble, it penetrates rapidly causing severe corneal injury and damage to the iris and lens. Ammonia takes less than a minute to penetrate the eye making the injury more difficult to ameliorate by subsequent irrigation.

2. Lye (NaOH)

Penetrates the eye nearly as fast as ammonia. Lye burns occur most often due to solid NaOH (used as a drain cleaner).

3. Potassium Hydroxide (KOH)

Penetrates the eye only slightly less rapidly than does NaOH and causes injuries of similar severity.

4. Magnesium Hydroxide (Mg(OH)$_2$)

It is present in sparklers and flares and the combination of thermal and alkali injury accounts for the severity of injury.

5. Lime (Ca(OH)$_2$)

Plaster, mortar, cement, whitewash is the most common cause of chemical injury in work place. It penetrates the eye relatively poorly due to the formation of calcium soaps on reacting with the epithelial cell membrane. These soaps precipitate and hinder further penetration. Therefore, injuries are less severe. However, corneal opacities caused by calcium hydroxide are visible before those as a result of ammonium or NaOH. In the Indian scenario, lime burns in children are commonly seen, also reported by Agarwal et al.[9] Bursting of cheap chuna packets (edible $CaOH_2$ paste), an additive to chewing tobacco as a household item was retrospectively evaluated in 21 children (25 eyes). The injury was severe with poor prognosis (grade IV in 23 eyes) with 17 eyes requiring surgical intervention. A warning on chuna packets for its potential dangerous nature is warranted.

6. Hydrofluoric Acid (HF)

It is a weak inorganic acid and a strong solvent. It is found in pure form (solutions ranging from 0.5% to 70% in strength) or mixed with other agents, e.g. nitric acid, ammonium difluoride and acetic acid. It penetrates easily due to its low molecular weight and small size and causes severe injury because of high degree of activity in dissolving cellular membranes allowing deep penetration.

7. Nitric Acid (HNO_3)

Injuries are similar to hydrochloric acid except epithelial opacities are yellow rather than the usual white color.

8. Methyl Ethyl Ketone Peroxide

It is used as a catalyst in various industries. Immediate and delayed corneal manifestations are seen. Exacerbations and remissions of limbal and corneal disease have been reported.

9. Household Detergent

Horgan et al[10] have highlighted the risk of alkali burns with liquid tablet washing detergent especially in children. Each tablet contains 50 mL concentrated alkaline detergent at a pH of 9. These products are designed to be placed directly in a washing machine and are interesting to young children. When squeezed hard enough or after softening with water they can burst leading to detergent being sprayed over the eyes and face. The authors have reported six cases in the age 8 months to 3 years over a 6-month period with bilateral injuries in three cases and significant conjunctival epithelial defects in four cases. All patients recovered completely with prompt irrigation and medical treatment.

10. Hydrogen Peroxide

It is an oxidizing agent that is used in a number of household products, including general-purpose disinfectants, chlorine-free bleaches, fabric stain removers, contact lens disinfectants and hair dyes, and it is a component of some tooth-whitening products. In industry, the principal use of hydrogen peroxide is as a bleaching agent in the manufacture of paper and pulp. Hydrogen peroxide has been employed medicinally for wound irrigation and for the sterilization of ophthalmic and endoscopic instruments. Hydrogen peroxide causes toxicity via three main mechanisms: (1) corrosive damage, (2) oxygen gas formation and (3) lipid peroxidation. Concentrated hydrogen peroxide is caustic and exposure may result in local tissue damage. It is allowed for use as a preservative in raw milk by small scale farmers in developing countries and reported cause accidental occular burns particularly in children in India.[11] Ocular exposure to 3% solutions may cause immediate stinging, irritation, lacrimation and blurred vision, but severe injury is unlikely. Exposure to more concentrated hydrogen peroxide solutions (> 10%) may result in ulceration or perforation of the cornea. There are rare cases of temporary corneal injury resulting from application of 3% solution to the eye (on contact lenses) including punctate staining of the cornea, decreased vision, corneal opacity and edema.

ACID INJURIES[2,6,7]

Most acid injuries are mild because the exposure is to weak acids or diluted strong acids. However, severe injuries do occur and are mostly associated with exposure to heavy metal acids such as chromic acid or mineral acids such as sulphuric, sulphurous or hydrofluoric acids. Unlike alkali injuries, the clinical picture resulting from a severe ocular acid injury is fairly constant regardless of the offending agent (Table 6.2.2).

1. Sulfuric Acid (H_2SO_4)

It is the most commonly encountered acid injury. It is a component of industrial cleaners and battery acid. It is an odorless, colorless oily liquid in its pure form.

Table 6.2.2: Common acids causing chemical injuries

Compound	Sources/uses
Sulfuric acid	Industrial cleaners, battery acid
Sulfurous acid	Fruit and vegetable preservatives, bleach, refrigerants (mixed with oil)
Hydrofluoric acid	Glass and silicone polishing and frosting, mineral refining, gasoline alkylation, production of organic fluorocarbons, semiconductors.
Acetic acid	Vinegar (4–10%), essence of vinegar (80%) or glacial acetic acid (90%)
Chromic acid	Chrome plating industry, cleaning agent

However, when even slightly contaminated by impurities, it becomes yellowish or brown and emits a foul odor. Sulfuric acid combines with water to produce heat resulting in thermal injury along with chemical burns. Most of the injuries, especially the more severe ones occur as a result of battery explosions. Hydrogen and oxygen are produced by electrolysis when sulfuric acid combines with water in the battery especially when the battery is charging. Inadvertent use of flame close to battery of inverter during power breakdown results in accidental battery explosions as the gaseous mixture explodes on contact with flame resulting in an injury, which is a combination of acid burns and contusions from particulate matter, lacerations and IOFB penetration.

2. Sulphurous Acid (H_2SO_3)

It is formed from sulphur dioxide by combination with corneal water. Contact is prolonged because of the hydrocarbon, resulting in severe tissue damage. It penetrates more easily as compared to other acids because of its high lipid and water solubility. SO_2 damages the corneal nerves resulting in corneal anesthesia. Initially, vision is not affected, but worsens gradually over hours to days. Damage is caused by sulphurous acid itself by denaturation of proteins and inactivation of numerous enzymes, causing the destruction of corneal tissues.

3. Acetic Acid (CH_3COOH)

Mild injury occurs with less than 10% contamination unless exposure is prolonged while higher concentrations cause severe injury.

4. Chromic Acid (Cr_2O_3)

Injury occurs by exposure to droplets of the acid in chrome plating industry and cleaning of glassware in labs. Chronic exposure produces chronic conjunctival congestion with brown discoloration of the epithelium in the interpalpebral fissure.

5. Hydrochloric Acid (HCL)

Used as 31–38% solution and in the pH balance of swimming pools as muriatic acid in weaker concentrations and school and college chemistry laboratories. Gas is irritant producing reflex tearing and preventing severe ocular damage. At high concentrations and prolonged exposures, liquid HCl may produce severe ocular damage.

6. Trichloroacetic Acid (TCA)

Trichloroacetic acid is frequently utilized for chemical peeling by physicians practicing dermatologic surgery. Thirty-five percent TCA may seep into the eye during a chemical peel. The patient may develop marked conjunctivitis and abrasions of the cornea.[12]

TOXINS

1. Petroleum Products

Petroleum products and other organic chemicals generally cause less severe injuries. The lacrimator chloroacetophenone in chemical mace (tear gas) causes mild to severe injury. Degree of severity is related to proximity of spray can to the eye, quantity of chemical entering the eye, duration of exposure, state of normal reflex mechanisms and other factors like mechanism of propelling the chemical as in solvent spray, pressurization or explosion. Epithelial defects, severe persistent stromal haze, edema secondary to endothelial damage and corneal neovascularization may result.

2. Mustard Gas

It has been used in chemical warfare. It is an organic molecule with a dual mechanism of action. It causes blistering of the skin and lungs and its interaction with moisture rapidly causes hydrolysis producing hydrocloric acid. Ocular effects are usually short lived and include conjunctivitis, pain, lacrimation, corneal ulceration and photophobia. Chronic effects are dry eye, conjunctival and stromal scarring and squamous metaplasia. Exposure to high concentrations may lead to blindness.

3. Color Powders Used During Celebration of Holi

Green/bluish-green holi colors have been reported[13] with a high incidence of ocular toxicity causing severe ocular irritation with epithelial defect upon exposure, though it does not penetrate through the cornea. In the eyewash fluid of four patients, high-performance liquid chromatography (HPLC) estimation confirmed the presence of malachite green which was responsible for its reported toxicity. Malachite green or 4-[(4-dimethylaminophenyl)-phenyl-methyl]-N,N-dimethyl-aniline was detected at different concentrations in *in vitro* and tissue retention studies revealed that increasing the contact time increases tissue concentration. After 2 minutes of exposure, the tissue concentration was significantly higher.

MECHANISM OF HEALING IN CHEMICAL INJURIES

Repair of Epithelium

Severely damaged epithelial cells desquamate from the cornea, exposing stromal tissue, which may opacify. Limbal conjunctiva and its vessels destroyed by chemical cauterization, allow transudation of proteins and PMN cells. The PMN cells collect in large numbers at the junction of normal and damaged epithelium. If undamaged limbal tissue persists, epithelial sliding over the burn site begins within 16 hours after injury. Sheets of cells may move together. Epithelial movement then stops by 72 hours. Although, the limbal area is only 24% that of the cornea, limbal cells can spread sufficiently to cover a total corneal defect.

When the burn is so severe that both corneal and limbal epithelium are lost, conjunctival epithelium serves as the source of healing. Conjunctival epithelium migrates over the burned cornea and the limbus must undergo both a morphological and a biochemical transformation called transdifferentiation. Loss of goblet cells, increase in density of epithelial cells and the formation of more hemidesmosomes takes place. However in these cases, re-epithelialization is delayed with persistence of goblet cells and recurrent epithelial erosions in addition to superficial and deep stromal vascularization.

Repair of Stroma

After corneal injury keratocytes from adjacent areas are mobilized to regenerate the injured stroma. These pluripotent cells secrete collagen, collagenase, glycosaminoglycan (GAG) ground substance and collagenase inhibitors and can phagocytose collagen fibrils. Ascorbate is a cofactor in hydroxylation of lysine and proline, the rate limiting step in collagen synthesis which may be hampered by decrease in aqueous ascorbate levels after severe burns resulting in corneal ulceration and perforation. Since collagen synthesis is maximum between 1 week and 8 weeks after burns with a peak at 3 weeks, corticosteroids must be limited after the 1st week in cases with severe burns as they interfere with keratocyte migration and collagen synthesis. Active corneal stromal ulceration takes place in the presence of persistent epithelial defect and degradation of the epithelial basement membrane by type IV collagenase. Type I collagenase production by keratocytes may be seen as early as 9 hours after injury, peaking at 2–3 weeks which corresponds to the period of maximal production and repair of collagen. The production of this enzyme is normally inhibited by epithelial cytokines. In presence of an epithelial defect, this inhibitory function is lost and the regenerating epithelium may rather stimulate collagenase activity.

Inflammation

Infiltration of the peripheral cornea with PMN and mononuclear cells starts within 12–24 hours after injury. In severe cases, a second wave of infiltration takes place at 7 days, peaking at 14–21 days. This infiltration persists in the presence of epithelial defect and/or necrotic conjunctiva. Persistent inflammation in turn prevents healing of epithelial defect and stimulation of keratocyte collagenase by mononuclear cells promotes sterile ulceration. Hence, therapeutic agents which act as anti-inflammatory agents can prevent the second wave and reduce the incidence of ulceration.

CLINICAL COURSE AND EVALUATION

Alkali Burns

Clinical findings present immediately after injury are related to area of involvement (extent of fluorescein staining), depth of penetration (loss of stromal clarity, limbal ischemia and/or necrosis of limbal and bulbar conjunctiva) and toxicity of the substance.

In recognition of the relationship of initial appearance to ultimate prognosis, Hughes[14] proposed a classification of alkali burns taking into account the epithelial defect and stromal opacity. Ballen and Roper Hall[14] modified this classification to include quantification of conjunctival and episcleral ischemia (area of whitening). Thoft[2] further classified injuries using a limbal stem cell injury based model. The latest classification by Dua et al[15] takes into account the extent of limbal involvement in clock hours and the percentage of conjunctival involvement (Figs 6.2.1 to 6.2.5).

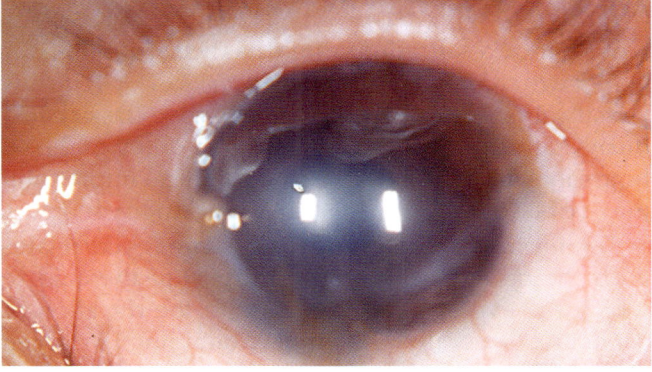

Fig. 6.2.3: Acute burns with only inferonasal epithelial defect and no limbal or conjunctival ischemia: grade I (both Roper Hall and Dua's classification)

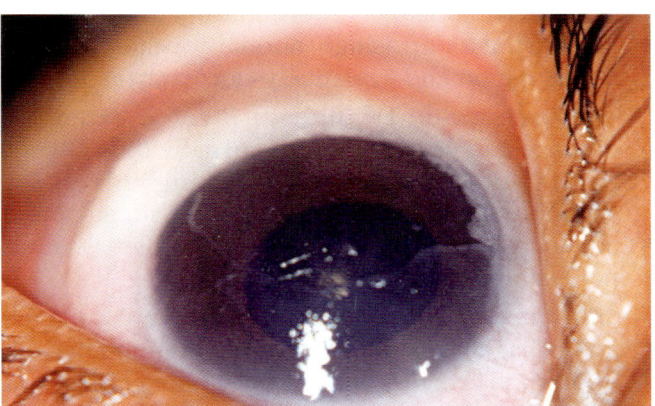

Fig. 6.2.1: Acute burns with total epithelial defect and intact limbus: grade 1 (both Roper Hall and Dua's classification)

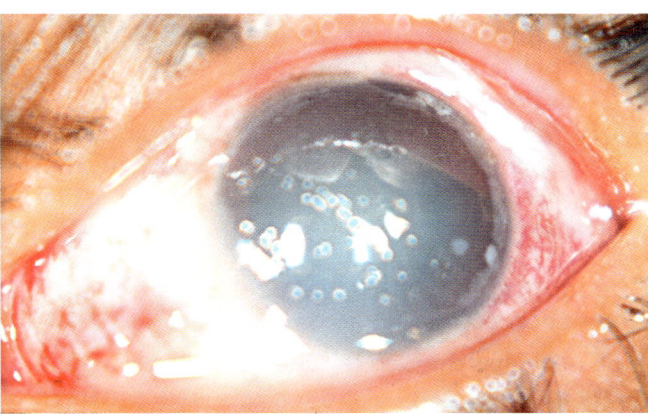

Fig. 6.2.4: Alkali burns acute stage with limbal and conjunctival ischemia from 4 o'clock to 12 o'clock with sectoral (inferonasal) corneal edema with total epithelial defect: grade IV by Roper Hall and grade V by Dua's classification. Guarded to poor prognosis

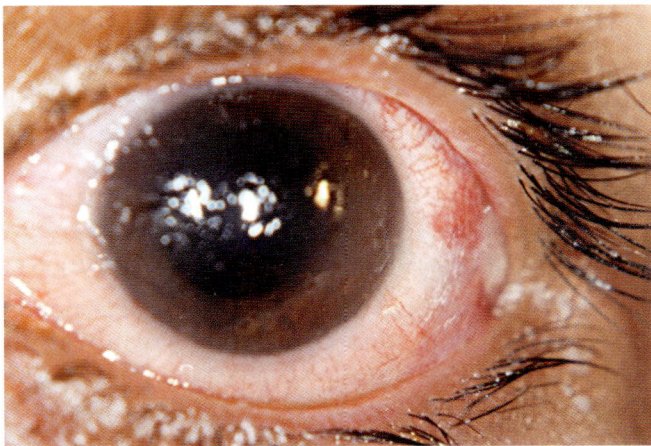

Fig. 6.2.2: Acute burns with only 50% epithelial defect and no limbal or conjunctival ischemia: grade I (both Roper Hall and Dua's classification)

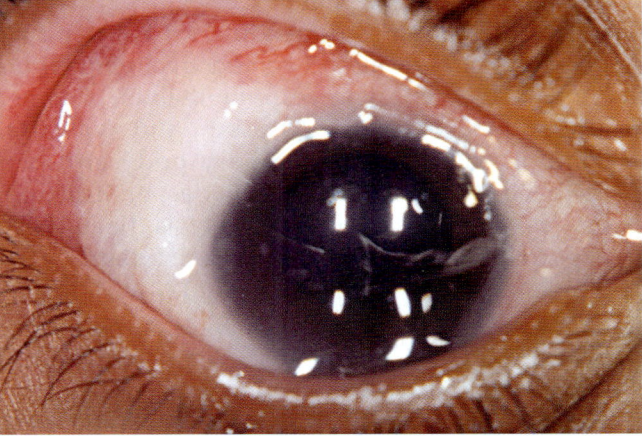

Fig. 6.2.5: Alkali burns acute stage with limbal and conjunctival ischemia from 5 o'clock to 12 o'clock with total epithelial defect: grade IV by Roper Hall and grade V by Dua's classification

Acid Burns

No specific classification system has been proposed for acid burns. However, a modification of Hughes classification of alkali burns can be used to classify acid burns.[8] In using the classification, a delay of 24–48 hours may be needed as the initial clinical impression may be better or worse than the actual injury.

For any acid, the degree of tissue damage correlates with the quantity and concentration of the acid to which the eye is exposed and with the duration of exposure. Generally, the fumes containing hydrogen ions and droplets of acidic solutions cause only minor injury; more severe injuries result from a direct splash. If the epithelium is intact, acids tend to cause severe tissue damage only if their pH is less than 2.5. If the epithelium is absent prior to exposure, acids at a higher pH can cause severe damage.

Clinical signs suggesting a poor prognosis after acid injury reflect the degree of acid penetration of the tissue. They include complete corneal anesthesia, conjunctival and episcleral ischemia, severe iritis and lens opacity.

Clinical Stages and Pathological Correlation of Alkali Burns

Mc Culley[2] has divided the clinical course of chemical injury into four distinct pathophysiologic and clinical phases: immediate, acute (day 0–7), early repair (day 7–21) and late repair (after day 21).

1. *Immediate phase:* As described in classification of chemical injuries.
2. *Acute changes:* Acute injury causes destruction of cellular membranes depending on the depth of penetration: corneal and conjunctival epithelium, keratocytes, corneal nerves, endothelium of cornea and blood vessels, cellular and vascular components of iris and ciliary body and lens epithelium. The damage to the deeper structures may not be apparent immediately as they may be obscured by the anterior stromal clouding.

   In the first few hours after alkali burns, IOP may be increased in a bimodal fashion, although the pressure is occasionally normal. Once this initial increase has passed, the pressure may fluctuate from glaucoma to hypotony for several days, depending on the balance between decreased aqueous humor production and decreased outflow. Grade I injury usually heals without incident during the acute phase. Grade II injuries have early re-epithelialization and slow recovery of stromal clarity. Grade III and grade IV injuries have little or no re-epithelialization with early keratocyte proliferation, inflammatory cell infiltration, little or no collagenase production and no corneal neo-vascularization.

3. *Early repair phase:* Epithelial migration continues in grade II injury but becomes alarmingly delayed in more severe injury. Ingrowth of vessels and invasion of the corneal stroma by inflammatory cells parallel the epithelial regrowth. The corneal opacity begins to clear and in mild to moderate cases may resolve completely during this period.

   Grade III injuries may show little or no re-epithelialization but a surprisingly normal appearance to the limbal region and a relatively clear cornea.

   Because grade IV injuries involve extensive damage and necrosis, there is usually little change in the clinical appearance during this phase especially if early necrotic tissue debridement and advancement of conjunctiva or tenon's tissue has not been performed early.

   Keratocyte proliferation with resultant collagen and collagenase production and inflammatory cell infiltration becomes very important for grade II and grade III injuries which have not been managed with aggressive anti-inflammatory therapy. Inflammation, loss of limbal blood supply and lack of vascularly derived collagenase inhibitor may result in evidence of anterior segment necrosis and sterile corneal ulceration even at an early stage in grade IV injuries.

4. *Late repair phase:* Based on the epithelial healing which has taken place so far, it is possible to classify the injury into a confirmed healing pattern. This classification can accurately predict the functional outcome in the absence of aggressive intervention and form the basis of recommendation for surgery.

Type I—normal epithelial recovery: Corresponds to grade I limbal stem cell injuries resulting in complete re-epithelialization by the beginning of this phase. Corneal epithelium is clinically and phenotypically normal. Goblet cell injury is unusual, but if present may result in abnormal mucus secretion with transient ocular surface wetting abnormalities and mild corneal epitheliopathy.

Type II—delayed differentiation: Corresponds to grade II limbal stem cell injuries. Sectoral epithelial defects in the quadrant with complete limbal stem cell loss may persist. The subsequent course will be one of delayed epithelialization and superficial vascular pannus. Greater likelihood of associated goblet cell dysfunction resulting in persistent ocular surface wetting abnormalities, which may persist for weeks or months after re-epithelialization is complete. Persistent epitheliopathy may result in subnormal vision for several months.

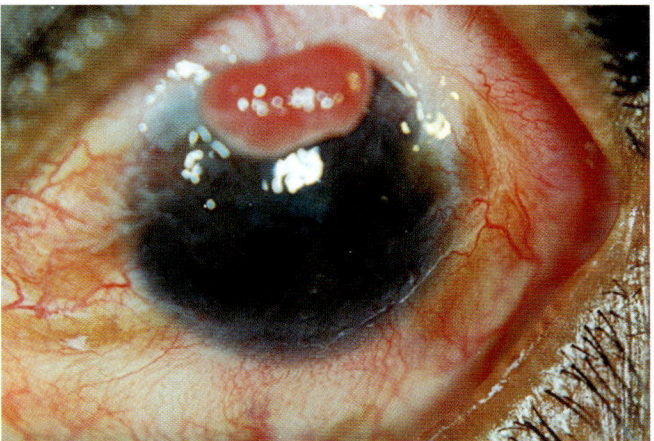

Fig. 6.2.6: Phase 4: alkali (cement) burns stage 4 (6 months postinjury) with limbal deficiency from 9 o'clock to 3 o'clock with granuloma pyogenicum at 12 o'clock

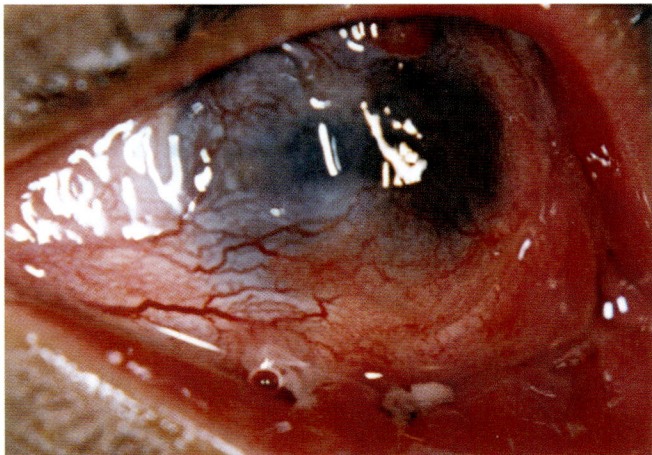

Fig. 6.2.7: Phase 4: severe conjunctival ischemia more than 270° from 4 o'clock to 12 o'clock with granuloma pyogenicum at 12 o'clock with scarred temporal cornea and conjunctival scarring leading to shelving of fornices (fair prognosis with ALT, AMT and PK)

Type III—fibrovascular pannus: Grade III injuries which have little or no re-epithelialization during the first 3 weeks after injury. In addition to progressive and complete fibrovascular pannus of the corneal surface, ocular surface abnormalities may be exacerbated by late progressive symblepharon formation, cicatricial entropion, trichiasis, additional corneal scarring (Figs 6.2.6 and 6.2.7).

Type IV—sterile corneal ulceration: In grade IV injuries, progressive sterile ulceration due to enzymatic destruction may have already been initiated in the early repair phase. Evidence of anterior segment necrosis, retrocorneal membranes, peripheral anterior synechiae, cataract, glaucoma, hypotony and phthisis bulbi may develop. Late sequelae of severe conjunctival injury are disorders of ocular surface wetting due to mucous membrane abnormalities, cicatrization of the conjunctiva with symblepheron and entropion formation. Even with aggressive management the final visual prognosis in grade IV injuries is poor.

Clinical Stages and Pathological Correlation of Acid Burns

1. *Immediate phase:* Immediate changes are similar to alkali burns with more severe appearance matching with the color of sulphuric acid, sulphurous acid, chronic acid and nitric acid.

2. *Acute phase (immediate to 1 week after burn):* Acids tend to penetrate more slowly than alkalis, causing a sharp demarcation of the injured area. Exposure of both conjunctival and corneal surface epithelia to acid results in coagulation of the cells and varying degrees of opacification become apparent within a few seconds after exposure. If the acid is concentrated or has a high protein affinity, coagulation and opacification are more pronounced. However, epithelium injured by either nitric or chromic acid will be yellow or brown, whereas following even severe HF acid injury, the epithelium is only minimally opaque.

Clinical manifestations of acid penetration include stromal granularity, stromal edema, ischemia, severe iritis and cataract formation. Except in the most severe cases, significant ischemia due to vascular endothelial necrosis or vascular thrombosis, as seen in alkali injuries, is not encountered. If the injury is mild, the epithelium regenerates

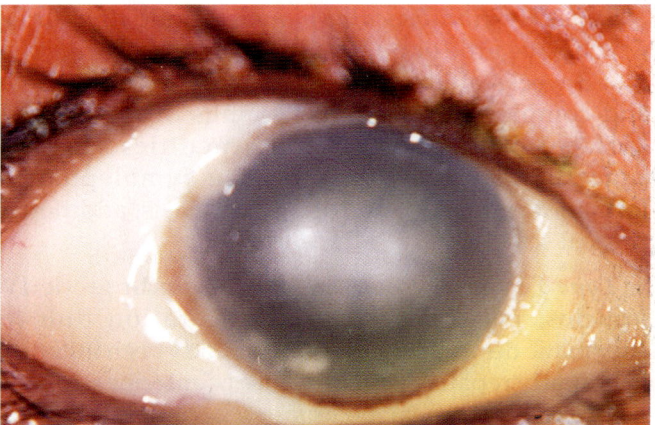

Fig. 6.2.8: Acid burns acute stage (a case of vitriolage) with 360° severe limbal and conjunctival ischemia with total cataract: grade IV by Roper Hall and grade VI by Dua's classification (very poor prognosis)

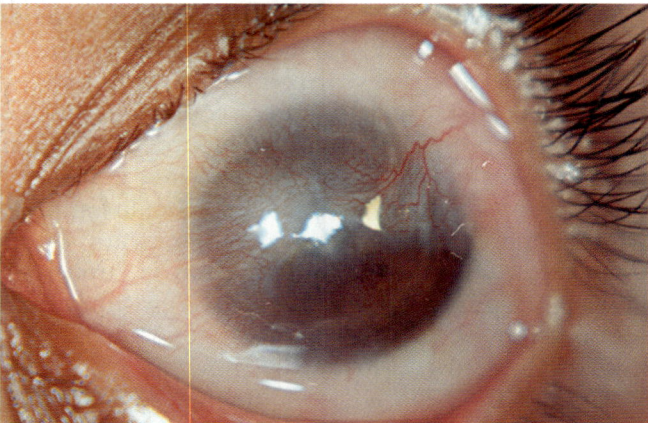

Fig. 6.2.9: Phase 4 acid burns (accidental injury in a laboratory) with conjunctival ischemia from 8 o'clock to 3 o'clock leading to superficial scarring of cornea superiorly. The conjunctiva and fornices are spared

within a few days and the eye recovers totally. After more severe injuries, the underlying stroma may have a grayish, ground glass appearance secondary to the direct action of the acid and to infiltration by inflammatory cells (Fig. 6.2.8). After sulfur dioxide or HF acid burns, the stroma may be damaged but there is minimal clouding of the tissue. Within minutes to hours of an acid burn, the conjunctiva becomes hyperemic and chemotic. Subconjunctival hemorrhage is not uncommon. Edema of the corneal stroma may also occur, but this does not necessarily indicate acid penetration into the stroma or the endothelium. Stromal edema can result from loss of the epithelial barrier to water flow. In the early phases after an acid burn, a mild reflex iritis is often present. During the first 24 hours after an acid injury, inflammatory cells infiltrate the corneal stroma through the limbus and the disrupted anterior surface. The intensity of the infiltrate is far less than that seen after an alkali burn. Within minutes after exposure to an acid, the IOP may increase in a manner similar to that seen after alkali burns. The IOP remains high for more than 3 hours and has less of a biphasic pattern than that encountered after alkali burns. A sustained increase in IOP occurs only if the hydrogen ions reach the AC.

3. *Early reparative phase (1–3 weeks):* Because most acid burns are mild, most patients recover by this stage. Moderate burns are generally followed by gradual repair of the damaged tissue and resolution of the inflammatory response. Approximately 2 weeks after the injury, the more severe acid burns are characterized by stromal ulceration and progressive corneal vascularization (Fig. 6.2.9).

4. *Late reparative phase and sequelae (3 weeks and longer):* All but the most severe injuries heal by 3 weeks after the burn. In those that do not, persistent and progressive stromal opacification and/or vascularization or corneal ulceration may develop. Stromal ulceration is relatively uncommon after acid burns. Retrocorneal membranes appear during the late reparative phase if the endothelium has been severely damaged. Other sequelae characteristic of this phase include recurrent epithelial erosions, persistent or recurrent iritis, delayed cataract formation, glaucoma and hypotony with subsequent phthisis bulbi. The mechanism of each is the same as described for alkali burns.

MANAGEMENT

Emergency Management of Chemical Trauma

Immediate Management[16]

1. *Irrigation* of the eye with copious amounts of fluids is of paramount importance in decreasing the severity of injury. Severe blepharospasm can be overcome by instillation of anesthetic drops and passive opening of eyelids. All aspects of conjunctiva

and cornea should be irrigated asking the patient to look in all directions. A cotton-tipped applicator soaked in ethylene diaminetetracetic acid (EDTA) 1% can be used to clean lime particles from the cul-de-sac or the eye can be irrigated with 0.01–0.05 M solution. According to the American National Standards Institute (ANSI) eye burns should be washed for 15 minutes with at least 500–1,000 mL of irrigating fluid which may be normal saline, ringer lactate, balanced salt solution (BSS) or BSS plus. Water should be avoided as it is hypo-osmolar and may increase corneal edema with diffusion of the chemical into the deeper layers of the cornea. A new amphoteric solution—0.4% diphoterine (pH 7.4 and osmolarity 820 mOsm/L) which binds both alkalis and acids is proposed for initial irrigation. Irrigation may be facilitated by implantation of a T-tube and use of an irrigating scleral lens. The effectiveness of irrigation can be assessed by using universal indicator paper to determine the pH of the tears in the conjunctival fornices. Irrigation should be continued as long as pH values remain outside the normal range. If pH remains elevated despite continued irrigation, double eversion of the lid should be done to look for retained particles which can be removed with a jeweler's forceps. If the injury includes an explosion as in case of a car battery, ocular integrity must be assessed prior to manipulation.

2. *Debridement:* Necrotic corneal epithelium, conjunctival and subconjunctival tissue should be debrided to remove a nidus of continued inflammation and the sustained release of proteolytic enzymes.

3. *Paracentesis:* Value of paracentesis and AC lavage during the first 2 hours after severe injury is not clear.

Patient Examination

Once a normal pH level is attained, a full ophthalmological examination is performed. Visual acuity is recorded for each eye. Pupil examination is performed, noting any irregular shape or sluggish response to light. An irregular response may indicate iris ischemia due to chemical coagulation of the blood vessels in the iris or in the ciliary vessels. The facial skin, eyelids, lashes, and lacrimal apparatus are examined for areas of lid burn, which can cause incomplete globe coverage, and for residual chemical particulate matter. A slit lamp examination is performed to detect

epithelial loss, corneal opacification, and limbal ischemia. A torchlight examination of the corneal surface is done to observe the luster of the epithelium. Injured epithelial cells lack their typical reflective luster, resulting in an irregular corneal light reflex from the ocular surface. Any gray or white areas of stromal opacification are noted by observing whether iris detail or pupillary border is apparent when looking through the cornea. Limbal ischemia is measured by the number of clock hours of blood vessel loss of the conjunctival tissues where it nears the peripheral edge of the cornea (Figs 6.2.10 to 6.2.13). A fluorescein staining of the ocular surface is then done

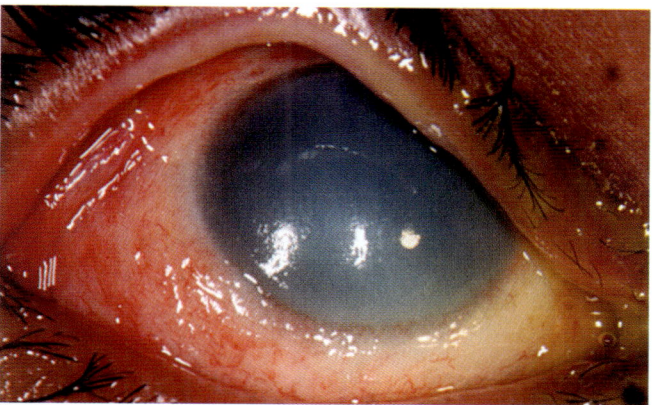

Fig. 6.2.10: Acid burns acute stage showing severe corneal edema with ground glass appearance and conjunctival ischemia of inferior 180°: grade IV by both Roper Hall and Dua's classification (moderate prognosis)

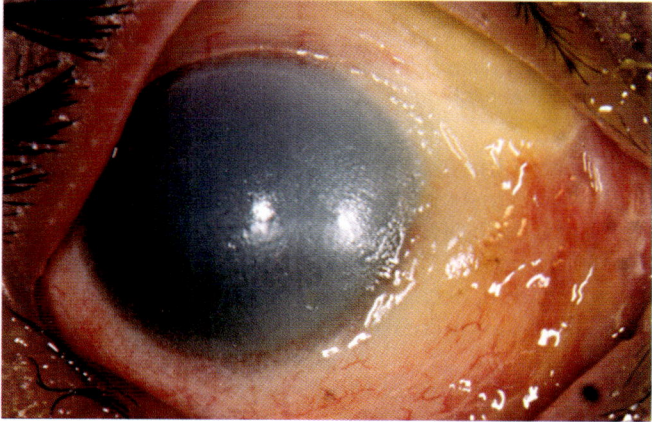

Fig. 6.2.11: With palpebral aperture widely opened showing superior conjunctival ischemia as well-grading worsens to grade V by Dua's classification

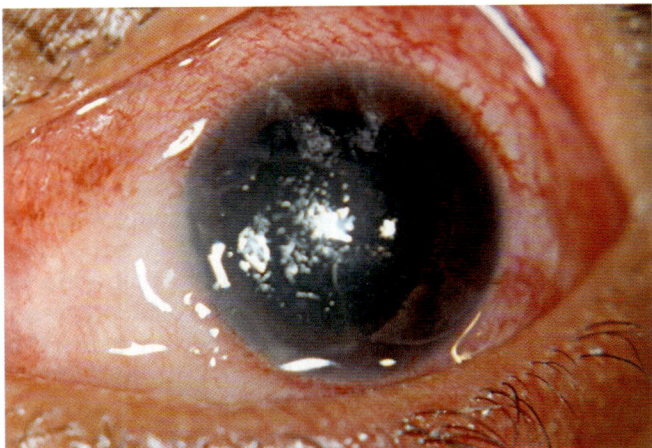

Fig. 6.2.12: Acute alkali burn with 4 o'clock hours limbal and conjunctival ischemia with localized epithelial defect corresponding to the area of limbal ischemia: grade II by Roper Hall and grade III by Dua's classification (good prognosis)

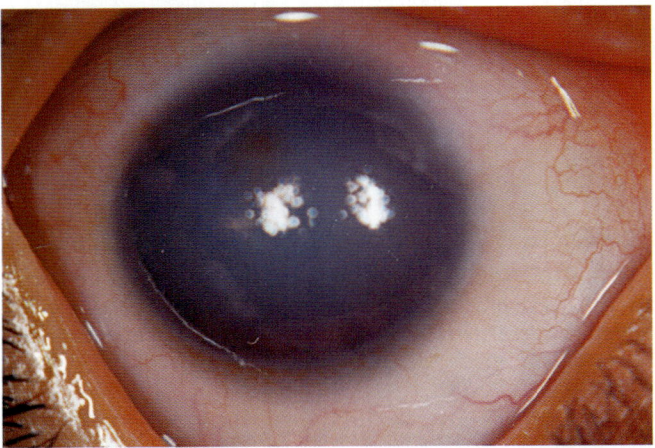

Fig. 6.2.13: Postoperative photograph of patient treated in the acute phase with amniotic membrane transplantation (AMT) with perilimbal hitching

to delineate the extent of corneal epithelial loss. IOP is measured instrumentally or digitally. The posterior segment is evaluated under dilatation with tropicamide or cyclopentolate. The use of phenylephrine is not recommended, because its vasoconstrictive properties may lead to an increased risk of ocular ischemia.

Medical and Surgical Management

Medical Management in Acute Phase

Aggressive medical management especially in grade I/II injuries ensures re-epithelialization of the cornea

and should start as soon as irrigation is complete. In grade III/IV injuries, medical management does not have much of a role and surgical intervention is required especially in grade IV injuries. Management of chemical injuries is an attempt to:

a. Promote complete re-epithelialization with normal corneal phenotypic transdifferentiation
b. Promote corneal repair and minimize ulceration
c. Control inflammation.

a. Promotion of Re-epithelialization with Transdifferentiation

1. *Tear substitutes:* Preferably preservative free tear substitutes with or without temporary/permanent punctual occlusion are of immense value. These should be continued even after complete re-epithelialization to prevent persistent epitheliopathy and to reduce the risk of recurrent erosions.

2. *Bandage soft contact lenses/collagen shields:* Protect the regenerating epithelium from the windshield-wiper effect of the lids and promote epithelial migration, regeneration of the basement membrane and epithelial stromal adhesion. However, they are poorly tolerated.

3. *Sodium hyaluronate:* Enhances the rate of epithelial migration following severe chemical injuries especially when combined with tenoplasty, may reduce conjunctival scarring and symblepheron formation.

4. *Investigational drugs:* Fibronectin (topical application has shown that it promotes re-epithelialization), epidermal growth factor (enhances the rate of epithelial migration following alkali injuries), retinoic acid (promotes transdifferentiation and probably goblet cell recovery, tear film stabilization and ocular surface wetting).

b. Promote Corneal Repair and Minimize Ulceration

1. *Ascorbate* used topically (10%) and systemically (2 gm QID) it can reduce the incidence of ulceration but does not prevent progression of established ulceration. In severe injuries, topical administration is superior to systemic administration as damage to ciliary body epithelium may reduce its active transport and concentration in the AC.

2. *Tetracycline derivatives* are efficacious in reducing collagenase activity and corneal ulceration probably

by chelation of zinc at the active site of the enzyme. They also inhibit PMN leukocyte activity. Doxycycline (100 mg BID) is more potent than tetracycline or minocycline.

3. *Collagenase inhibitors:* These include cysteine, acetylcysteine (mucomyst), sodium EDTA, calcium EDTA and penicillamine. Only acetylcysteine (10% and 20%) is available for clinical use. It is unstable, must be kept refrigerated and has to be replaced weekly, penetrates poorly into the stroma, has to be applied frequently and is relatively toxic.

c. Control Inflammation

1. *Corticosteroids:* They reduce initial inflammatory cell infiltration and ameliorate the second wave infiltration which begins at 7 days and peaks between 14 days and 21 days. They inhibit stimulation of keratocyte collagenase production by mononuclear leukocyte cytokines and stabilize PMN leukocyte cytoplasmic and lysosomal membranes. They also impair stromal wound repair by inhibiting keratocyte migration and collagen synthesis. The deleterious effects become evident after 10–14 days when corneal repair processes begin. The suppression of keratocyte collagen synthesis may offset the anti-inflammatory effect and collagenase inhibition resulting in corneal ulceration. Hence, their anti-inflammatory effect must be maximized in the first 7–10 days of injury and the dose can be tapered/discontinued at the earliest sign of corneal thinning.

Progestational steroids: Less potent anti-inflammatory agents but have a minimal effect on collagen synthesis and stromal wound repair. They also inhibit neovascularization. Topical, subconjunctival or systemic medroxyprogesterone (provera) may be started at 7–10 days of injury when corticosteroids are tapered/discontinued to suppress inflammation without inhibiting stromal healing.

2. *Nonsteroidal anti-inflammatory drugs (NSAIDs):* Reduce inflammation but the effect on collagen synthesis and stromal wound repair, neovascularization and collagenolytic activity is not known.

3. *Citrate:* It is a calcium chelator which decreases the membrane and intracellular calcium levels of PMN leukocytes. It inhibits collagenase and significantly reduces ulceration if administered early. Topical administration (10%) is superior to oral route.

Surgical Therapy

Ocular surface transplantation techniques are important for immediate re-establishment of limbal vascularity, to provide a proximate source of epithelium and limbal cells and as an anatomic barrier to keep adhering surfaces apart. In late cases, surgical intervention is required for re-estabilishment of conjunctival fornices, epithelial surface and normal apposition of the lids and globe.

a. Promotion of Re-epithelialization with Transdifferentiation

1. *Conjunctival/Tenon's advancement (tenoplasty):* It is based on the principle of using vital connective tissue to establish limbal vascularity and to provide a proximate source of epithelium for the denuded ocular surface. This may reduce the development of type IV healing pattern in severe burns. This technique has been reported to be useful in preventing anterior segment necrosis and sterile ulceration, but is less successful in complete recovery of the epithelial surface. The technique has been described by Teping and Reim.[17] All necrotic conjunctival and episcleral tissue is excised followed by blunt separation of Tenon's tissue from the globe and extraocular muscles (up to the equator). This flap with its carefully preserved vascular supply is advanced to the limbus and tightly sutured to the episclera. Its surface should be smooth to allow conjunctival epithelium to slide on it.

2. *Limbal stem cell transplantation (LSCT):* This is the only technique to re-establish a normal corneal phenotype in grades III/IV injuries at an early stage. The technique has been described by Kenyon and Tseng[18] (modified from Thoft's technique of conjunctival transplantation). Two crescents of peripheral corneal limbal epithelium with corresponding section of conjunctiva are harvested from the contralateral normal or less injured eye of the patient (autograft) or from a close relative (allograft) (Fig. 6.2.14). The graft should extend approximately 0.5 mm into the clear cornea centrally and 2 mm into the bulbar conjunctiva peripherally with a depth of 150 µm (calibrated diamond blade is preferred to achieve the desired depth). The initial incision is at the clear corneal edge to avoid visual obscuration by blood if conjunctiva is incised first.

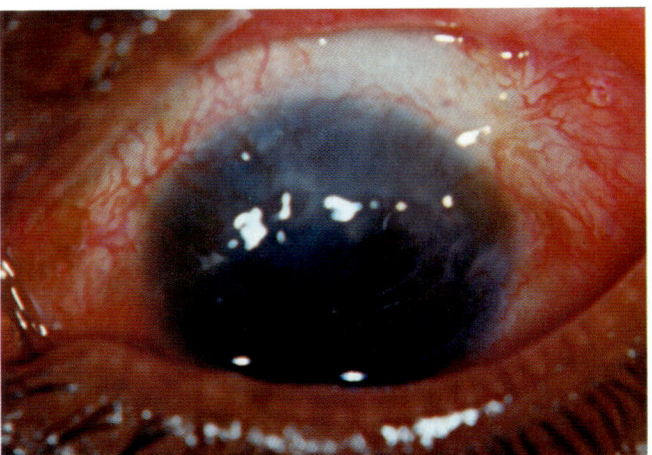

Fig. 6.2.14: Operated conjunctival—limbal autograft at 12 o'clock postoperative photograph of patient in Fig. 6.2.10

The second incision is made along the conjunctival margin and the intervening tissue is dissected free. The donor site can be left open as it heals spontaneously. The lenticules are sutured at the corneal margin with 10-0 nylon and at the conjunctival margin with 8-0 vicryl. A TBCL is placed to protect the grafts and allow re-epithelialization. Instead of two semicircular grafts, four lenticules can also be used.

In grade IV injuries, a tenoplasty either as a preparatory procedure or in conjunction with limbal stem cell transplantation (LSCT) is a must to establish vascularity for the grafts. Control of ocular inflammation and attachment of the lenticules to vascularized conjunctiva are important for successful transplantation. In most cases after allograft limbal transplant (ALT) re-epithelialization occurs within the first few weeks and epithelium is stable with good adhesion. When performed as a delayed procedure, as was being done previously, a superficial keratectomy is also required. Now, it is being done as early as 3 weeks after grade III injury to allow a healing similar to grade II injury. However, in the acute stages role of LSCT is not very well established due to inflammation and ischemia which may prevent uptake of the graft. In grade IV injury, the best possible outcome may be a type III healing pattern.

ALTs from live-related donor or cadaveric or cultured limbal stem cells (if suitable living donor is not available) are used for bilateral burns. But,

the chances of rejection are high of which is not prevented even with the use of systemic immuno-suppression. In the future, development of monoclonal antibodies to human limbal stem cells may allow harvesting of small numbers of limbal stem cells in eyes with incomplete but severe burns. Cell culture and intermediate animal transfer may be used before retransplantation in the original eye.

3. *Amniotic membrane transplantation (AMT):* It alone can be performed in the acute phase or it can be combined with ALT in the early or late reparative stages in severe cases.[19] Amniotic membrane does not express HLA-A/B/DR antigens and hence immunological rejection does not occur. It has anti-fibroblastic properties, serves as an anatomic barrier to keep adhering surfaces apart; the stromal matrix excludes inflammatory cells and contains various forms of protease inhibitors which reduce stromal inflammation. It is anti-angiogenic and inhibits neo-vascularization. It is believed to have anti-microbial properties. It also serves as a transplanted basement membrane and promotes epithelial migration, reinforces epithelial-stromal adhesion, promotes epithelial differentiaton and prevents epithelial apoptosis. Because of these properties amniotic membrane has been used in cases with persistent epithelial defects and as an alternate to conjunctival flaps. It has analgesic and anti-fibroblastic properties and suppresses subconjunctival fibrosis. It is believed that when used at an early stage AMT promotes ocular surface healing by decreasing the duration and severity of leucocyte infiltration and protecting the proliferating epithelial stem cells. In mild to moderate burns AMT alone rapidly restores both corneal and conjunctival surfaces. In severe cases, it restores the conjunctival ocular surface without formation of symblepheron and reduces limbal stromal inflammation but does not prevent limbal stem cell deficiency. Amniotic membrane can be used a circular patch covering the cornea and limbus. The membrane is transferred to cover the surface defect of the recipient eye with the basement epithelial surface facing up, i.e. the amniotic membrane surface is away from the cornea. The edges are sutured to the less damaged conjunctival surface with episcleral hitching woth 8-0 vicryl suture (Fig. 6.2.15). In severe cases, the whole ocular surface from lid margin to lid margin is covered with fornix forming sutures and a

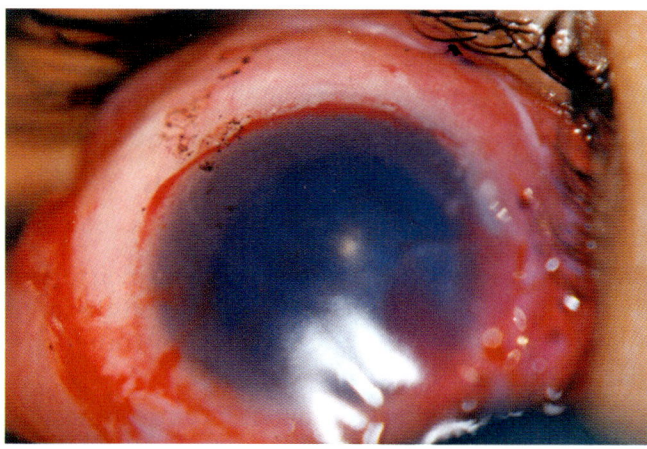

Fig. 6.2.15: Postoperative photograph of patient treated in the acute phase with AMT with perilimbal hitching

symblepheron ring is fitted over it. The membrane disintegrates on its own over a period of 7–20 days. Arora et al[20] have reported the outcome of fresh amniotic membrane for ocular surface reconstruction in acute chemical burns performed within 3 weeks of the injury. All patients in their series had immediate pain relief postoperatively with re-epithelialization and improved vision. None of the eyes showed corneal perforation. However, Dua et al[21] reported failure to restore the ocular surface or preserve the integrity of the globe in severe acute burns.

4. *Conjunctival transplantation:* Its role is largely confined to advancement with tenon's capsule with LSCT in acute burns to re-establish limbal vascularity.

5. *Keratoepithelioplasty:* It was described by Thoft in severe bilateral burns as an alternate to conjunctival transplantation. The procedure is technically difficult and results are poor. The initial procedures to restore the ocular surface used allogenic corneal donor limbal epithelium taken on thin crescents of stroma. Large diameter PK (11–12 mm) may provide a more favorable tissue for transfer and migration of limbal stem allografts and visual recovery than either keratoepithelioplasty or allograft LSCT alone. The main disadvantage of this procedure is eventual rejection.

b. Promote Corneal Repair and Minimize Ulceration

Progression to corneal thinning and perforation is common after grade III/IV injuries. Treatment is aimed at providing tectonic support (cyanoacrylate glue and tectonic PK) and ocular surface repair (tenoplasty, LSCT and large diameter therapeutic PK).

1. *Tenoplasty:* Vascularly derived collagenase inhibitors may prevent collagenolytic-related ulceration of the corneal stroma.

2. *Limbal stem cell transplantation:* Re-establishment of an intact epithelium arrests fibroblast collagenase production by cytokines and excludes PMN leucocytes thus supporting repair and minimizing ulceration.

3. *Large diameter therapeutic PK:* Favorable results have reported in both acute and chronic severe burns.[22]

4. *Cyanoacrylate glue:* This is reserved for impending perforations or actual perforations of 1 mm or less.[23] Glue is applied to the area and TBCL is placed over it. The glue can be left till it loosens spontaneously as re-epithelialization occurs or it can be removed when inflammation has subsided and neovascularization has taken place.

5. *Tectonic keratoplasty:* May be required for large perforations with or without iris prolapse. A small graft is preferred, cyanoacrylate glue may be required as an adjunct to prevent leaks at the graft-host junction or if thinning progresses with impending perforation within the graft itself. Large diameter therapeutic PK may be preferable as it may provide a tissue for transfer and migration of limbal stem allografts and visual recovery.

c. Late Rehabilitation

If conjunctivalization of the ocular surface is present despite early LSCT, a superficial keratectomy with ocular surface transplantation techniques can be done at later stages.

1. *Limbal stem cell transplantation:* In cases with superficial scarring and opacification, LSCT with superficial keratectomy may provide a dramatic improvement in corneal clarity. When deeper involvement is present, additional deep/lamellar keratoplasty (DLK)/PK may be needed with ALT. The prognosis for long-term graft survival is improved in these cases.

2. *Conjunctival transplantation:* Bulbar conjunctiva may be used to release adhesions as in symblepheron, cicatricial entropion, fornix fore-shortening, restriction of ocular movements, trichiasis, distichiasis and to relieve ocular surface keratinization and vascularization. It is used mainly in unilateral or asymmetric bilateral burns.[24]

3. *Mucus membrane grafts:* Mucosal tissue may be useful in reconstruction of the fornix and restoration of normal lid-globe apposition but does not provide source of epithelial regeneration. It is used in bilateral cases where contralateral conjunctiva is not available. Buccal/nasal mucosa may be used. Nasal mucosa may restore some mucus secreting capabilities of the ocular surface because of its goblet cells which may improve the prognosis for a subsequent PK.

4. *Penetrating keratoplasty:* Prognosis is favorable only if ocular surface can be rehabilitated by LSCT, conjunctival or mucus membrane transplants. Fresh donor material with intact epithelium is essential along with efforts to protect the epithelium intraoperatively. Oversized donor button with interrupted suturing technique may be used in vascularized corneas. In patients with dry eye punctual occlusion preoperatively or tarsorrhaphy intraoperatively can be performed.

5. *Keratoprosthesis:* It is indicated in bilateral severe injuries with irreparable ocular surface damage or when corneal transplants are repeatedly rejected.

Recommended Treatment

In the early management except grade IV injuries, medical therapy should be emphasized. In grade IV injuries, necrotic tissue debridement and tenoplasty is necessary. At the end of acute stage, LSCT should be considered if there is evidence of limbal ischemia.

Immediate treatment: Irrigation, debridement, paracentesis.

Acute phase
Grade I: Topical lubricants, corticosteroids, prophylactic antibiotics and antiglaucoma and cycloplegics if required.

Grade II/III:
1. Topical corticosteroids every 4–6 hourly
2. Sodium ascorbate (10%) 2 hourly topically
3. Sodium citrate 10% 2 hourly topically
4. Sodium ascorbate 2 g orally QID
5. Doxycycline 100 mg orally BID
6. Antiglaucoma and cycloplegics as required.

Grade IV: All of the above with tenoplasty.

Early repair phase
Grade I: Following complete re-epithelialization topical medication is tapered gradually and then discontinued. Topical lubricants may be continued for discomfort and PED.

Grade II: If re-epithelialization is incomplete, topical steroids, topical/systemic sodium ascorbate, topical/systemic tetracycline and topical citrate may be tapered.

Grades III/IV: Topical steroids should be discontinued or tapered with careful monitoring for corneal thinning and can be replaced by topical medroxyprogesterone or NSAIDs. Topical/systemic sodium ascorbate, topical/systemic tetracycline and topical citrate should be continued.

Late repair phase
Type I: Topical lubricants (preferably preservative free) may be continued for discomfort and persistent epitheliopathy.

Type II: Even with complete re-epithelialization prolonged lubrication may be needed for persistent epitheliopathy. Retinoic acid (0.01%) HS may be used for goblet cell dysfunction. Medroxyprogesterone 1% may be used for persistent inflammation and/or vascularization.

Types III/IV: LSCT or large diameter therapeutic PK should be considered for continued absence of epithelialization (Fig. 6.2.16). Topical/systemic sodium ascorbate, topical/systemic tetracycline, medroxyprogesterone or NSAIDs and topical sodium citrate should be continued post-surgery till re-epithelialization is complete.

Ocular chemical burns can be devastating and its sequelae can result in permanent blindness. Public education is an important factor in the prevention and early management of alkali injuries. Industrial safety precautions including eye protection gear and availability of equipment for immediate irrigation of the eye can improve the final outcome in many accidental burns.

Guidelines for Management of Chemical Burns

Irrigate immediately
↓

Acute phase: assess epithelial defect, conjunctival ischemia, corneal haze, limbal ischemia, retained particles, lid status, AC reaction, digital tension

Grade I	*Grade II/III*	*Grade IV*
Topical lubricants	Topical lubricants	Same as grade II/III
		With tenoplasty
Corticosteroids	Corticosteroids	
Antibiotics	Antibiotics	
Cycloplegics	Cycloplegics	
Antiglaucoma	Antiglaucoma	
	Sodium ascorbate topical/oral	
	Sodium citrate topical	
	Doxycycline	

↓

Early repair phase (2 weeks): assess epithelial defect, conjunctival ischemia, corneal haze, limbal ischemia, lid status, digital tension
↓

Taper steroids, if conjunctival ischemia and necrosis, symblepheron formation consider AMT
↓

Late repair phase (4–6 weeks): assess healing pattern
↓

Type I/II	*Type III/IV*
Re-epithelialization complete	Conjunctivalization
↓	Symblepheron
Lubricants	Corneal haze
	↓
	Consider LSCT with/without AMT/superficial keratectomy/ DLK/PK

REFERENCES

1. Parrish CM, Chandler JW. Corneal Trauma The Cornea, 2nd ed, In: Kaufman HE, Barron BA, Mc Donald MB. Published by Butterworth–Heinemann 1998:633–72.
2. Wagoner MD. Chemical injuries of the eye: Current Concepts in Pathophysiology and Therapy. Surv Ophthalmol 1997;41(4):275–313.
3. D Morgan S. Chemical burns of the eye, causes and management. Br J Ophthalmol 1987;71:854–7.
4. Griffith GA, Jones NP. Eye injury and eye protection: a survey of the chemical industry. Occup Med (Lond) 1994; 44(1):37–40.
5. Saini JS, Sharma A. Ocular chemical burns—clinical and demographic profile. Burns 1993;19(1):67–9.
6. Smolin and Thoft's The cornea, Scientific foundations and Clinical Practice Ed. 4th ed. Foster CS, Azar DT, Dohlman CH pub by Lippincott Williams and Wilkins 2005 Pfister RR Chemical trauma 2005:781–796.
7. Pfister DR, Pfister RR. Acid Injuries of the Eye. 1277–84. ed by Krachmer JH, Mannis MJ, Holland EJ, Cornea 2nd ed, Elsevier Mosby; 2005;1:1277–84.
8. Pfister RR, Pfister DR. Alkali Injuries of the Eye. 1285-94. ed by Krachmer JH, Mannis MJ, Holland EJ, Cornea 2nd ed vol 1 pub Elsevier Mosby 2005.

9. Agarwal T, Vajpayee RB, Sharma N, Tandon R. Severe ocular injury resulting from chuna packets. Ophthalmol 2006;113(6):960–961.

10. Horgan N, McLoone E, Lannigan B, et al. Eye injuries in children: A new household risk. *Lancet*. 2005;366:547–548.

11. Arora R, Sharma N, Sachdev R, et al. Common household items causing ocular injury. Accepted for publication in Cornea 2010.

12. Fung JF. Chem inj to the eye front from trichloroacetic acid. Dermatol surg 2002;28:609–610.

13. Velpandian T, Saha K, Ravi AK, Kumari SS, Biswas NR, Ghose S. Ocular hazards of the colors used during the festival-of-colors (Holi) in India—malachite green toxicity. J Hazard Mater 2007;139(2):204–8.

14. Roper Hall MJ. Thermal and chemical burns: Trans Ophthalmol Soc UK 1965;85:631–53.

15. Dua HS, King AJ, Joseph A. A new classification of ocular surface burns. Br J Ophthalmol 2001;85:1379–83.

16. Kuckelkorn R, Schrage N, Keeler G, et al. Emergency treatment of chemical and thermal eye burns. Acta Ophthalmol Sc and 2002;80:4–10.

17. Reim M, Teping C. Surgical procedures in the treatment of most severe eye burns. Revival of the artificial epithelium. Acta Ophthalmol Suppl 1989;192:47–54.

18. Kenyon KR, Tseng SCG. Limbal autograft transplantation for ocular surface disorders. Ophthalmology 1989;96:709–722.

19. Lee SH, Tseng SCG. AMT for persistent epithelial defects and ulceration. Am J Ophthalmol 1997;123:303–12.

20. Arora R, Jain V, Mehta DK. Amniotic membrane transplantation in acute chemical burns. Eye 2005; 19(3):273–8.

21. Dua HS. Failure of AMT in the treatment of acute ocular burns. Br J Ophthalmol 2001;85:1065–69.

22. Redbrake C, Buchal V, Reim M. Keratoplasty with a sclera rim after most severe eye burns. Klin Monatsbl Augenheilkd 1996;208:145–51.

23. Thoft RA. Conjunctival transplantation. Arch Ophthalmol 1977;95:1425–1427.

24. Togle JA, Kenyon KR, Foster CS. Tissue adhesive arrests stromal melting in the human cornea. Am J Ophthalmol 1980;89:795–802.

6.3 OCULAR INJURIES DUE TO PHYSICAL AGENTS

• Prerna Agrawal • DK Mehta

Mechanical trauma and chemical injuries have been responsible for blindness and visual morbidity. Physical agents are also responsible for ocular damage that may be temporary or long lasting. Visible and invisible spectrum of light and irradiations may damage the eye from corneal epithelium to retinal layers (Fig. 6.3.1 and Table 6.3.1).

IONIZING RADIATIONS AND EYE DAMAGE

X-rays and other radiation have been responsible to have caused collateral damage while there wide spread usage in different situation have been very useful. Ocular injuries due to these physical agents may effect lids, conjunctiva and lens.

a. *Lids:* The skin of lids is thinnest in our body next to prepuce, so it is particularly succeptible to damage by X-rays. These radiations can cause loss of lashes with scarring that can result in ectropion or entropion of lid margins. Watering and lacrimation is a common complaint that is difficult to address in a good number of cases.

b. *Conjunctiva:* Prolonged chronic exposure of conjunctiva to ionic radiation leads to loss of goblet cells and scarring of the conjunctiva that affect the mucinous layer of tear film resulting into dry eyes.

c. *Lens:* The adverse effect of X-ray on lenticular transparency radiation in a dose of 500–800 R is well documented. It can cause cataract sometimes with a delay of several months to a year before cataract

Table 6.3.1: Parts of the eye at risk from different wavelengths

Wavelength eye range	Eye component	Effect
180–315 nm (UV-B, UV-C)	Cornea	Photokeratitis equivalent to sunburn
315–400 nm (UV-A)	Lens iris	Photochemical cataract (clouding of lens), iritis
400–780 nm (visible)	Layers of retina	Photochemical damage to the retina, rays are maximally absorved by RPE, and macular xanthophil
780–1,400 nm (near IR)	Lens retina	Cataract, retinal burn
1.4–3.0 μm (IR)	Anterior chamber, cornea, lens	Aqueous flare (protein in the aqueous humor, cataract, corneal burn)
3.0 μm to 1 mm	Cornea	Corneal burn

appears and one may not relate the development of opacity to previous X-ray exposures.

ULTRAVIOLET RADIATION AND OCULAR INJURIES

The Cornea Absorbs Most UV Radiation (UVR)

The association between UV-B exposure and photo-keratitis, or snowblindness, has been established. UVR damage to the corneal epithelium is cumulative. Ozone in the atmosphere effectively filters most of the harmful UVR of wavelengths shorter than 290 nm; natural UV sources, such as the sun, rarely cause injury after short exposures. Exposure to the sun on highly reflective snow fields at high elevation can lead to direct corneal epithelial injury which is known as snow blindness.[1]

Artificial sources of UVR also cause corneal damage. Injury from a welder's arc commonly is known as flash burn, welder's flash, or arc eye. Other sources of UVR injury include sun tanning beds, carbon arcs, photographic flood lamps, lightening, electric sparks, and halogen desk lamps.

Prolonged exposures to UVR can lead to chronic solar toxicity, which is associated with several ocular

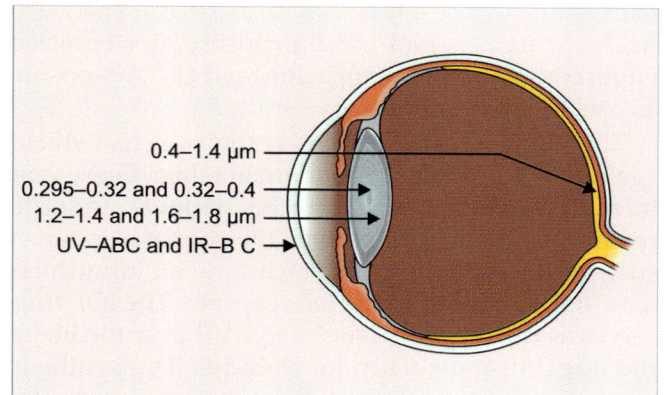

0.4–1.4 μm
0.295–0.32 and 0.32–0.4
1.2–1.4 and 1.6–1.8 μm
UV–ABC and IR–B C

Fig. 6.3.1: Parts of the eye at risk from different wavelengths

surface disorders (e.g. pinguecula, pterygium, climatic droplet keratopathy, squamous metaplasia, carcinoma). Pterygium is common in nasal side because of prolonged toxin exposure in lacus lacrimalis. The only ocular cancer associated with UVR is epidermoid carcinoma of the bulbar conjunctiva, which occurs with increased frequency in the tropics and subtropics and has been experimentally replicated in animal models using UVR. Rarely, retinal absorption of visible to near-infrared (400–1,400 nm) radiation from welding arcs can lead to permanent, sight-threatening injury.

Photophthalmia may be caused by exposure to short wavelength UV rays either reflected from snow surface (snow blindness) or from other sources (welding or short circuiting of high tension electric current). The essential pathology is desquamation of corneal epithelium causing multiple erosions. Symptoms appear after latent period of 5–6 hours of exposure. Healing occur by epithelium regeneration since Bowman's membrane is intact no opacity is left behind.

Pathophysiology: UV rays irritate the superficial corneal epithelium, causing inhibition of mitosis, production of nuclear fragmentation, and loosening of the epithelial layer. An inflammatory response occurs, which causes edema and congestion of the conjunctiva and a stippling of the corneal epithelium. SPK is a nonspecific corneal condition associated with multiple ocular disorders. It is characterized by small pinpoint defects in the superficial corneal epithelium, which stain with fluorescein. If superficial punctate keratitis (SPK) is severe, it may be followed by total epithelial desquamation, with conjunctival chemosis, lacrimation and blepharospasm. Re-epithelialization usually occurs within 36–72 hours, and long-term sequelae are rare. This SPK contrasts with the more severe effects frequently encountered with corneal damage caused by alkaline or strongly acidic chemicals.

Diffuse uptake of fluorescein stain as seen in ultraviolet keratitis (Fig. 6.3.2).

In general, ocular pain and decreased visual acuity occurs 6–12 hours after the injury. This lag time involves an unexplained pattern of corneal sensory loss and return and is thought to indicate a probable photochemical injury rather than a thermal injury to the cornea.

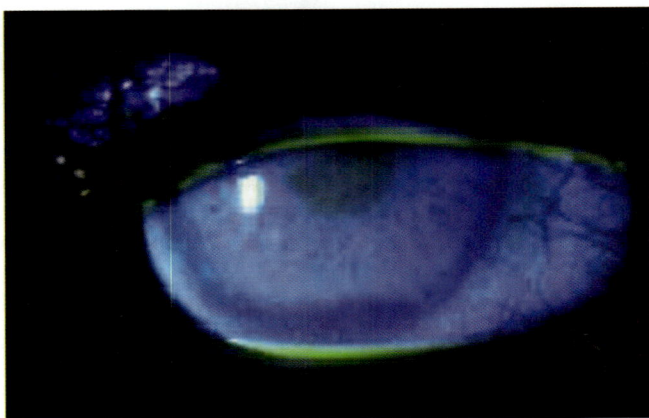

Fig. 6.3.2: Fluorescein stain showing diffuse stainning of cornea

The outdoor workers with high solar exposure have an approximate threefold risk of developing pterygium (a fleshy growth on a normally clear cornea) and a sixfold risk of having climatic droplet keratopathy (a deposition of altered proteins on the superficial cornea leading to opacification) of cornea.

Effects on the Lens

There is a proven association between UV-B exposure and development of cataract. But, UV exposure is supposed to be risk factor in development of cataract. One study examined 838 watermen who worked on the Chesapeake Bay, Maryland, USA (latitude 37° N), and showed a clear, consistent relationship between the development of cortical cataract and estimated ocular solar UV-B exposure. A doubling of exposure increased the risk of cortical cataract by a factor of 1.6. No evidence was found for a threshold level of sun exposure either in terms of irradiance, duration of exposure or age. There was no association between nuclear cataracts and UV-B exposure, nor between either cortical or nuclear opacities and UV-A exposure as concluded from the above study.[2-5]

The native crystalline lens is the principal shield against UVR, damage to the human retina. Every year in the US, more than 1 million patients undergo removal of the natural lens in the course of cataract surgery (phakectomy), at which time an intraocular lens (IOL) is placed in the lens capsule. The IOL thus serves as the principal barrier to UVR over the life of the implant, potentially for decades. The synthetic organic molecules of which IOLs are composed offer little UV protection unless ultraviolet-absorbing chromophores are incorporated into the lens material during manufacture. However, chromophores are alkenes potentially subject to radiolytic degradation. It is unknown whether ionizing radiation at clinical doses (e.g. to the brain or in the head-and-neck region) affects the UV-absorbing capacity of chromophore-bearing IOLs and consequently exposes the retina to potentially chronic UV damage. In addition, the polymers of which IOLs are composed are themselves subject to radiation damage, which theoretically might result in optical distortion in the visible light range. This suggests the selection of blue light-filtering IOLs for patients of any age, but especially for pediatric and presbyopic lens exchange patients with a longer pseudophakic life. Without clinically substantiated potential risks, these patients should experience the benefit of overall better quality of vision, reduced glare disability at least in some conditions, and better protection against retinal phototoxicity and its associated potential risk for age-related macular degeneration (AMD).[3-5]

Effects on the Retina

Unprotected exposures to the sun or solar eclipses may cause solar retinitis. There is no clear cut association between solar UV-B exposure and any effect on macular degeneration. Incidence of intraocular malignant melanoma has been linked with sunlight exposure. The macula in the aphakic eye may be at risk from solar UVR exposure following cataract surgery. The natural crystalline lens absorbs all incident UV-B and almost all UV-A radiation and concern has been expressed that some types of implanted thin plastic intraocular lenses may not provide adequate UV protection to the retina. There is no clear association of retinal damage and UV-B exposure.

A male welder who had been working in an industrial machine plant for more than 20 years experienced acute intense pain in his left eye with continuous lacrimation while performing arc welding in 1997. Later in 1997, at the age of 39 year, macular edema was found in his left eye. He was diagnosed with macular degeneration (MD) of the left eye in 2002, and with right eye MD in 2004. Radiation in the visible and near infrared (IR) spectra penetrates the eye and is absorbed by the retina, possibly causing thermal or photochemical damage. Such retinal damage may be permanent and, therefore, sight-threatening.[6] The

young age and history of an acute painful eye injury are not consistent with AMD but rather is likely maculopathy caused by welding arc exposure. Occupational welders exposed to a welding arc environment have a higher risk of phototoxic maculopathy than nonwelders, as diagnosed most effectively using OCT. Although the anterior portion of the eye is the most susceptible to UV damage, the retina is at risk to the longer UV wavelengths that propagate through the ocular media. Some phototoxicity may be counteracted or reduced by dietary intake of antioxidants and protective phytonutrients.

INJURIES DUE TO VISIBLE RADIATION (LIGHT)

Visible light penetrate fully to retina, cause thermal, mechanical and photic injuries. RPE absorbs light and converts it into heat that causes photocoagulation of retinal tissues. These injuries are usually caused by lasers used in therapy which increases the temperature in retina by 10–20°C. Mechanical injuries are caused by sonic shock waves produced from Q-switched or mode-locked laser which disrupt retinal tissue. Prolonged exposure to intense light cause varying degree of damage at macula. It is most commonly caused by sun gazing but prolonged exposure to welding arc can also cause retinal damage with consequent permanent decrease in visual acuity. The intensity of light, length of exposure and age all are important factors in determining the retinal damage. Natural lens absorbs most of the harmful rays, so people who have previously undergone cataract surgery are more at risk.

INJURIES DUE TO INFRARED RADIATION

Visible spectrum has IR accompaniment and intense bright visible light initiates the protective ocular responses like constriction of pupil, blink and reflex closure of eyes and blepharospasm. Effect on eyelid-blink reflex protects the eye and also spread tear film on anterior surface of eye for better protection. IR exposure and damage is often prevented by this mechanism. But, ocular exposure to IR rays in absence of visible spectrum does not initiate these responses and this leads to structural and functional damage.

Absorption of IR radiation by aqueous humor-leads to increase in temperature this rise in temperature raises the temperature of ocular components most notably lens. Iris pigment heavily absorbs IR and prolonged IR may result in low grade iritis, constriction of pupil and formation of aqueous flare.[7]

Effect on lens: A number of reports suggested that glassblowers and furnace workers had a higher incidence of cataracts than unexposed population.[7-9] There is not any specific type of cataract, true capsule exfoliation being only the specific sign. Cataract formation is due to direct absorption of IR in the lens or is secondary to heating of the aqueous humor and iris by absorption of IR.[10,11] This suggest photochemical type of lens damage with a constant dose relationship based on reciprocity between time and frame power[11] has shown that acute high level exposures direct to the iris can produce cataracts in the areas of the lens behind the exposed iris presumably through heat transfer. However many factors such as heredity, race, drug use, disease and immunological and nutritional factors can predispose toward cataractogenesis or be synergistic among themselves or with other factors.

Effect on retina: Absorption of shortest IR wavelengths differs only slightly with that of visible radiation. There are no specific effects of IR radiation on retina apart from thermal effects that are usually attributed to visible radiation.

SOLAR RETINITIS

Solar retinitis is a type of retinal ocular hazard that follows direct or indirect viewing of the sun. It is also known by names of photic retinopathy, eclipse retinopathy, solar retinopathy and foveomacular retinitis. It can occur in those individuals who view eclipse without protective eyewear and persons who gaze at sun. It is also seen in military persons who fly aircraft close to sun and also common with sun bathers.

Symptoms associated with the retinopathy include metamorphopsia, micropsia, central scotoma, paracentral scotoma, chromopsia, photophobia, an after image and decreased vision. Usually, it is a bilateral condition but unilateral cases do occur. In mild cases, a yellow spot may be detected in fovea on fundoscopy that is surrounded by a gray zone from within a few days of photic injury after watching solar eclipse.

The symptoms appeared at various intervals usually within 1–4 hours of looking at eclipse. The onset was insidious in cases of sun gazing and the duration of development of symptoms could not be ascertained. The symptoms were closely related to the severity of the fundus lesion. In grade I the usual symptoms were metamorphopsia, micropsia, photophobia and glare and diminution of vision. In grade II, there was blurring of vision, fogging and translucid scotoma. In grade III and IV, absolute and positive scotoma with gross diminution of vision occurred. The ocular findings recorded in different grades were as under:

- *Grade I:* The macula was apparently normal.
- *Grade II:* The macula was congested and was surrounded by an edematous area of retina.
- *Grade III:* A greyish white patch surrounded the fovea which was surrounded in turn by a black pigmentary ring.
- *Grade IV:* Macular cyst/macular hole and gross pigmentary changes.

The severity of lesion was dependent on amount of visual energy absorbed. It is suggested that amblyopic eye resists the visual energy stimulus or else there is lack of concentration of visual energy at the macular area either through a defective focusing mechanism or through lack of normal visual chemical substance. The basic pathologic defect in solar retinitis is probably identical to central angiospastic retinopathy, i.e. a vasospasm and diminution of retinal nutrition in that area cause ischemia. In all cases of grade I and II and some cases of grade III, the retro-bulbar injection of 1 mL of priscol was the treatment of choice. Priscol probably acts by vasodilation and improves nutrition of retina that pretreatment with ketamine-xylazine anesthesia protects retinas against light damage, reducing photoreceptor cell death. These data support the notion that anesthesia with ketamine-xylazine provides neuroprotective effects in light-induced cell damage The current treatment revolves around anti-inflammatory regimes rather than vasodilators.

LIGHTNING RETINOPATHY

Lightning maculopathy describes acute visual loss and macular changes that occur after one is injured by lightning. Lesions described include macular edema, macular hole, cyst, or a solar retinopathy-like picture, cataract, retinal detachment, retinal artery occlusions, and relative afferent pupillary defect.[12] Visual recovery often occurs over time, even with severe maculopathy. High-dose intravenous methylprednisolone treatment may play a role in recovery of vision, because its use has been associated with reversal of lightning-induced blindness.[13]

OPERATING MICROSCOPE PHOTOTOXICITY

Operating microscope phototoxicity has been associated with multiple surgical factors, including increased microscope brightness, wavelength of light exposure, prolonged surgical duration, and surgical technique.[14] Although the duration of surgery has decreased with phacoemulsification, phototoxic retinal lesions still may occur. Retinal phototoxic lesions after short-duration cataract surgery (defined as surgery less than 30 minutes) were associated with a final refraction within 1.0 D of emmetropia and with diabetic retinopathy.[14] The risk of photic damage may increase after IOL insertion, which can focus the incoming light on the retina; however, photic injury has been described without IOL insertion. Patient susceptibility factors include increased body temperature and blood oxygenation, chorioretinal pigmentation, pre-existing maculopathy, pupillary dilatation, diabetes mellitus, retinal vascular disease, deficiencies of either ascorbic acid or vitamin A, and hydrochlorothiazide use.

The risk of photic damage may increase after IOL insertion, which can focus the incoming light on the retina; however, photic injury has been described without IOL insertion. Patient susceptibility factors include increased body temperature and blood oxygenation, chorioretinal pigmentation, pre-existing maculopathy, pupillary dilatation, diabetes mellitus, retinal vascular disease, deficiencies of either ascorbic acid or vitamin A, and hydrochlorothiazide use.

LASER EXPOSURE/IRRADIATION

Laser instruments are used in all areas of human activity. Use of lasers in different fields carry its own advantages but it may also lead to accidental injuries. These injuries are mostly retinal because of the concentration of visible and near infrared radiation (400–1,400 nm, retinal hazard region) on retina. Mostly these radiations are absorbed by melanin pigment in RPE. Retina is most vulnerable to laser radiation which are used in dermatology. The nature and severity if retinal injury depends on duration of laser and amount of energy transferred. Retinal injury may cause sudden loss of vision that may improve over a period of few weeks and sometimes it is associated with late complications.

UV and far IR spectrum are absorved by anterior segment of eye causing damage to cornea and lens. IR radiations are very dangerous because only the visible light initiates blink reflex. People who are exposed to high power Nd:YAG laser (1,064 nm) donot experience pain and indication of retinal damage is from pop or click sound due to very high temperatures generated at RPE level (actually retina was heated above 100°C) resulting in immediate creation of blind spot. Most commonly accidental injuries with laser use are seen in military. Adherence to safety practices effectively prevents accidental laser induced ocular injuries. Protection should be given to all persons in the laser-operating room including the patient, laser operator, assistants, and observers. Laser radiation predominantly causes injury via thermal effects. Moderate to high powered lasers can cause injury to the eye.

Lasers can cause *complications* or *incidents*, depending on whether the undesirable effect is within or outside the area of treatment. There is no treatment in medicine which does not expose the patient to some risk of complication. Even though lasers can be considered particularly safe instruments, their rate of complications is not zero. One can only hope to reduce their frequency by better training of doctors and improvements in the knowledge of laser effects on tissue. On the other hand, the rate of incidents must be, and is for most of the time, nil. These are incidents which are concerned with problems of safety. Their prevention is achieved through a good knowledge of their causes and the application of measures which allow them to be avoided.

There are two possible types of incident: (1) those related to the laser beam itself (optical risks) and (2) those due to other causes (nonoptical hazards).

DAMAGE MECHANISMS IN LASER EXPOSURE

Laser can cause damage to biological tissues by various mechanisms. Denaturation of proteins occur due to rise in temperature which cause thermal damage to biological tissue. Laser light also triggers photochemical reactions which are more common with short wavelength and UV. Ultra-short pulses can also exhibit self-focusing in the transparent parts of the eye, leading to an increase of the damage potential compared to longer pulses with the same energy.[7]

The skin is usually much less sensitive to laser light than the eye but excessive exposure to UV light from any source (laser or non-laser) can cause short- and long-term effects similar to sunburn, while visible and IR wavelengths are mainly harmful due to thermal damage.[4]

Lasers potentially usable for keratorefractive surgery have wavelength in UV range and lasers used in argon laser trabeculoplasty have wavelength in visible spectrum.

Laser Pointer and Ocular Trauma

The use and availability of laser pointers to the general public has become quite common. There is a potential for misuse of and inadvertent ocular exposure to these handheld lasers. As well, the emitted red beam may produce visual distraction or simulate a weapon-aiming beam. There are very few reports of presumed retinal damage caused by laser pointers.[15-18] The mechanism of injury is not clear, but it appears due to thermal chorioretinal damage, because the longer red 650 nm or 635 nm wavelength light emitted from a laser pointer should not produce significant retinal phototoxicity.[19] Damage manifests as transient visual abnormalities and macular RPE disturbances that correspond to window defect hyperfluorescence on fluorescein angiography.[15] Acute uniocular reduction in vision to 20/40 with two small pericentral scotomata and a hypopigmented ring-shaped foveal lesion was described in a 19-year-old woman after deliberate staring into a commercial class II laser pointer for 10 seconds. Visual acuity improved to 20/20 and visual field returned to normal within 8 weeks, but a subjective decrease in brightness and foveal RPE disturbances persisted. Retinal injury was not demonstrated in three patients after class IIIA laser pointer retinal exposure (parameters 1 mW, 2 mW, or 5 mW for up to 15 minutes' duration to foveal and juxtafoveal locations) prior to enucleation for uveal melanoma. Other than transient after images for minutes, there was no specific laser-induced ocular damage noted with ophthalmoscopy, angiography, or histology.[20] Thus, it appears to be difficult to produce ocular injury with a laser pointer without deliberate inappropriate, prolonged, foveal exposure. Factors such as patient age, pre-existing maculopathy, and clarity of the ocular media likely play a role in determining retinal susceptibility to damage.

Laser pointers are effective tools when used properly. The following considerations should be observed when using laser pointers:

- Never look directly into the laser beam
- Never point a laser beam at a person
- Do not aim the laser at reflective surfaces
- Never view a laser pointer using an optical instrument, such as binocular or a microscope
- Do not allow children to use laser pointers unless under the supervision of an adult
- Use only laser pointers meeting the following criteria
  - Labeled with food and drug administration (FDA) certification stating "Danger: Laser Radiation" for class IIIR lasers or "Caution: Laser Radiation" for class II pointers.
  - Classified as class II or IIIR according to the label. Do not use class IIIb or IV products.
  - Operates at a wavelength between 630 nm and 680 nm.

Has a maximum output less than 5 mW, the lower the better.

Lasers and Aviation

Since November 19, 2004 there have been over 2,800 incidents of lasers directed at aircraft within the US which led to an inquiry in the US Congress.[5] Laser exposure may create dangerous conditions such as flash blindness, if this occurs during a critical moment in aircraft operation, the aircraft may be endangered. Some individuals experience an involuntary sneezing fit when exposed to a sudden flash of light.

Specific symptoms of laser injury, when there is exposure to a visible laser beam, one can detect bright color flash of the emitted wavelength and after image of its complimentary color. When there is some retinal damage due to laser, there is difficulty in detecting blue and green colors secondary to cone damage. Invisible carbon dioxide laser beam causes burning pain at the site of exposure on cornea and sclera. Q switched Nd:YAG laser beam is invisible and causes no pain, so it is more dangerous as it initially goes unnoticed, mostly it is diagnosed by pop sound at the time of exposure. The pop sound emmited by lasers indicates very high energy entering the eye and requires reduction in energy in further shots.

Laser classification: Lasers have been classified by wavelength and maximum output power into four classes and a few subclasses since the early 1970s. The classifications categorize lasers according to their ability to produce damage in exposed people, from class I (no hazard during normal use) to class IV (severe hazard for eyes and skin). There are two classification systems, the "old system" used before 2002, and the "revised system" being phased in since 2002.

Lasers and laser systems are classified by their ability to cause biological damage to the eye or skin during use. Purchased lasers are labeled and classed by manufacturers to comply with requirements of the Federal Laser Product Performance Standard. Lasers which are modified in ways which may change the classification provided by the manufacturer must be reclassified by the Laser Safety Officer in accordance with ANSI Standard Z-136.1–1993, "American National Standard for the Safe Use of Lasers."

Class I Lasers

Lasers or laser systems incapable of producing damaging radiation during intended use are class I lasers. These lasers are exempt from any controls or administrative requirements during normal use. Most class I laser systems contain embedded lasers of a higher class, however. Alignment and service procedures for embedded class II, III, or IV lasers require appropriate control and administrative procedures appropriate to the class during these functions.

Class II Lasers

Class II lasers (low power) are lasers emitting radiation in the visible portion of the spectrum. Even though the power of these lasers is such that they will normally be protected by a physiological aversion response (blink reflex), personnel should wear laser eyewear for protection. The class II maximum permissible exposure limits can be exceeded if the beam is viewed directly for extended periods.

Class III Lasers

Class III lasers and laser systems (medium power) produce radiation that can cause eye damage when viewed directly, or when a specular reflection is viewed. A diffuse reflection is usually not a hazard.

Class IV Lasers

Class IV lasers and laser systems (high power) produce radiation that may be dangerous to the eye even when viewing a diffuse reflection. The direct beam can produce skin damage and can also be a fire hazard.

Many laser systems contain embedded lasers which are more hazardous (of higher class) than the system. Alignment or service procedures for embedded lasers must be conducted in accordance with requirements appropriate for the class of the embedded laser.

Lasers or laser systems that are modified in ways that may alter the hazard of the emitted radiation must be reclassified by the laser safety officer (LSO) in accordance with ANSI Z-136.1–1993. The reclassification will usually be from a lower to a higher class. Although modifications of laser systems which provide additional safety features may result in a lower classification.

Multiwavelength Lasers

Laser classification will be based on the most hazardous possible configuration for a multi-wavelength laser or laser system.

Eye Safety and Technical Considerations

Maximum permissible exposure (MPE), is the level of exposure of laser radiation to a person which does not have hazardous effects in the eye. MPE level depends on laser wavelength, exposure time and pulse repetition. The MPE is usually expressed either in terms of radiant exposure in J/cm^2 or as irradiance in W/cm^2 for a given wavelength and exposure duration. If person is exposed to laser energy above MPE, it results in biological tissue damage. Generally, longer the wavelength, the higher the MPE the longer the exposure time, lower the MPE.

The nominal hazard zone (NHZ) is the physical space in which direct, reflected or scattered laser radiation exceeds the MPE. LSE must be worn within NHZ. When lasers are used in dermatologic procedures, the entire room should be considered within NHZ as laser fiber can be directed anywhere in the room.

Safety Measures
General Precautions

Everyone who uses a laser should be aware of the risks. This awareness is not just a matter of time spent with lasers; to the contrary, long-term dealing with invisible risks (such as from infrared laser beams) tends to reduce risk awareness, rather than to sharpen it.

- Adequate eye protection should always be required for everyone in the room if there is a significant risk for eye injury.
- Never point a laser in someone's eyes, even low power hand held units can cause eye damage due to the focusing effect of the lens in the eye.
- Never project un-scanned beams into an audience.
- Never deflect laser beams with hand held mirrors as they are difficult to control and can direct beams in unexpected ways causing eye damage.
- Do not use mirrors or watch crystals to deflect static beams at shows as you can cause eye damage to yourself or other spectators.
- Watches and other jewelry that might enter the optical plane should not be allowed in the laboratory.
- Never float Mylar coated balloons at shows into the beam paths above the audience as they can deflect laser beams into people's eyes.
- Never track a moving vehicle such as a car or aircraft with a laser—even a very low power hand held HeNe laser or diode based laser pointer. With higher power units you may temporarily blind the operator or destroy their night vision. The effect is similar to having your picture taken with a flash camera in a dark room. There is no permanent damage but your vision is disrupted and there is an after image of the flash that persist for some seconds. Even low power lasers may cause a distraction to the driver/pilot leading to an accident.
- Optical experiments should be carried out on an optical table with all laser beams travelling in the horizontal plane only, and all beams should be stopped at the edges of the table. Users should never put their eyes at the level of the horizontal plane where the beams are in case of reflected beams that leave the table.
- High-intensity beams that can cause fire or skin damage (mainly from class IV and ultraviolet lasers) and that are not frequently modified should be guided through tubes.
- Alignment of beams and optical components should be performed at a reduced beam power whenever possible.

Protective Eye Wear

Selection of specific eyewear[21] in laser area

1. Laser wavelength at which protection is afforded.
2. Optical density (OD) of the LSE for the wavelength being used. OD refers to the ability of a material to reduce laser energy of a specific wavelength to a safe level below the MPE. It can be expressed by the following formula:

$$OD = \log 10 \ (E_i/E_t)$$

E_i = incident beam irradiance (W/cm^2) for a "worse case exposure"

E_t = transmitted beam irradiance (MPE limit in W/cm^2)

The required OD for any given laser can be determined by:

a. Calculation
b. Consulting nomograms or tables (e.g. ANSI 136.1 guidelines)
c. Consulting the laser manufacturer.

The OD of the LSE will decrease if the LSE is damaged. The damage threshold refers to the maximum protection that the LSE will provide for at least 5–10 seconds following noticeable melting.

Protective Eyewear

Protective eyewear in the form of spectacles or goggles with appropriately filtering optics can protect the eyes from the reflected or scattered laser light with a hazardous beam power, as well as from direct exposure to a laser beam. Eyewear must be selected for the specific type of laser, to block or attenuate in the appropriate wavelength range (Fig. 6.3.3).

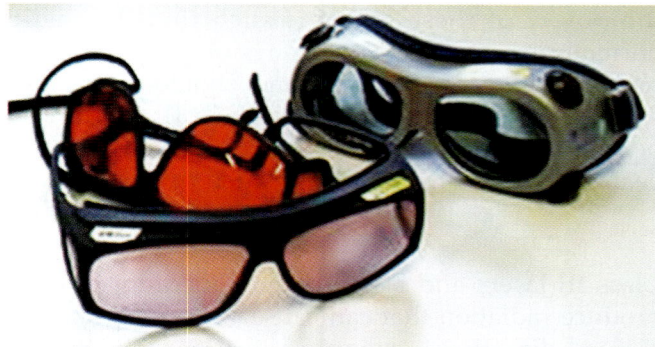

Fig. 6.3.3: Protective glasses

Laser Goggles

- Tightly fitting goggles
- Big enough to accommodate prescription glasses under them
- Constructed with frame vents to minimize lens fogging.

Spectacles

- Seperate lenses with side sheilds
- These glasses should be available easily vision-correcting prescription eye glasses to avoid the exposure to the ammetropic patients.

Wraps

Wraps are light and made of one lens for both eyes.

Other Safety Measures Interlocks and Automatic Shutdown and Laser Safety Officer

Some systems have electronics that automatically shut down the laser under other conditions.

In many jurisdictions, organizations that operate lasers are required to appoint a LSO. The LSO is responsible for ensuring that safety regulations are followed by all other workers in the organization.

Practical Pearls in Laser Eye Safety[21]

1. *Laser warning signs* must be placed at the entrance to laser operating rooms.

2. Only those individuals who are adequately *educated in laser safety should be allowed entry in laser rooms*. Each laser facility must develop its own safety procedures to be enforced by an appropriately trained LSO for the facility.

3. As LSE often looks alike in style and color, it is mandatory to *check the wavelength and optical density* imprinted on each pair of LSE prior to its use.

4. *Color coding* of the laser handpiece and LSE may help to minimize confusion especially in facilities where multiple laser wavelengths are available.

5. *LSE should not move between laser rooms,* nor should they be carried in laboratory coat pockets between use.

6. LSE can be very expensive, so proper care and handling is mandatory. The integrity of the LSE must be *inspected regularly* since small cracks or loose fitting filters may permit the laser beam to reach the eye directly.

7. The *patient's eyes must always be protected* from laser energy. If the patient is awake, appropriate opaque "mini" goggles must be worn. Great care must be taken to avoid accidentally exposing the straps of the patient goggles to laser light, since this can ignite them.

8. Whenever laser energy is used in the immediate vicinity of the eye (treating eyelids) a *stainless steel or lead eye shield* should be positioned on the surface of the orbit after the application of a topical ophthalmic local anesthetic. Plastic patient eye shields cannot be expected to withstand the thermal and mechanical effects of pulsed lasers, and should never be used.

REFERENCES

1. Ultraviolet Keratitis. Author: Reed Brozen, MD; Chief Editor: Rick Kulkarni, MD

2. Diffley BL. Solar ultraviolet radiation effects on biological systems. Phys.Med.Biol. 1991 vol 36(3):299–328. Regional medical Physics Department, Dryburn Hospital, Durham DHI 5TW,UK

3. Mainster MA, Turner PL. Blue–Blocking IOLs decrease photoreception without providing significant photo-protection. Surv Ophthalmol 2010;55(3):272–89.

4. Mainster MA and Turner PL. Blue light's benefits Vs blue blocking intraocular lens chromophores. Graefes Arch. Clin Exp. Ophthalmol. 2012;250(8):1247–48. Published online 2011 August7.doi.10.1007/s00417-011–1749.

5. Ellerin BE, Nisce LZ, Roberts CW, Thornell C, Sabbas A, Wang H, Li PM, Nori D.The effect of ionizing radiation on intraocular lens. Int J Radiat Oncol Biol Phys. 2001 1;51(1):184–208

6. Kim EA, Kim BG, Yi CH, Kim IG, Chae CH, Kang SK. Macular degeneration in an arc welder. Ind Health. 2007; 45 (2):371–3.

7. Fischer, FP et al. Uber die zur Schadigung des Auges notge Minimal-quantitat von ultravioletem and infraotem Licht (On the minimum amount of ultraviolet and infrared light required to damage the eye).Archiv fur Augenheikunde, 1935;109:462–67.

8. Mackenzie WA. A practical treatise on diseases of the eye.: Philadelphia, PA, Blanchard & Lee, PP 1985.

9. Meyhofer W. Quoted by Turner HS. The interaction of infrared radiation with the eye: a review of the literature. Columbus, OH, Ohio State Research Foundation, 1970.

10. Pitts DG, Cullen AP. Determination of infrared radiation levels for acute ocular cataractogenesis:.Von Graefes Archiv fur Klinische and experimentelle Ophthalmologie, 1981;217:285–297.

11. Wolbarsht ML. Damage to the lens from infrared; Proceedings of the Society for photo-optical and Instrumentation Engineers. 1980;229:121–142.

12. Lee MS, Gunton KB, Fischer DH, Brucker AJ. Ocular manifestations of a remote lightning strike retina.; Am J Ophthalmol. 2002;22: 808–10.

13. Norman ME, Younge BR. Association of high-dose intravenous methylprednisolone with reversal of blindness from lightning in two patients. Ophthalmology. 1999;106:743–5.

14. Kleinmann G, Hoffman P, Schechtman E, Pollack A. Microscope-induced retinal phototoxicity in cataract surgery of short duration. Ophthalmology. 2002;109:334–8.

15. Sell CH, Bryan JS. ,Maculopathy from handheld diode laser pointer. Arch. Ophthalmol. 1999; 117:1557–8.

16. Zamir E, Kaiserman I, Chowers I. Laser pointer maculopathy. Am. J Ophthalmol. 1999;127:728–9.

17. McGhee CNJ, Crain JP, Moseley H. Laser pointers can cause permanent retinal injury if used inappropriately. Brit J Ophthalmol. 2000;84:229–230.

18. Mainster MA, Timberlake GT, Warren KA, Sliney DH. Pointers on laser pointers. Ophthalmology. 1997; 104:1213–4

19. Mainster MA, Reichel E. Transpupillary thermotherapy for age-related macular degeneration: long-pulse photocoagulation, apoptosis and heat shock proteins. Ophthalmic Surgical Lasers. 2000;31:359–73.

20. Robertson DM, Lim TH, Salomao DR, et al. Laser pointers and the human eye: a clinicopathologic study. Arch Ophthalmol. 2000;118:1686–91.

21. Laser Safety and the Eye, Hidden Hazards and Practical Pearls Osama Bader and Harvey Lui. From the Lions Laser Skin Centre, Division of dermatology. Vancouver Hospital and Health Sciences Center and University of British Columbia, Vancouver, BC Presented at the American Academy of Dermatology, Annual meeting Poster Session, Washington DC. Febuary 10–15, 1996.

Posterior Segment Trauma

• R Kim • Manish Tandon

POSTERIOR SEGMENT TRAUMA

Introduction

Ocular trauma is one of the leading causes of uniocular visual loss and is associated with socioeconomic loss. Lack of unambiguous terminologies related to trauma is one of the major factors in description of eye injuries and causes communication errors. Hence, a standard classification for ocular trauma was proposed by Ocular Trauma Society Group to categorize the ocular injury at the time of initial patient examination.[1] This classification has been designed for the use of ophthalmic and non-ophthalmic personnel who care for patients with ocular injuries and conduct research on ocular injuries Fig. 7.1.1.

OPEN GLOBE INJURIES

Pathophysiological Basis of Ocular Wound Healing[2]

Open globe injury causes break in blood ocular barrier and inflammation which is potentiated by the loss of blood ocular barrier. Inflammation causes release of cytokines and growth factors which exert effect on adjacent retinal pigment epithelium (RPE) fibroblasts and glial cells. The RPE exacerbates the contractile forces that develop as a result of fibroblastic activity. When this fibroblastic activity reaches a critical level it overcomes the forces between RPE and neural retina thus causing tractional retinal detachment (RD) (Fig. 7.1.2).

Histopathology of Eye in Penetrating Eye Injury[3]

The histopathology of eye in penetrating eye injury in experimental conditions on rhesus monkey eyes is

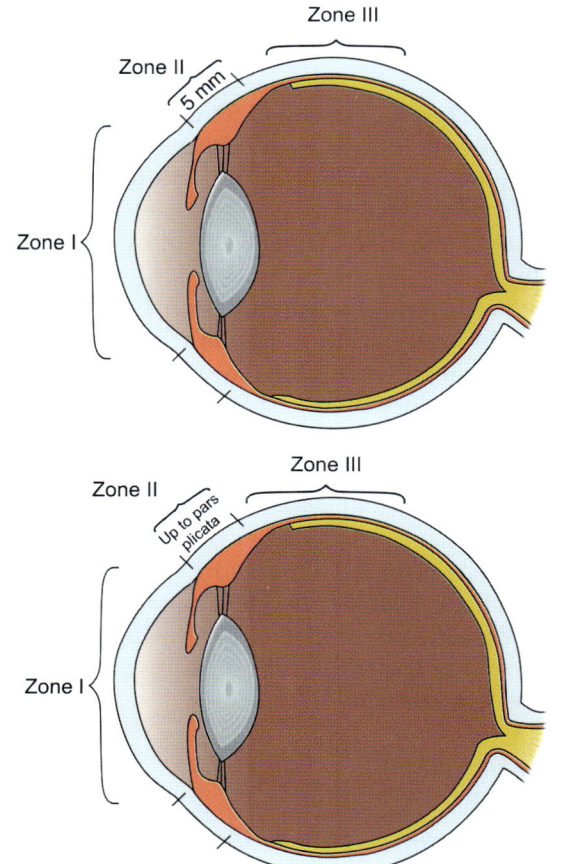

Fig. 7.1.1: Zones of injuries

also applicable to human eyes. The characteristic findings were intraocular fibrosis with the formation of cyclitic membranes and epiretinal and subretinal

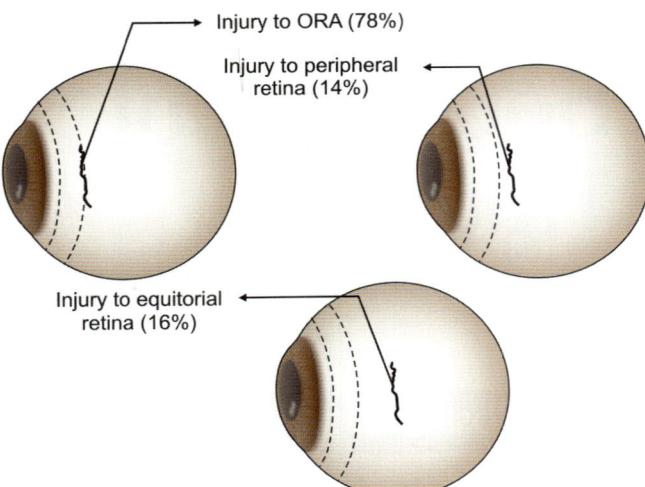

Fig. 7.1.2: Chances of (RD) secondary to ocular trauma at different location[4]

3. *Inflammatory cells:* These are the earliest cells to be involved due to breakdown of blood retinal barrier. The effect is the recruitment of other inflammatory cells and collagen formation. The cellular and humoral immune response to retinal antigens following RD and proliferative vitreoretinopathy in experimental conditions point toward an association of autoimmunity being involved but clear evidence is lacking.

4. *Glial cells:* These contribute to proliferative vitreo-retinopathy (PVR) membranes and are derived from Müller cells or retinal astrocytes.

5. *Tenon fibroblasts:* They have a role in PVR development in trauma with scleral wound and vitreous hemorrhage.

6. *Myofibroblasts:* These originate from fibroblasts and RPE cells. They have an important role in wound contraction in granulation tissue.

membrane. The progression to fibrous in growth from a wound occurs only in eyes with blood in vitreous. The intravitreal fibroblastic proliferation has origin mainly from stroma of ciliary body and choroids at the wound and also from non-pigmented ciliary epithelium.

Fibroblastic response starts within 4 days after the injury and forms cyclitic membrane by 6 weeks.

Epiretinal membranes have been noted to form by 4 weeks after injury over peripheral retina anterior to the equator. These epiretinal membranes originate from fibrous in growth as well as from glial cells.

The subretinal membranes originate from RPE and glial cells.

Also, it has been shown in animal models that the maximal chances of RD are when injury to ora serrata occurs (78%) as compared to injury through equatorial retina (16%) and peripheral retina involving ciliary body and ora serrata.

Cellular Constituents to Formation[5] of Epiretinal Membranes

1. *Retinal pigment epithelium:* The RPE have a special property of migration, proliferation and alteration of their phenotype to become macrophage, fibroblast and have myofibrillary morphology.

2. *Growth factors:* The growth factors like hepatocyte growth factor have effect on RPE with an epithelial to mesenchymal morphological transformation.

Pathogenesis of Epiretinal Membrane (Fig. 7.1.3)

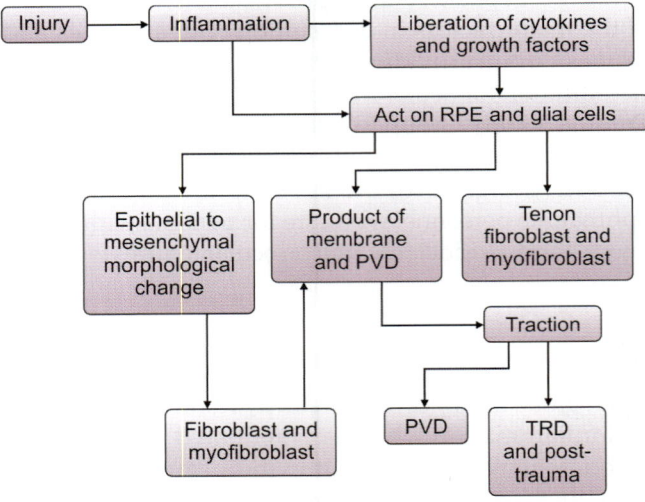

Fig. 7.1.3: Development of epiretinal membrane

Anatomic Changes in Posterior Segment Secondary to the Effect of Trauma

1. Posterior vitreous detachment (PVD)[6]
2. Tractional retinal detachment (TRD) and posterior tractional PVR[7]
3. Traumatic endophthalmitis
4. Intraocular foreign body (IOFB)

Posterior Vitreous Detachment (Fig. 7.1.4)

Breakdown of blood ocular barrier leads to migration of macrophages and leakage of serum component into the vitreous cavity. Macrophages release enzymes and lyse vitreous gel and vitreoretinal bond. Cleavage may occur at following locations:

a. Between cortical vitreous and internal limiting membrane (ILM) (most common)
b. Within outer cortical vitreous
c. Rarely in the ILM.

TRD and Posterior Tractional Proliferative Vitreoretinopathy

Traumatic wound healing process leads to TRD in open globe injuries (as described before).

Traumatic injury particularly with intraocular hemorrhage causes inflammation and breakdown of blood retinal barrier with expression of cytokines and growth factors. These cytokines and growth factors in turn affect RPE and glial cells which have contractile properties and on contraction cause TRD. Experimental models in rhesus monkeys suggest epiretinal membrane (ERM) is common in both in periphery and on the posterior pole.

ERM connects to bridge formed by glial processes which traverse through ILM to neural retina. When it contracts the normal adhesion breaks and TRD occurs. In primates, PVD occurs and any anteroposterior traction is precleuded. But at vitreous base, the vitreous is tightly adherent and traction in the periphery induces RD which commences in the periphery.

Posterior traumatic PVR causes severe vision loss. The frequency of PVR is maximal with perforating injuries (43%) followed by rupture of the globe (21%) and penetrating injury (15%) and IOFB (11%).

Risk factors for PVR

1. More common in males
2. Perforating injuries
3. Preoperative visual acuity ($< = 5/200$)
4. Anterior and posterior segment of the eye involvement
5. Wound size (more than 10 mm)
6. Retinal detachment
7. Intraocular inflammation
8. Choroidal hemorrhage

Last two are independent risk factors:

Average interval between injury and PVR development:

1. Perforating injury (1.3 months)
2. Rupture (2.1 months)
3. IOFB (3.1 months)
4. Penetrating injury (3.2 months).

Traumatic Endophthalmitis[8]

In 2–48% eyes develop this devastating complication. The prognosis get poorer with cuture positive cases. Most common organisms and gram-positive (*Staphylococcus species* predominate). 8–25% have gram-negative organism (*Escherichia* and *Bacillus species* are the most common).

Risk factors for development of endophthalmitis

1. IOFB
2. Systemic disease (e.g. diabetes mellitus)
3. More than 50 years
4. Delay in seeking medical attention
5. Delay in treatment

The details of management are discussed elsewhere (Chapter 7.5).

Intraocular Foreign Body (IOFB)[9]

Retained IOFB occurs in 5–40% of all penetrating injuries (the details are discussed elsewhere).

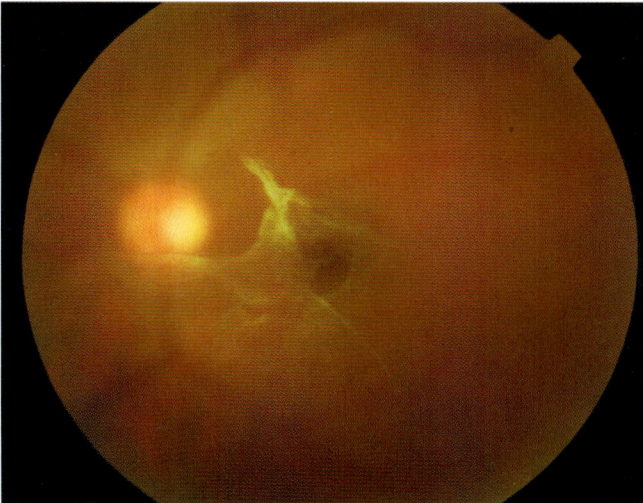

Fig. 7.1.4: Posterior vitreous detachment (PVD)

Treatment of Open Globe Injuries

Surgical Management

The principle of management is primary repair with or without vaginectomy as a part of enlate in nutrition.

Goals of vitrectomy

a. Removal of all blood and vitreous scaffold
b. Lowering the load of pathological stimulant of wound healing.

Removal of the blood and vitreous leads to less reaction and hence less chances of development of PVR and TRD.

Timing of surgery

There are two schools of thought:

1. Early intervention
2. Late intervention.

1. **Early intervention:** This implies that the surgery is undertaken within 48–72 hours of injury.[10]

   Advantages:

   a. Less inflammation
   b. Less inflammatory mediators
   c. Immediate repair of retinal tears and detachment.

   Disadvantage:

   Intraoperativley, severe hemorrhage may occur due to uveal congestion.

2. **Late intervention:** The surgery is undertaken after 5–7 days (within 2 weeks) of injury.[11] We prefer early intervention because of the advantages.

   Advantages:

   a. Proper evaluation of patient is possible
   b. Spontaneously, PVD occurs in a week's time
   c. Less chances of hemorrhage intraoperatively.

Addition of buckling depends on surgeons choice an operative skill to remove near complete vitreous. Breaks can be lasered or cryoed but cryo causes more inflammation so it is best avoided except for unavoidable circumstances (e.g. very anterior break).

Pharmacological Treatment

The goals of medical management are:

a. Inhibition of PVR[12]
b. Inhibition of inflammation[13]
c. Inhibition of growth factors[14]
d. Inhibition of intracellular signal pathways.[15]

Treatment options that are available

1. *Steroids:* The mode of action is decrease in inflammation.
2. *Anticancer drugs (5 FU, cyclosporin):* These medicines reduce cellular proliferation but toxicity is the disadvantage and effects are transient.
3. Mytomycin (MMC), hypericin (targets protein kinase-C) and Taxol (acts on retinal cells and inhibits migration and proliferation) are a good substitute and have less toxicity.
4. *Prinomastat:* PVR can be decreased by this drug which is a matrix metalloproteinase inhibitor.
5. Suramin blocks binding of growth factors and amide bonds.
6. Hepatocyte growth factor is inhibited by NK-4.
7. Proteinkinase-C and mitogen activated protein-kinase (MAPK) are critical signaling pathways for RPE proliferation and migration and may be amenable to be targeted.
8. Neutralizing antibodies to transforming growth factor and platelets derived growth factor against RPE mediated retinal contraction is also under research.

Gene Therapy

PVR can be prevented by gene transfer of soluble transforming growth factor β-2 receptors via adenovirus vector.[16]

Trasduction of nonsuicide genes and antisense sequences alter the effect of cytokines, metallo-proteinases and production of collagen which have important role in PVR. But, the gene therapy as of now is mostly futuristic and further research is needed.

Summary of Open Globe Injury

- Open globe injury are major cause of ocular morbidity
- RD following penetrating injury most frequently occurs due to traction as a part of wound healing response
- Blood in vitreous is risk factor for TRD and PVR
- Vitreous surgery remains the mainstay in removing the scaffold of proliferation
- In future, pharmacologic approaches for inhibition of cellular proliferation and inhibition of growth factors may have an important role in prevention of PVR and TRD
- Alteration of cell function by gene therapy is under research.

CLOSED GLOBE INJURY

The manifestation of closed globe injuries are varied from being no or very subtle anatomic and functional manifestations to total loss of vision.

The impact of ocular trauma is compounded by socioeconomic loss and rehabilitation.

Types of Closed Globe Injury[17]

1. *Blunt injury:* Diffuse injury and has worst outcomes.

2. *Lamellar or lacerating injuries:* These are elocalized injuries and can be dealt with primary repair. The visual outcome depends on whether visual axis is involved or not and whether any cocomitant retinal, choroidal or optic nerve injury is present or not.

3. *Supeficial foreign bodies:* These injuries occur when the foreign body has not penetrated the full thickness of ocular coat. The treatment is removal of the foreign body and visual prognosis depends on involvement and extent of visual axis and other associated ocular injuries.

Epidemiology

Ocular trauma not only has an enormous impact on the personal and socioeconomic status of an individual but also the effect is compounded to growth of society as most common age group to be affected is the youth. In USA, it is second to cataract in the most common cause of visual impairment. Incidence has increased from one million to 2.4 million cases per year in USA.[18]

Risk Group

1. Young males
2. Violent behavior
3. Sports like base ball, soccer or boxing.

Clinical Presentations

a. Commotio Retinae

Also known as Berlin's edema and was first described by Berlin in 1873.[19]

Mechanism of Injury

Commotio retinae occurs due to contrecoup injury where damage occurs opposite to the site of impact. The line of forces which form, travel through the eye causing maximum damage at tissue interfaces.[20]

Clinical Features

a. Transient focal or extensive area of gray white opacification of retina at deep sensory level due to disruption of photoreceptor outer segments and damage to RPE (Figs 7.1.5 and 7.1.6).

b. Hemorrhage where may be preretinal, intra-retinal or subretinal

c. May be associated with choroidal rupture.

d. Visual acuity may vary from being normal to total loss of central vision if macula or optic nerve is involved, and depending on the severity of traumatic insult the visual decline may be transient or permanent.

e. After resolution (usually 3–4 weeks) no clinical findings may be seen or RPE migration or

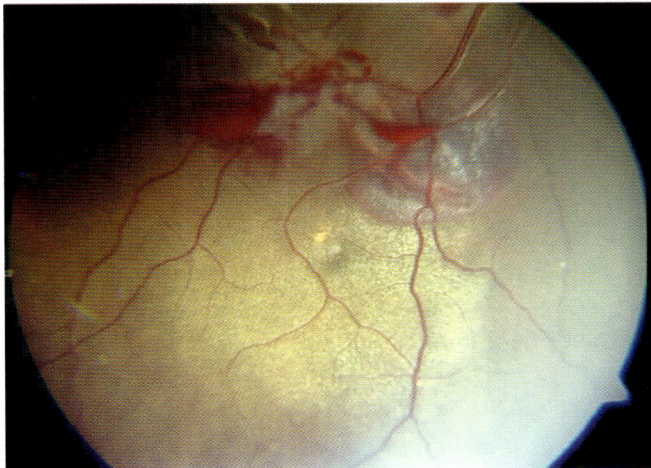

Fig. 7.1.5: Choroidal rupture with commotio retinae

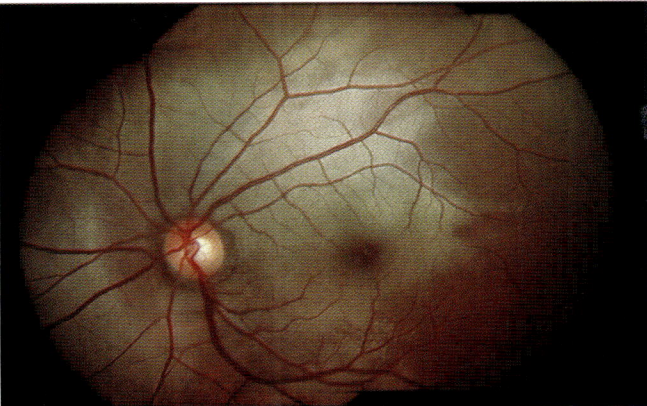

Fig. 7.1.6: Commotio retinae

hyperplasia may be noted, that may or may not be associated with foveal atrophy.

f. Full or partial thickness macular hole may develop.

Management

A careful evaluation of the eye is a must to find other sites of injury especially scleral rupture which may be difficult to diagnose but if seen needs to be closed at the earliest.

Indications for Exploration of Scleral Rupture

a. Visual acuity (less than or equal to perception of tight (PL)
b. Intraocular pressure (IOP) (< 5 mm Hg)
c. Hemorrhagic chemosis
d. Abnormally deep or shallow anterior chamber
e. Hyphema
f. Irregular pupil
g. Afferent pupillary defect
h. Media opacity with no view of fundus with indirect ophthalmoscopy.[21]

b. Traumatic Optic Neuropathy[22-24] and Optic Nerve Avulsion

The optic nerve may be damaged in its course from orbit to the brain. The most common location of injury to the optic nerve is in the optic canal.

Clinical Features

a. Decreased visual acuity of varying severity depending on the extent of optic nerve injury.
b. Decreased brightness sense.
c. Decreased color differentiation.

Signs of Optic Canal Fracture

1. Loss or sluggish pupillary reaction.
2. Wound on the lateral aspect of brow.
3. Nasal bleed.

Diagnosis of Optic Canal Fracture

Neuroimaging is essential and computed tomography (CT) scan is modality of choice.

Management

In management of optic nerve injury, it is wise to follow the hippocratic adge "to do no harm".

The modalities of management are:
1. Observation.
2. Medical management by intravenous steroids.
3. Surgery for decompression of optic canal.

Treatment Protocol

1. Prompt and correct diagnosis.
2. If orbit is tense canthotomy and drainage of subperiosteal hematoma if present.
3. Intravenous methylprednisolone 30 mg/kg as loading dose and 5.5 mg/kg/hour as maintenance dose.
4. Surgical decompression of optic canal if no response comes in 48 hours of starting intravenous methylprednisolone.
5. If vision and other symptoms improved shift to oral steroids after 48 hours but if visual deterioration is noted reinstitute intravenous methylprednisolone and consider surgical decompression.

Optic Nerve Avulsion/Anterior Indirect Traumatic Optic Neuropathy (Fig. 7.1.7)[25,26]

In this condition, the optic nerve is disinserted from retina, completely or patially choroid, vitreous and lamina cribrosa is retracted from the scleral rim (check nomenclature).

Types of Optic Nerve Avulsion[27]

1. Complete.
2. Partial: Occurs when the object intrudes between globe and orbital wall and displaces the eye.

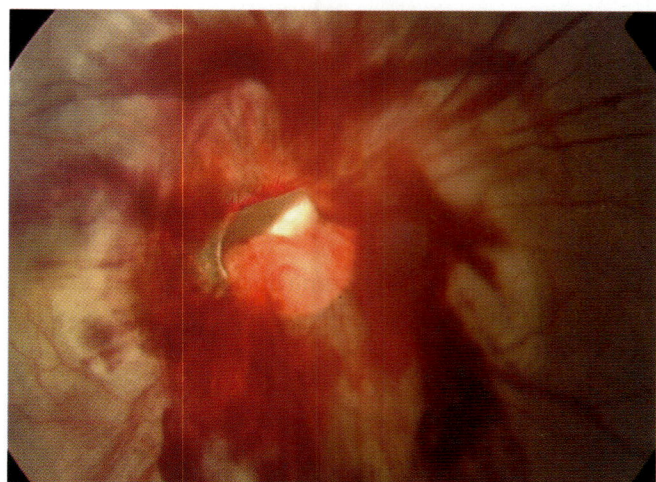

Fig. 7.1.7: Complete optic nerve head avulsion

Details partial and complete disinsertion and neuropathy as such optic nerve sheath hemorrhage.

Mechanism of Injury

The hypothesis for the explanation of optic nerve avulsion are as follows:

1. Sudden extreme rotation of globe—causing pull on the optic nerve.
2. Sudden increase in intraocular pressure which forces optic nerve out of scleral canal.
3. Sudden anterior globe displacement (mechanics of disinsertion like velocity of global movement and optic nerve follow through).

Clinical Features

1. Complete avulsion of the optic nerve leads to a blind eye with dilated pupil.
2. Partial avulsion leads to variable degree of vision loss and sectorial defects. There may be relative afferent papillary defect (RAPD) or hemianopic pupil. Absolute visual field defect corresponding to the area of disinsertion of the optic nerve in cases of partial optic nerve avulsion.
3. Usually associated with hyphema or vitreous hemorrhage.
4. If the media is clear, then fundus appearance is striking "hole or cavity where optic disk has retracted into its dural sheath".

Treatment

Prognosis in both cases is poor. No medical or surgical treatment is effective and the final visual acuity is poor. Early diagnosis saves the patient undergoing unnecessary investigations and interventions.

The partial optic nerve avulsion has a better prognosis depending on the presenting visual acuity sectorial vision island may be restored in occasional case.

Diagnosis

The diagnosis of optic nerve avulsion is usually radiological if the media is not clear.

B-scan: This shows widening of the optic nerve with or without fluid in subtenon space (Fig. 7.1.8).

Computerized tomography (CT) scan: The findings in CT scan are variable thickening of optic nerve sheath complex. The separation of optic nerve is suggested

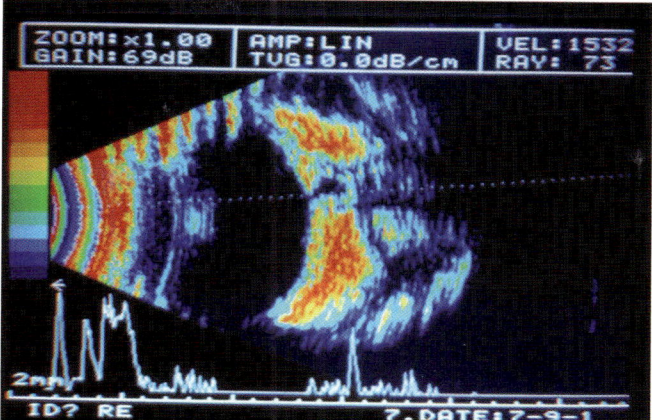

Fig. 7.1.8: Complete ONH avulsion showing discontinuity at ONH with fluid in subtenon space

by the hypolucency at the junction of nerve and globe with linear hyperlucency a little posteriorly which signifies retrodisplacement of lamina cribrosa.

Magnetic resonance imaging (MRI): This may also be of help in diagnosis of optic nerve avulsion. An 18 channel head coil is effective for routine orbital imaging including optic nerve head avulsion evaluation. Complete optic nerve head avulsion is seen as a discontinuity along the course of optic nerve and partial optic nerve avulsion is seen as increase in thickening and intraneural bright signal with or without perineural edema.

c. Choroidal Rupture

Described by Von Graefe in 1854.[28] It is a condition where tears in "choroid, Bruch's membrane and RPE occur resulting from blunt ocular trauma and associated with subretinal or sub-RPE hemorrhage (Figs 7.1.9 and 7.1.10) which may obscure visualization of the size of the rupture". The mechanism of choroidal rupture is primarily mechanical but vascular damage may also have a role. Any patient was choroidal rupture should be followed up regularly until the blood in subretinal and sub-RPE level absorbs and a clear extent of choroidal rupture can be seen.

Types of Choroidal Rupture (Fig. 7.1.11)

a. *Direct:* Rupture occurs at the site of impact and is parallel to ora.
b. *Indirect:* Rupture occurs posterior and away from the site of impact and crescentric in shape and oriented concentric to optic nerve.

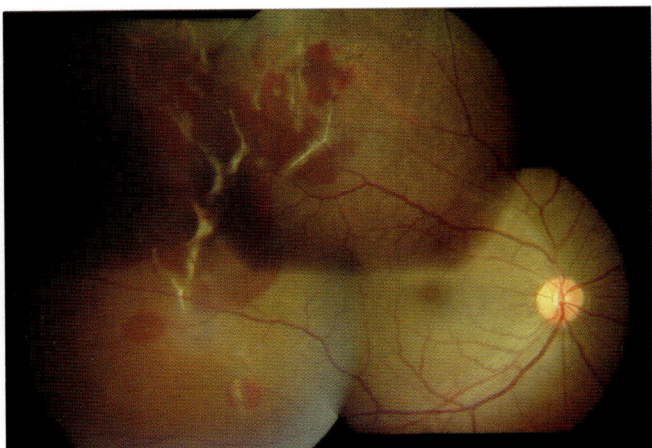

Fig. 7.1.9: Multiple choroidal ruptures with subretinal and preretinal bleed

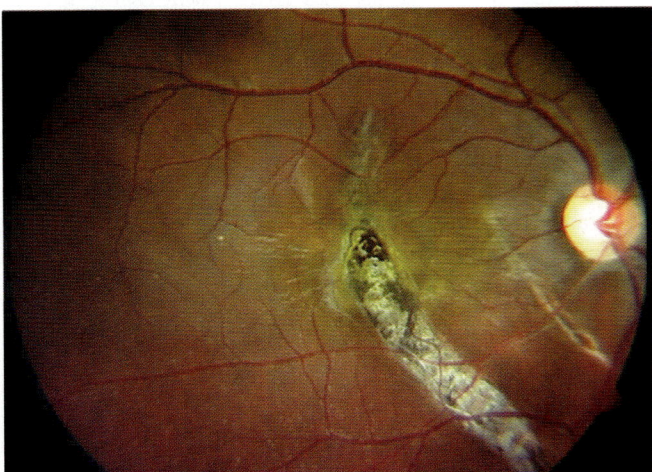

Fig. 7.1.10: Healed choroidal rupture

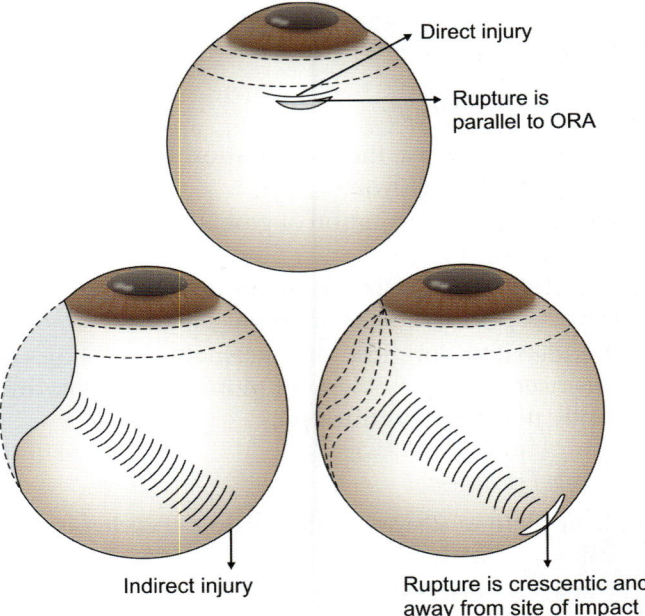

Fig. 7.1.11: Choroidal rupture

patients are at higher risk for choroidal rupture as the Bruch's membrane is fragile inherently.

Clinical Features

a. Visual deterioration if it involves the macula. In this scenario the immediate vision loss is due to inner retinal injury and hemorrhage rather than direct foveal damage.

b. Hemorrhage which may be pre retinal, sub-retinal and sub-retinal pigment epithelial.

c. Choroidal neovascular membrane (CNVM) is the most serious complication associated with choroidal rupture. It develops in about 15–30% cases.[29] The patients of choroidal rupture involving the macula are to be followed by Amsler Grid.

Risk Factor for Development of CNVM in Choroidal Rupture[30]

a. Distance of rupture from the center of fovea < 1,500 μ.

b. Length of rupture ≥ 4,000 μ.

c. *RPE status:* Patients with RPE diseases are more likely to develop CNVM.

d. *Duration:* First year incidence is 82% after the end of second year it falls to 18%.

Indirect choroidal ruptures are four times commoner than direct form.

Patients with angiod treat are at higher risk for choroidal rupture.

Mechanism of Injury

When there is sudden compression and hyperextension of globe the sclera is protected by virtue of its tensile strength and retina escapes the injury due to its elasticity, but Bruch's membrane ruptures as it lacks tensile strength and is inelastic. Angioid streak

Angiographic Features of Choroidal Rupture

- *Fluorescein angiography:* This investigation may not be of much use in acute presentation due to blocked fluorescence secondary to hemorrhage. When the blood at subretinal and sub-RPE level absorbs then we can see choroidal filling delay corresponding to the shape of rupture which is seen as hypofluorescent streak in the early phase and hyperfluorescent streak corresponding to rupture in the late phase.
- *Indocyanine green angiography:* This investigation is better in cases of acute injuries as it can depict the choroidal lesion hidden behind the subretinal and sub-RPE hemorrhage as hypofluorescent streak in early phase that becomes pronounced in middle and late phase and sometimes delayed filling of choroidal veins on subtraction indocyanine green (ICG) angiography.

Diagnosis of CNVM in Choroidal Rupture

The diagnosis of CNVM is confirmed by angiographic tests that show leak (Figs 7.1.12 and 7.1.13) and OCT that shows serous detachment of neural retina (Fig. 7.1.14) or may show intraretinal edema or a combination of both. OCT has a supportive value in primary diagnosis but can be used to monitor the regression of CNVM post-treatment.

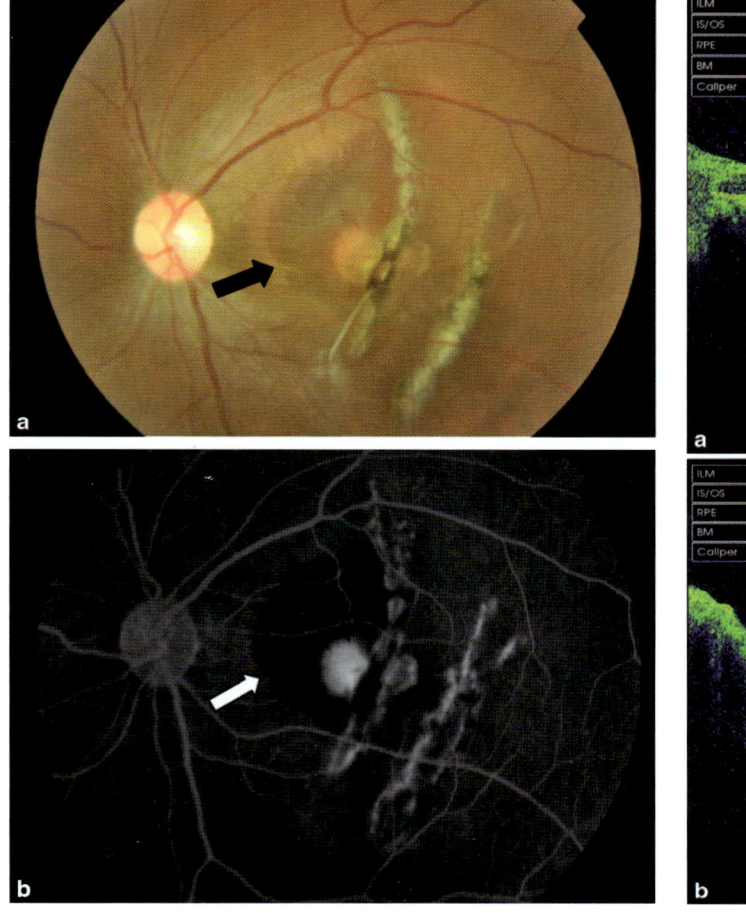

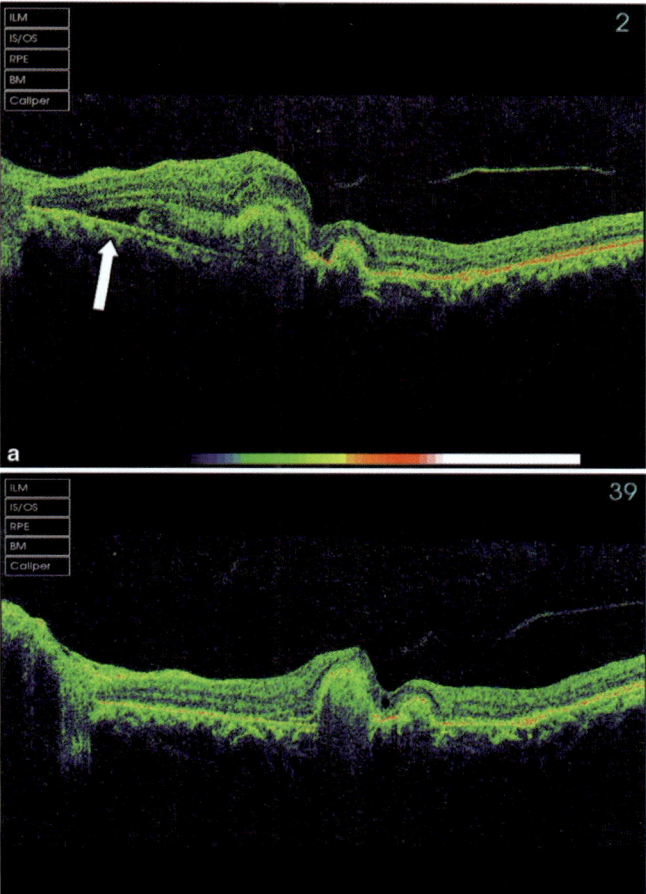

Figs 7.1.12a and b: In the fundus photochoroidal rupture scars with subretinal hemorrhage (black arrow) involving the fovea (a). The corresponding FFA image shows leak due to CNVM and the area of subretinal hemorrhage shows blocked fluorescence (white arrow) (b).

Figs 7.1.13a and b: (a) Shows a small pocket of subretinal fluid (white arrow) with (CNVM) juxtafoveal; (b) the pocket of subretinal fluid has disappeared post-treatment with anti-VEGF with regression in the activity of CNVM

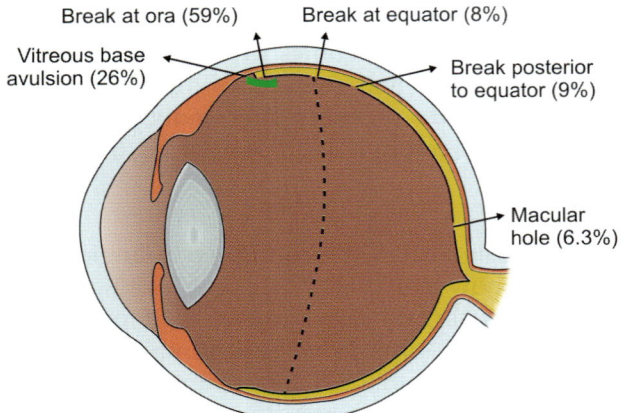

Break at ora (59%)   Break at equator (8%)
Vitreous base avulsion (26%)   Break posterior to equator (9%)
Macular hole (6.3%)

Fig. 7.1.14: Location of traumatic retinal tears and detachments

Management of CNVM Associated with Choroidal Rupture

Extrafoveal CNVM can be treated with laser photocoagulation.[31] For juxtafoveal and subfoveal CNVM the treatment of choice nowadays is anti-vascular endothelial growth factor (anti-VEGF). Though photodyanamic therapy has been tried before but the recent trend is to use anti-VEGF. In its natural history the CNVM secondary to choroidal rupture, has chances for spontaneous regression and the visual acuity stabilizes at 0.18 on average.

As described by Goldberg et al chorioretinal anastamosis may develop at the site of choroidal rupture.

Treatment and Prognosis of Choroidal Rupture

Choroidal rupture if not associated with other ocular complications like retinal tear or detachment is managed conservatively. The visual prognosis depends on whether the macula is involved in choroidal rupture, or optic nerve is damaged concurrently.

d. Traumatic Chorioretinal Rupture (Scleropetaria)

This condition is also known as chorioretinitis proliferans, retinitis sclopetaria, acute retinal necrosis and chorioretinitis rupture.[32,33] The condition was first described by Goldzieher in 1901.[34] It is an uncommon presentation in non-penetrating ocular trauma. As it is a traumatic and non-inflammatory condition better term to use is "traumatic chorioretinal rupture". Simultaneous trauma of choroid and retina results when high velocity missile (e.g. bullet) passes adjacent to the globe but does not penetrate the eye.

Mechanism of Injury

Shockwaves of high velocity object cause rapid globe deformity resulting in stress on retina, choroid, sclera and posterior vitreous cortex.[35] The tensile strength of the sclera protects it, and rupture of retina and choroid occurs. Simultaneous retraction of choroid and retina at the site of break reveals bare sclera.

Types

1. Direct (coup) injury
2. Indirect (contracoup) injury.

1. Direct Injury

In this, structures are damaged on the path of the missile.

2. Indirect Injury

The damage occurs at a point which is remote from the point of contact. The trauma may be so severe that only one large lesion involving both areas may be seen. Immediately after the injury, extensive vitreous hemorrhage, retinal or subretinal hemorrhage may obscure the fundus view. Later when blood clears, healed white proliferative scar with RPE degeneration is noted (fibroblastic activity occurs between 4 days and 14 days and scar founds between 3 weeks and 4 weeks).

Factors affecting the extent of chorioretinal rupture

a. *Proximity of the foreign body to the globe:* Nearer the foreign body more is the energy transfer and more is the damage.
b. *Size of the object:* Larger the size more the damage
c. *Velocity of the object:* More the velocity, more is the energy transfer and more is the damage.

Treatment

The proliferation of the fibroblasts does not usually cause RD as the retina and choroid are firmly adherent to sclera. Hence, treatment modalities like laser, cryo and scleral buckling are not indicated. Occasionally, pars plana vitrectomy for unresolving vitreous hemorrhage may be indicated especially in young patients.

Prognosis

It is poor if macula or optic nerve is damaged.

Traumatic Retinal Tears and Detachment
(Figs 7.1.14 and 7.1.15)

In young males with traumatic RD, 70–80% are secondary to blunt injury.[36,37] The presentation varies from immediate (12%) to 2 years (40–80%). The most common area for retinal break is ora (59%) followed by ora and equatorial area (23%). Vitreous base is avulsed in about 26% cases.

Clinical Sign

1. Peripheral commotio retinae
2. Choroidal ruptures
3. Retinal or vitreous hemorrhage.

Mechanism of Injury[38]

Anteroposterior compression of the globe, with lateral expansion of the equatorial area leads to traction at the vitreous base. The hypothesis for traumatic RD secondary to blunt ocular injury has been gives as follows:

Retinal break occurs because of the direct contusion and subsequent retinal necrosis or vitreoretinal traction due to globe expansion.

Traumatic vitreous syneresis overlying the break may happen immediately or months after the blunt injury and liquid vitreous may dissect under retinal break causing RD (Fig. 7.1.14).

Treatment

- Laser barrage around the break or dialysis area so that the detachment does not progress.

- Cryopexy around the break or dialysis area if lasers are not possible as in cases with vitreous hemorrhage.

- Scleral buckling can be done when the extent of RD is large and laser or cryopexy may not be of benefit to the patient or the laser barrage or cryopexy have failed.

- Pneumatic retinopexy can also be tried in very limited subgroup of patients with single superior break.

f. Retinal Dialysis and Irregular Retinal Breaks

Retinal dialysis occurs in 84% RD following blunt injuries.[39] Most common site is superonasal quadrant[40] (46% of blunt injuries) (Fig. 7.1.16). Patients with myopia are more susceptible to RD caused by blunt injury.[41,42] As vitreous is more formed in young patients, RD caused by dialysis advance slowly especially in cases with inferior dialysis, and hence signs of chronicity like demarcation line and intraretinal cysts are common in this scenario.

Irregular retinal breaks form in the areas of contusion which undergoes hemorrhagic necrosis of choroid and secondary fragmentation of retina in area with no vitreous attachment. Most common site is inferotemporal quadrant where maximum direct[41] trauma occurs. Irregular retinal breaks form within 24 hours of injury and liquefaction of overlying vitreous is necessary for the formation of RD.

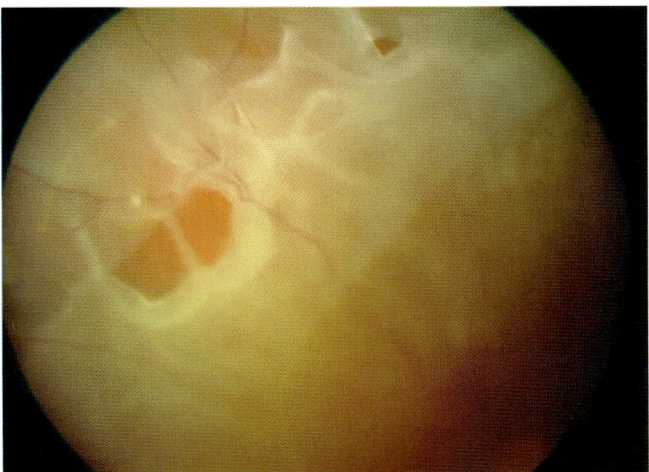

Fig. 7.1.15: Retinal tears

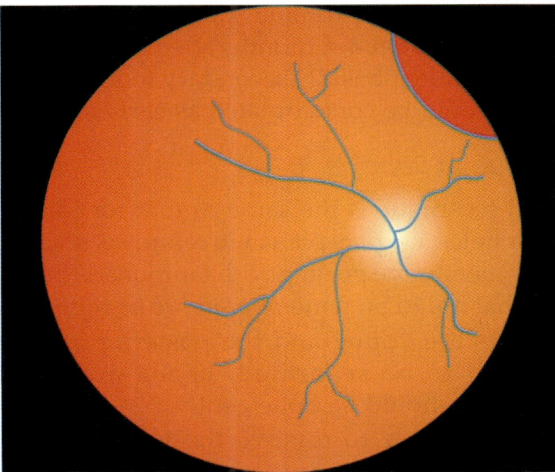

Fig. 7.1.16: Dialysis is most common in superonasal quadrant

Treatment Modalities

The treatment modalities include:
- Laser barrage
- Cryo
- Scleral buckling.

g. Traumatic Macular Hole

Blunt ocular trauma account for 9% of full thickness macular holes[43] are secondary to ocular trauma. The associated injuries that can be present are commotio retinae, choroidal rupture, subretinal hemorrhage, retinal dialysis and angle recession.

Mechanism of Injury

The pathogenesis of traumatic macular hole is unknown but few hypothesis that are given are as follows:
1. Post-contusion necrosis
2. Subfoveal hemorrhage leading to degeneration
3. Acute vitreoretinal traction as a result of contrecoup injury.[44]

Clinical Features

1. The visual acuity varies from 20/80 to 20/400.
2. The hole size is 300–500 μ.
3. The hole is sharply defined though rarely margins may be varying.
4. Surrounding cuff of neurosensory detachment.

Timing for surgery: Different schools of thoughts are there regarding timing of repair for traumatic macular holes. Yamada et al[45] showed traumatic macular holes may spontaneously close between 3 weeks and 6 months after initial trauma. Hence the surgery is to be undertaken after 4–6 months after trauma. In cases where the patient has RD secondary to macular hole, surgery should be contemplated as early as possible.

Technique of Repair[46]

Surgical technique is the same as that for idiopathic macular holes, i.e. pars plana vitrectomy with internal limiting membrane peeling with tamponade but a few points that are to be remembered are as follows:
- Patients are young and the posterior hyaloid is difficult to be separated, hence during PVD induction should be done gently.
- It is preferable to remove the internal limiting membrane, and any associated epiretinal membrane should also be removed along with it.

- In those patients who may not be able to maintain prone position as in very young children silicon oil may be used as tamponade, but this procedure will require an additional surgery for silicon oil removal later.

Indirect Closed Globe Ocular Injuries in Posterior Segment

1. Purtscher's retinopathy and Purtscher's like retinopathies
2. Terson's syndrome
3. Shaken baby syndrome
4. Valsalva retinopathy
5. Fat embolism
6. Whip lash retinopathy.

1. Purtscher's Retinopathy and Purtscher's Like Retinopathies (Fig. 7.1.17)

Classical Purtscher's retinopathy is multiple patches of superficial whitening of retina with retinal hemorrhage surrounding hyperemic optic nerve head in patients with head trauma.[47] The Purtscher's like retinopathy has been described with other causes like chest compression, acute pancreatitis, child birth, connective tissue disorders (e.g. SLE), amniotic fluid embolism and retrobulbar anesthesia.

Pathogenesis

It is not clear but injury induced compliment activity has been implicated as a cause which leads to granulocyte, aggregation and leucoembolization.[48,49]

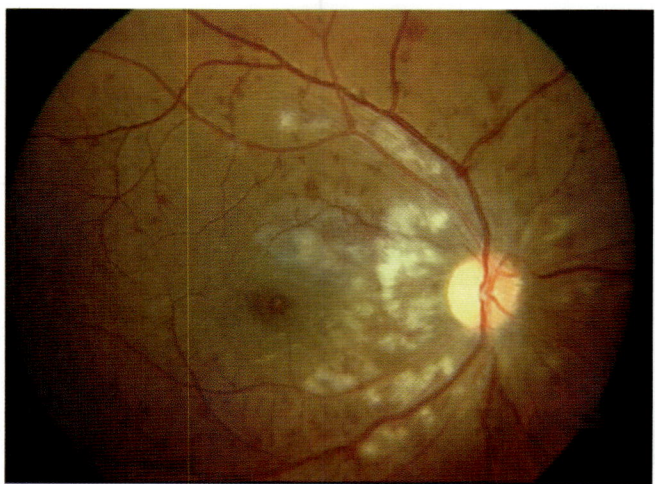

Fig. 7.1.17: Purtscher

This process in turn occludes smaller arterioles such as those in the peripapillary area.

Clinical Features

Sudden visual deterioration of varying level.

Management

Treatment of the etiological factor.

Prognosis

Although retinal findings disappear but patient may be left with visual field defect because of optic nerve atrophy in about 50%.

2. Terson's Syndrome (Fig. 7.1.18)

Original description of this condition was given by Littin (1881)[50] and repeated by Terson (1900).[51] This is the condition of intraocular hemorrhage with subarachnoid hemorrhage. The incidence of this condition is 3–8% in subarachnoid hemorrhage cases.[52] The affected persons are in the age group of 30–50 years. The most common cause is ruptured intracranial aneurysm. Bilateral ocular involvement is common.[53]

The blood accumulates between internal limiting membrane and posterior hyaloid face and may break through into vitreous cavity which provides a scaffold for cellular proliferation and development of elevated epiretinal membrane.

Pathogenesis

Acute increase in intracranial tension leads to transmission down into intravaginal space of optic nerve. The venous stasis via compression and stretching of intraorbital veins which in turn increases intraocular venous pressure causes distension and rupture of fine papillary and retinal capillaries which causes vitreous hemorrhage.

Treatment

Observation up to 3 months but if the blood does not clear vitrectomy. In children, early surgery is to be considered to decrease the chances of development of amblyopia.

Prognosis

Prognosis is good and 81% of cases achieve a visual acuity of more than 20/30.[54]

3. Shaken Baby Syndrome

This term is also known as "battered child syndrome" and was described in 1964 by Kifthey.[55] The age group affected is less than 3 years with majority in the first year.

Mechanism of Injury

Head results from sudden rotational deceleration with forceful striking of head against a surface.[56]

Systemic Features

1. Bradycardia, apnea, decrease body temperature
2. Hypotony, lethargy and seizures
3. Failure to thrive
4. Signs of intracranial hypertension
5. Skin bruises
6. Spiral fracture of long bones
7. Intracranial hemorrhage.

Ocular Features

a. Periorbital injection (ecchymosis and edema).
b. Anterior segment shows hyphema, angle recession, cataract.
c. *Retinal findings:* Retinal hemorrhages (55–95%), cotton wool spots, vitreous hemorrhage, RD, hemorrhagic schisis cavities and optic atrophy.

Diagnosis

A high index of suspicion is needed and CT scan can be done for diagnosis of fractures.

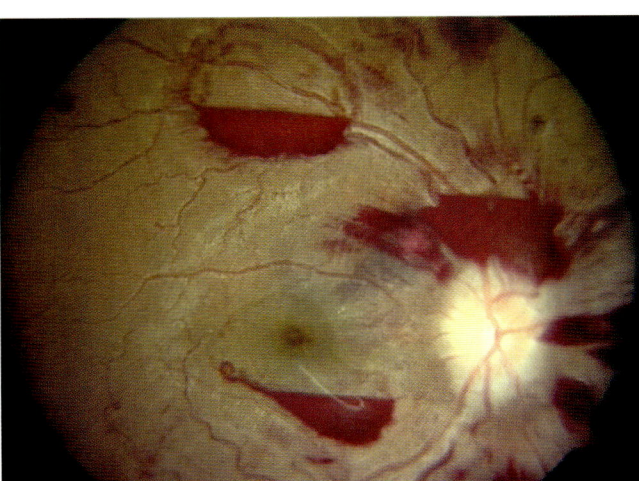

Fig. 7.1.18: Terson's syndrome

Management

In patients who have dense vitreous hemorrhage vitrectomy should be performed after confirmation of retinal function by electroretinography. Also always to be remembered is general overall health of the child as they may have severe neurological damage.

Prognosis

Some degree of permanent visual loss remains if macula, optic nerve, occipital cortex damage occurs and their combination has an even poorer prognosis.

4. *Valsalva Retinopathy* (Figs 7.1.19a and b)

It is a condition of preretinal hemorrhage with history of increased intrathoracic pressure caused by forceful exhalation against a closed glottis, e.g. coughing, vomiting and sneezing.[57]

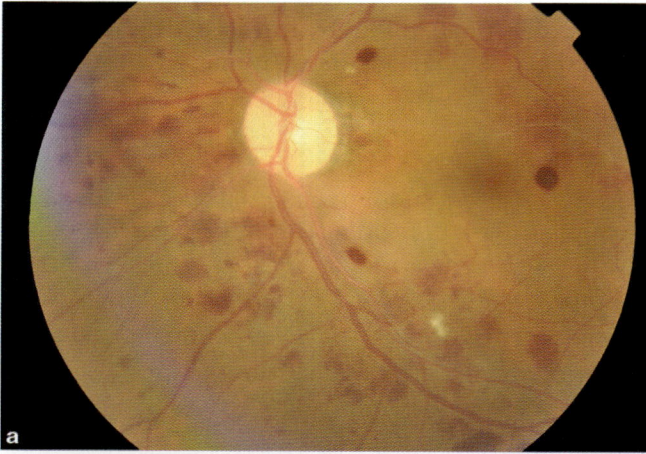

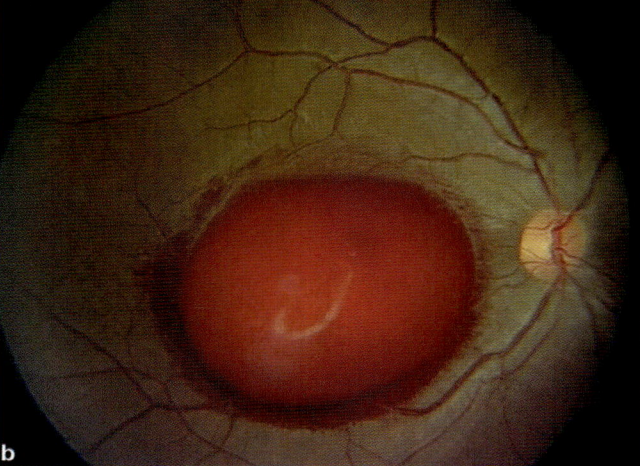

Figs 7.1.19a and b: Valsalva retinopathy

Clinical Features

Decreased visual acuity which is secondary to hemorrhagic detachment of internal limiting membrane and preretinal hemorrhage with or without vitreous hemorrhage.[58] Gass described circumscribed round or dumbbell shaped, bright red mound of blood under internal limiting membrane at or near macula which may get dehemoglobinized in sometime.

Prognosis

Visual prognosis is good as the hemorrhage clears without sequelae and laser or surgical intervention is rarely needed. For selected group of cases neodymium:yttrium aluminium garnet (Nd:YAG) laser can be used to disrupt the preretinal hemorrhage into the vitreous cavity so that absorption of the hemorrhage occurs faster associations with familial retinal artery tortuosity.[59]

5. *Fat Embolism*

This is condition is associated with the fracture of medullated bones.[60] Retinal changes are seen in 60% of the patients who meet the diagnostic criteria of fat embolism syndrome, but only in 5% of patients with fracture of long bone without other systemic signs.[61]

Systemic Features

Petechial rash over the skin, respiratory distress and central nervous system involvement. This condition can be fatal in 20% cases.

Ocular Features

The classical findings are of bilateral cotton wool spots. Multiple patches of superficial whitening of retina with retinal hemorrhage surrounding hyperemic optic nerve head (the hemorrhages are smaller, less numerous and more peripheral as compared to Purtscher's retinopathy).

Management

Currently, no treatment is available for the ocular manifestations, and only systemic condition is to be taken care of.

Prognosis

Prognosis is good and most patients have a good visual recovery. Some complain of permanent scotoma.

6. Whip Lash Retinopathy

This injury is caused by extreme flexion-extension of head in neck without direct eye injury (e.g. automobile accidents).[62]

Mechanism of Injury

Traction at the vitreoretinal interface due to sudden flexion-extension of the neck.

Clinical Features

Bilateral, mild decrease of visual acuity $< = 20/30$.

Ocular Findings

Grayish swelling of the fovea. Foveal pit size is 50–100 μ. A shallow PVD may also be evident.

Prognosis

Visual acuity improves in a few days and no treatment is needed.

Lens displacement: Subluxation and dislocation: traumatic dislocation and subluxation often needs the attention of posterior segment surgeon and the management of such cases is a joint approach.

Posterior Segment Approach in Dislocated Lens

Indications:

a. Posterior dislocation of lens causing inflammation and or mechanical trauma
b. Non-clearing vitreous hemorrhage
c. Retinal detachment
d. Retinal dialysis.

Surgical choice is pars-plana vitrectomy with pars-plana lensectomy.

Points to be remembered while performing lensectomy:

1. Avoid making sclerotomies in weak/traumatized areas.
2. Soft nucleus can be easily aspirated with vitrectomy cutter.
3. Hard nucleus requires phacofragmentation and careful handling of nucleus.
4. Nucleus has to be freed of surrounding vitreous before removal.
5. Perfluorocarbon liquid (PFCL) usage is important to avoid inadvertent damage to retina in case of hard nucleus.
6. Vitreous hemorrhage—discussed elsewhere.
7. Commotio retinae—discussed elsewhere.
8. Retinal detachment and macular hole—discussed elsewhere.

REFERENCES

1. The ocular trauma classification group. A system for classifying mechanical injuries of the eye (globe). Am J Ophthal. 1997;123:820–831.
2. Posterior segment trauma: open globe Ryan 4th ed.
3. Cleary PE, Ryan SJ. Histology of wound, vitreous and retina in experimental posterior penetrating eye injury in Rhesus monkey. Am. J Ophthal. 1979;88:221–231.
4. Hsu HT, Ryan SJ. Experimental retinal detachment in the rabbit: Penetrating ocular injury with retinal laceration. Retina 1986;6:66–69.
5. Rentsch FJ. The Ultrastructure of pre-retinal macular fibrosis. Graefes Arch. Clin. Exp Ophthalmol. 1977; 203:321–337.
6. Gregor Z, Ryan SJ. Combined posterior contusion and penetrating injury in pig eye. II. Histological features. BJO. 1982;66:799–804.
7. Cardillo JA, Stout JT, et al. Post traumatic proliferative vitreoretinopathy. The epidemiological profile, onset, risk factors and visual outcome. Ophthalmology. 1997; 104:1166–1173.
8. Bruton GS, Topping TN, et al. Post traumatic endo-phthalmitis. Arch ophthalmol. 1984;102:547–550.
9. Jonas JB, Knorr HLJ. Prognostic factors in ocular injuries caused by intraocular or retrobulbar foreign bodies. Ophthalmology 2000;107:823–828.
10. Coleman DJ. Early vitrectomy in management of severely traumatized eye. Am J Ophthal. 1982;93:543–551.
11. de Juan E Jr, et al. Timing of vitrectomy after penetrating ocular injury. Ophthalmology. 1984; 91:1072–1074.
12. Fastenberg DM, et al. The role of cellular proliferation in an experimental model of massive periretinal proliferation. Am J ophthal. 1982; 93:565–572.
13. Tano Y, et al. Inhibition of intraocular proliferation wit intravitreal corticosteroids. Am J ophthal. 1980; 89:131–136.
14. Jabolonski MM, et al. Investigating the mechanism of retinal degeneration with antisense oligonucleotides. Doc Ophthalmol.2001; 102:179–196.
15. Hinton DR, et al. Mitogen activated protein kinase activation mediates PDGF directed migration of RPE cells. Exp Cell Res 1998; 239:11–15.
16. Oshima Y. Gene transfer of soluble TGF-Beta Type II receptor inhibits experimental proliferative vitreoretino-pathy. Gene Ther. 2002;9:1214–1220.
17. The ocular trauma classification group. A system for classifying mechanical injuries of the eye (globe). Am J Ophthal. 1997;123:820–831.
18. White ME Jr, Morris R, et al. Eye injury: prevalence and prognosis by setting. South med. J 1989;82:151–158.
19. Berlin R. Zursogenauten commotio retinae. Klin Monastbl augenheilkd. 1876;1:785–796.
20. Walter JR. Coup-contrecoup mechanism of ocular injuries. Am J Ophthal. 1963;56:785–796.

21. Kylastra JA, Lamkin JC, et al. Clinical predictors of scleral rupture after blunt ocular trauma. Am J Ophthal. 1993; 115:530–535.

22. Fujitani T, Inoue K. Indirect tr. Optic neuropathy-visual outcomes of operative and non-operative cases. Jpn J Ophthal. 1986;30:125–134.

23. Lessell S. Indirect Optic Nerve trauma. Arch Ophthal. 1989;107:382–386.

24. Steinasapirk D, et al. Traumatic Optic Neuropathy. Survey ophthal. 1994;38:487–578.

25. Foster BS, et al. Optic nerve avulsion. Arch Ophthal. 1997;115:623–630.

26. Wlliam DF, Mieler WF, et al. Post segment manifestation of ocular trauma. Retina. 1990;10:535–544.

27. Sanborn GE, Gonder JR. Evulsion of optic nerve. A clinico pathological study. Can J ophthal. 1984;19:10–16.

28. Von Graefe A. Graefe. Zwei Falle von Ruptur der choroidea Arch. Ophthal. 1854;1:402–403.

29. Smith RE, et al. Late macular complications of choroidal ruptures. Am J Ophthal. 1974;77:650–658.

30. Seretan M, Sickenberg M, et al. Retina. 1998;18:62266.

31. Smith RE, et al. Late macular complications of choroidal ruptures. Am. J. Ophthal. 1974; 77:650–658.

32. Bloom MA, Ruiz RS, et al. Acute retinal necrosis. Annal. Ophthalmol.1979;11:723–728.

33. Dubovy SR, Guyton DL, et al. Clinico pathological correlation of chorioretinitis scleropetaria. Retina. 1997; 17:510–520.

34. Goldzieher W. Bietrage zur pathologie der orbitalen Schussverletzungen Z Augenhielkd. 1901;6:277–285.

35. Martin DF, Awh CC, et al. Treatment and pathogenesis of traumatic choriroratinal rupture (scleropetaria). Am J Ophthal. 1994;117:190–200.

36. Giovinazzo VJ, Yannuzzi LA, et al. The ocular complications of boxing. Ophthalmology. 1987;94:587–596.

37. Malbran E, Dodds R, et al. Traumatic retinal detachment. Mod Probl. Ophthalmol. 1972;10:479–489.

38. Eagling EM. Ocular damage after blunt trauma to the eye:its relationship to the nature of injury. BJO. 1974; 58:126–140.

39. Dumass JJ. Retinal detachment follwing contusion of the eye. Int. Ophthal. Clinics. 1967; 7:19–38.

40. Hagler WS. Retinal dialysis: A statistical and genetic study to determine pathogenic factors. Trans Am. Ophthalmic Soc. 1980; 78:686–733.

41. Dumas JJ. Retinal detachment following contusion of the eye. Int Oph Clin. 1967; 7:19–38.

42. Goffstein R, Burton TC. Differentiating traumatic from nontraumatic retinal detachments. Ophthalmology. 1982; 89:361–368.

43. Rubin JS, Glaser BM, et al. vitrectomy, fluid gas exchange and transforming growth factor ?-2 for treatment of traumatic macular holes. Ophthalmology.1995;102:1840–1845.

44. Gass JDM. Stereoscopic atlas of macular diseases: Diagnosis and treatment, 4th Edition. St. Louis: Mosby; 1997.

45. Yamada H, Sakai A, et al. Spontaneous closure of traumatic macular hole. Am J Ophthal. 2002; 134:340–347.

46. Pieramici DJ. Ophthal Clin North Am. 2002; 15:225–234.

47. Purtscher O. Angiopathica retinae Traumatica: Lymphorrhagien des Augengrandes. Arch. Ophthal. 1912; 82:347–371.

48. Jacob HS, Goldstein IM, et al. Sudden blindness in acute pancreatitis: possible role of compliment induced retinal leucoembolism. Arch Int Med. 1981;141:134–136.

49. Jacob HS, Craddock PR, et al. Compliment induced granulocyte aggregation:an unsuspected mechanism of disease. North Eng J Med. 1980;302:789.

50. Litten M. Uber Einge vom allgemein-klinischen Standpunkt aus interessante Augenveranderungen. Berl Klin Wochenschr. 1881;18:23–27.

51. Terson A. del'hemorrhagie dans le corps vitre au cours de l'hemorrhagie cerebrale. Clin Ophthalmol. 1900;6:309–312.

52. Kuhn F, Morris R, et al. Tersen syndrome: results of vitrectomy and significance of vitreous hemorrhage in patients with sub-arachnoid hemorrhage. Ophthalmology. 1998;105:472–477.

53. Schultz PN, Sobol WM, et al. Long term visual outcomes in Tersen syndrome. Ophthalmology. 1991;98:1814–1819.

54. Kuhn F, Morris R, et al. Tersen syndrome: results of vitrectomy and significance of vitreous hemorrhage in patients with sub-arachnoid hemorrhage. Ophthalmology. 1998;105:472–477.

55. Kifthey GT. Jr. The eye of the "Battered Child". Arch. Ophthalmol. 1964;72:231–233.

56. Duhaime AC, Christian CW, et al. Non accidental head injury in infant- The "Shaken-Baby" syndrome. N. Eng. J. Med. 1998;338:1822–1829.

57. Duane TD. Valsalva hemorrhagic retinopathy. Trans Am. Ophthalmol. Soc. 1972;70:298–313.

58. Gass JDM. Stereoscopic atlas of macular diseases: Diagnosis and treatment. 4th Edition. St. Louis: Mosby; 1997.

59. Goldberg ME, Pollack IP, Green WR. Familial retinal arteriolar tortuosity with retinal hemorrhage. Am J Ophthalmol 1972;73:183–191.

60. Zeuker FA. Beitrage zur anatomie und physiologie de lunge, Dresden. 1861. J. Braunsderf.

61. Chuang EL, Miller FS III, Kalina RE. Retinal lesions following long bone fractures. Ophthalmology 1985; 92:370–374.

62. Kelly JS, Hoovei RE, et al. Whiplash maculopathy. Arch. Ophthalmol. 1978;96:834–835.

7.2 TRAUMATIC VITREOUS HEMORRHAGE

• DK Mehta • Piyush Mishra

INTRODUCTION

Vitreous hemorrhage is defined as presence of extravasated blood within the space outlined by the internal limiting membrane of the retina posteriorly and laterally, the nonpigmented epithelium of the ciliary body laterally and the lens zonular fibers and posterior lens capsule anteriorly.

Trauma causes vitreous hemorrhage in 12–18.8% cases.

Hemorrhage in all spaces (Burger's space, canal of petit, cloquet's canal and bursa premacularis) except the canal of Hannover and in space generated by a posterior vitreous detachment (retrohyaloid and subhyaloid) are considered in vitreous hemorrhage.

It may not be possible to clinically distinguish hemorrhage between the internal limiting membrane and the nerve fiber layer (subinternal limiting membrane) from retrohyaloid (subhyaloid) hemorrhage and hence the former is also considered to be a vitreous hemorrhage.[1]

The bleed in the vitreous after an injury form a silk like veil present as thicker ochre membrane within 24 hours. The macrophages released on 5th day are followed by liberation of red blood cell (RBC) from the clot in 7 days. The vitreous liquefaction starts in about 2 weeks and lysis gets initiated by macrophages and giant cells in 3 weeks time. In 5–8 weeks after injury ocular macrophages and formation of pseudo-membrane becomes more prominent due to decrease in debris and new macrophages and RBC. Most of the debris is removed and remaining blood products may remain unaffected in the later course. Hemosiderin (iron) release following ocular trauma initiates the process of sineresis by generating free hydroxyl radicals that cause hyaluronic acid depolymerization ending into collapse of hylorunate-collagen matrix framework. By 18 months the vitreous strands get broken and process of syersis is complete.[2-4]

The vitreous has low thromboplastic activity and low coagulability. There is abundance of platelet aggregation along with rich collagen presence and enhanced clotting mechanism add to clot formation. The process gets complicated further by lattice arrangement of collagen fibers resisting free diffusion of RBC and fibrin initiating the compartmentalization of clots. Slow lysis of fibrin due to plasminogen activator levels and cross linking of vitreous resists plasmic digestion and poor polymorphonuclear adds to reluctance to absorption of blood products and extracellular lysis of blood cells results into slower clearance of vitreous.

Clinical Features

Patient with acute vitreous hemorrhage complain of visual haze, floaters, smoke signals, photophobia and perception of shadows and cobwebs.

INTEGRAL HEMORRHAGE

Features depend on the amount of blood in the vitreous cavity.

Profuse vitreous hemorrhage is diffuse anteriorly and centrally; obscuring the view of peripheral retina and ora.

Slit lamp—extensive hemorrhagic debris in the anterior vitreous and on posterior lens capsule.

Blood in the formed vitreous clots rapidly (due to platelet activation by collagen) and finger like projections can be seen from the site of bleeding into the vitreous gel.

Blood generally remains stationary in the vitreous cavity except to the extent that the formed vitreous gels it moves with movement of globe.

Blood in formed vitreous gel tends to stay longer and resolve more slowly.

Organized vitreous hemorrhage appears as yellowish fluffy vitreous opacity and dense yellowish and white vitreous membranes.

PRERETINAL/SUBHYLOID HEMORRHAGE AND SUB-ILM HEMORRHAGE

Subhyloid hemorrhage is located between internal limiting membrane of the retina and detached posterior hyaloid membrane. Blood in this location does not clot, moves freely on ocular or head movements and settles down on gravity forming a boat-shaped figure in the normal vitreous. However, the same may be altered in vitreoretinal adhesions. It may have different shades of red and graywhite depending on the duration of bleed, ocular and body mobility and sedimentation of RBCs disintegrating blood products. This blood may settle down as layers of RBCs and plasma. Since the subhyaloid space is limited by vitreous base anteriorly thus a peripheral rim of retina can be well-visualized on indirect ophthalmoscope.

Bleeding in this location resolves and resorbs rapidly (due to close proximity of blood to retina and retinal circulation).Visual impairment in the patient with pre-retinal hemorrhage is dependent on the amount of bleeding, position of the patient and location (involvement of macular region).[3,5]

Sub-ILM hemorrhage in trauma can be seen as relatively well defined deep bleed with overlying shining reflex. The blood is under tension and does not shift with changes in the position of patient's head as observed in subhyaloid hemorrhage but hemorrhage may become little more mobile when it breaks through the ILM into subhyloid space. Sub-ILM hemorrhage in some instances can spare the central fovea as ILM has attachment plaques to the remainder of retina only in the central fovea[6] and peripheral to the posterior pole.

SEQUELAE FOLLOWING VITREOUS HEMORRHAGE

Vitreous membranes outside the clot may get formed as a result of inflammation incited by the presence of iron (ferrous iron) and macrophages in the vitreous cavity. These membranes may lead to traction on vitreoretinal interfaces and can lead to RD.[1]

Vitreous undergoes liquefaction and some times cholesterol deposits may be seen after a resolved hemorrhage.

Hemoglobin spherules are a term given to a rare occurrence of brown-colored aggregation of hemoglobin, instead of break down of hemoglobin to ferritin.

Cylindroid structures may get formed in the vitreous as result degenerative scintilans influence of degradation products of hemoglobin (vitreous cylinders).

Iron is liberated during catabolism of hemoglobin (Hb) which is toxic to the retina especially the photoreceptors and Müller's cells. This may finally lead to permanent retinal damage and hemosiderosis bulbi.

Iron related toxicity becomes clinically manifest in extensive long-standing vitreous hemorrhage.[1]

Acute iron toxicity causes pyknosis and degeneration of photoreceptor cells, along with inner retinal edema.

Iron in its ferrous form, binds to acid mucopolysaccharides at posterior hyaloid face, perivascular tissue, optic nerve head, and trabecular meshwork. Toxic effects are first noted around these structures. Choroid and ciliary muscle remain largely unaffected.

Patients may complain of decreased vision especially at night and xanthopsia. Peripheral field show constriction and later the central field may also get involved.

In cases of subretinal hemorrhage, damage to photoreceptor is extensive, with signs of choroidal inflammation on histopathology. It is observed that a small cloud of vitreous turbidity follows in deep subretinal hemorrhage leading to retinal necrosis and increased permeability allowing RBC to cross the intact ILM. This observation may necessitate the early displacement of the blood to prevent retinal damage and visual deficit.

PROLIFERATIVE RETINOPATHY IN VITREOUS HEMORRHAGE

Hb or iron in the vitreous may cause fibrovascular or glial proliferation internal to the retinal internal limiting membrane with secondary RD.

The degree of retinal proliferation is dependent on the amount of bleed.

Direct stimulation of fibrovascular elements by iron or possible deletion of an inhibitory factor which normally prevents the growth of fibrous tissue was responsible for the observed proliferations.

Once preretinal proliferations are established recurrent bleeding may cause vitreous collapse with traction on newly formed and normal vessels and subsequent recurrent hemorrhage which may perpetuate and repeat the problems.[2,4,7]

GLAUCOMA RELATED TO VITREOUS HEMORRHAGE

1. *Ghost cell glaucoma:* Following vitreous hemorrhage, fresh RBC (biconcave, pliable cells) degenerate into ghost cells (smaller, khaki colored, spherical, and more rigid cells) usually in 1–3 weeks. Ghost cells contain intracellular, denatured Hb adherent to the red cell membrane (Heinz body).

Ghost cells pass forward into the anterior chamber after disruption of the anterior hyaloid face after accidental trauma cataract extraction or vitrectomy. Being more rigid and less pliable than fresh RBC, ghost cells can lower the aqueous outflow much more significantly.

Clinical features: AC is deep and filled with multiple, small, tan colored cells. Angle is open, with a discolored trabecular. Mesh work ghost cells form a typical tan colored precipitate inferiorly which mimics hypopyon also called as hemophthalmitis.

If fresh RBC also coexist, a double-layered precipitate of light khaki on top of red is present (Candy Stripe sign).

2. *Hemolytic glaucoma:* Trabecular meshwork is obstructed by RBC debris, free Hb and Hb laden macrophages.

Clinical features are indistinguishable from ghost cell glaucoma.

3. *Hemosiderotic glaucoma:* This rare condition may present years after recurrent vitreous hemorrhage. Mucopolysaccharides of the trabecular meshwork have a high affinity for iron and this high concentration of iron may damage endothelial cells in the human trabucular meshwork, which may cause secondary degenerative changes such as sclerosis and obliteration of the interorbicular spaces.

Investigations

A detailed history and general physical examination should be done in each. Mode of injury may indicate the source of the bleed. History of ocular or systemic disease especially diabetes, hypertension, trauma, retinal break or detachment in the other eye, family history of detachment may also be pertinent.

Careful Ocular Examination

Base line visual acuity and projection of rays.

Corneal status: Corneal edema, opacities and any evidence and squeal of trauma.

Pupil examination for light reflex and relative afferent papillary defect.

Iris examination for rubeosis, synechiae, tears or hole (may indicate a penetrating ocular injury), sectoral ischemia or atrophy.

Intraocular pressure (IOP) recording during the follow-up periods.

Gonioscopy: Angle study may reveal angle recession/tears ot the root of iris in early stages and show closure/vascular proliferation for in long standing cases.

Indirect ophthalmoscopy is a must for detailed fundus examination to determine whether the underlying retina is attached or detached whether bleeding is from a retinal tear or neovascular frond. Scleral depression is necessary to reveal any breaks or detachment extending in to that area. Judicious use of scleral depression in open globe injuries after repair of the open globe is important (avoid in first 3 weeks)

Fluorescein angiography has a limited role in early stages of vitreous hemorrhage due to trauma.

Ultrasonography is very important tool in assessing retinal status and presence of IOFB in most cases of intense vitreous hemorrhage. Extent of vitreous detachment, and fibrovascular status in a long standing case can also be revealed.

Electrophysiological tests in the presence of dense vitreous hemorrhage, traditional means of measuring electroratinogram (ERG) amplitude with conventional intensity light stimulus can lead to erroneous conclusion with regard to retinal function. Reduced or absent ERG amplitudes when elicited by conventional light sources in the presence of dense vitreous hemorrhage could be attributed either to retinal pathology or to an ineffective stimulus caused by the filtering effect from vitreous blood. Therefore, a bright flash ERG is done. An a-wave increase of 100 µV or greater successfully predict the presence of a normal functioning retina.

MANAGEMENT OF VITREOUS HEMORRHAGE

Observation: Patient with fresh vitreous hemorrhage and on ultrasonography (USG) attached retina are asked to rest with head in elevated position, can be evaluated.[8,9]

Eyes with attached retina and known cause, which not require treatment, are evaluated after 3–4 weeks.

Medical Measures

Oral vitamin C may be given for faster clearance as it is said to induce liquefaction and loss of gel structure. Oral use of collosol iodine is purely empirical.

Fibrinolytic agents: Streptokinase and strepto-dorinase injections in the vitreous have shown a good response in clearing of intravitreal leaks in early cases but the response is often accompanied by severe inflammatory response. Use of chymotrypsin, trypsin and urokinase do not have significant response in long-standing cases. The use of fibrinolytic agents have not gain much popularity.

Pure ovine hyaluronidase (Vitrase R.) assisted liquefaction of vitreous may some time may help in clearing of dense vitreous hemorrhage with no initial visibility. Pure ovine hyaluronidase (Vitrase R.) multinational randomized controlled clinical trial has shown statistically significant results in 4 weeks old hemorrhages with vision less than 6/60. It is not indicated in organized vitreous hemorrhage and in RD.

Hemolytic agents: Agents like surfactants (spooning, phenylhydralazine) and anti-Rh IG (In Rh + patients) causing hemolysis may help in faster clearance. While ultrasonic radiation also may have similar effects these modalities are not are not welcome since breakdown products may be toxic to retina causing permanent damage to photoreceptors.

Use of agents like IL-1 may enhance phagocytosis and may give significant effects in clearing of the bleed but the risk of raised tension resulting from increase numbers of big phagocytes (after engulfing RBC) in intermediate stages of vitreous hemorrhage needs to be carefully observed.

CRYOTHERAPY AND DIATHERMY

Blood resorption from vitreous is mainly limited by rate of intravitreal hemolysis, fibrinolysis, phagocytic activity, vitreous liquefaction. These procedures though are effective in checking the fresh bleed but they may help in enhancing hemolysis, fibrinolysis, liquefaction of vitreous and thus helping the phagocytosis resulting into faster clearing of the hemorrhagic vitreous.

Anterior Retinal Cryotherapy

Slow clearance of the blood and blood products is responsible for low grade vitritis and uveitis. The substances may have a toxic effect on photoreceptors and IOP may rise due to clogging of trabecular meshwork. Anterior retinal cryopexy may be considered after 6 weeks if there is no significant clearance of otherwise dense hemorrhage. However, Associated Retinal Consultants (ARC) promote formation of preretinal fibers and contraction of vitreous gel and may cause tractional RD cryotherapy.

Cryotherapy should not be performed in eyes with tractional detachment. Also, it can lead to formation of vitreous membranes.

The best indication for ARC would be post-vitrectomy eyes with recurrent vitreous hemorrhage from sclerotomy sites or from early anterior hyaloid proliferation.

Posterior Hyaloidotomy

Hemorrhage located between ILM and hyloid membrane near the fovea and a bleed trapped between in ILM and nerve fiber layer and subhyloid hemorrhage may be annoying due to significant vision drop soon after the injury and collection of blood products

Neodymium-doped: yttrium aluminium garnet (Nd: YAG) laser disrupts ILM and releases blood into vitreous cavity. This reduces the density of trapped collected blood and allows for better diffusion in the vitreous cavity followed by gravitation off the macula increasing the area for absorption in a big way partially compensating for relative slow phagocytosis expected with in the vitreous gel.

VITRECTOMY

In traumatic vitreous hemorrhage physiological goals are removal of core vitreous, thus removing the scaffold for possible future intraocular proliferation and the excision of media opacities in general and blood in particular, which are stimulants for proliferation and scaring.

Anatomical goals are removal of damaged lens, if present; the excision of vitreous hemorrhage, relief of vitreous traction and closure of all retinal breaks and associated detachments.

Vitrectomy; the surgical evaluation of the vitreous bleed may have to be done in lesser number closed globe injury since most eyes are otherwise healthy and respond to spontaneous clearing.[10,11]

Preoperative evaluation of vitreous hemorrhage:
- Recent visual acuity
- Relative afferent papillary defect
- Intraocular pressure
- Rubesis iridis
- Lenticular opacities
- Ultrasound to evaluate for RD and associated PVR changes, PVD, IOFB, areas of vitreoretinal adhesions
- Flash VEP and bright flash ERG for prediction of visual potential.

Management of Vitreous Hemorrhage

Simple vitrectomy is needed in case of dense hemorrhage with in 3 months if it does not show signs of good clearance. The pars plana vitrectomy gives better results after spontaneous PVD which may be seen in 2 weeks time and induction of PVD is an important step in other step in other cases. PFCL injection after clearing the vitreous helps in moving the blood from post pole? Macula and a soft brush/cannula can be used in removing the collected blood safely away from macula. Removal of PFCL and fluid gas is required at the end of procedure. The procedure can be further facilitated in submacular hemorrhage by tissue plasmin activator (tPA25-100 mg in 0.1–0.2 mL) in subretinal space. The risk of retinal detachment and PVR are more common apart from nearly 45 minutes of extra-time needed for the lysis process to be completed and injection of expansile gas (0.3–0.4 mL SF6) is usually required in more refractory cases when tPA is used. Finer instruments through smaller multiple retinotomies may give better outcome.

Localization of a break in all cases with or without detachment is vital. Careful peroperative retinal periphery examination through the clear media and tacking all breaks (pre-existing/iatrogenic) is the key for good outcome. Extent of macula off and its duration may be a deciding factor for final visual outcome.

Late surgery has a poor outcome due to pre-existing fibrosis and compromised posterior pole status and lenticular damage adds to the visual results extensive subretinal fibrosis and traction may not respond well surgery even after multiple retinotomies.

Sutureless vitrectomy, early vitreoretinal surgery using 25/23 gauge instruments gives very satisfying results in early cases trauma.

It has been shown that 25 GA. Surgery is ideal for vitreous hemorrhage, rhegmetogenous retinal detachments and giant breaks, and is applicable for diabetic traction RD with modest amount of epiretinal membrane as well.

Buckling: External support is not required in most cases of cases of simple vitrectomy but it is more rewarding to put an encirclage after vitrectomy in a long-standing vitreous hemorrhage and multiple breaks.

Internal temponade: Internal temponade is needed preoperatively and postoperatively only in bad proliferative cases.

Lensectomy: Lensectomy may be necessary if lenticular opacity does not allow a clear visualization of vitreous cavity. Sometimes, lensectomy may be performed in the same sitting with anticipated progression of the cataract after surgery. IOL can also be implanted in the same sitting after satisfactory completion of vitreous clearing. Lenses with 4+ nuclear sclerosis can be removed by limbal extraction and tight closure of the wound preferably with interrupted sutures.

Final outcome of vitreous hemorrhage: In closed globe injuries, absorption of blood from vitreous cavity can be expected faster if IOPs are kept controlled and inflammation checked B-scan evaluation on regular intervals can guide timings of surgical intervention. The prognosis is usually favorable in timely intervention. Vitreous hemorrhage in open globe has a unfavorable outcome.

REFERENCES

1. Abok K, Blomquist E, Ericsson J, Brunk U. Macrophage radiosensitivity in culture as a function of exposure to ionic iron. Virchows Arch B Cell Pathol Incl Mol Pathol. 1983;42(2):119–29.
2. Benson WE, Wirostko E, Spalter HF. The effects of inflammation on experimentally induced vitreous hemorrhage. Arch Ophthalmol. 1969;82(6):822–6.
3. Burke JM. Vitreal superoxide and superoxide dismutase after hemorrhagic injury: the role of invasive cells. Invest Ophthalmol Vis Sci. 1981;20(4):435–41.
4. Forrester JV, Lee WR, Williamson J. The pathology of vitreous hemorrhage. I. Gross and histological appearances. Arch Ophthalmol. 1978;96(4):703–1.
5. Butner RW, McPherson AR. Spontaneous vitreous hemorrhage. Ann Ophthalmol. 1982;14(3):268–70.
6. Harvey Lincoff etal.Pathogenasis of the Vitreous cloud Emanating from Subretinal Hemorrhage Arch Ophthal 2003;121:91–96.
7. Dana MR, Werner MS, Viana MA, Shapiro MJ. Spontaneous and traumatic vitreous hemorrhage. Ophthalmology. 1993;100(9):1377–83.
8. Ferrone PJ, de Juan E Jr. Vitreous hemorrhage in infants. Arch Ophthalmol. 1994;112(9):1185–9.
9. Greenwald MJ, Weiss A, Oesterle CS, Friendly DS. Traumatic retinoschisis in battered babies. Ophthalmology. 1986;93(5):618–25.
10. Masahito Ohji. Yoshihito,Atsushi Hayashi, John M.Lewis, Yasuo Tano Neumatic displacement of subretinal hemorrhage without tissue plasmin activator Arch Ophthalmol,1998;116;1326–1332.
11. Goff MJ, McDonald HR, Johnson RN, et al. Causes and treatment of vitreous hemorrhage. Compr Ophthalmol Update. 2006;7(3):97.

7.3 RETAINED INTRAOCULAR FOREIGN BODY

• R Kim • Manish Tandon

INTRAOCULAR FOREIGN BODIES (IOFBs) AND PERFORATING INJURIES

Introduction

Whenever ocular or periocular tissues are lacerated the ophthalmologist must suspect the presence of an IOFB unless proven otherwise.[1] The optimal management depends on a few factors like accurate localization of the foreign body (FB), knowledge of its composition, shape and size. Also defining the extent of ocular and orbital trauma is important so as to plan the management of FB, keeping in mind the technical expertise required.[2,3] The medicolegal implications are also to be kept in mind while managing the cases of retained IOFBs.

Types of Foreign Bodies

1. *Metallic:* These are the most common types of IOFBs. The most common metallic foreign body is iron followed by lead, copper, zinc, silver and nickel.
2. *Nonmetallic:* Most common nonmetallic foreign body is glass followed plastic, cilia and wood.
3. *Organic:* Soil and plant materials constitute this group of IOFBs.
4. *Rare materials:* Bentonite (material used for dental surgery), pencil lead graphite and color pencils.

Risk Factors for Intraocular Foreign Bodies

1. *Open globe injuries:* 18–41% of this group of ocular injuries are associated with IOFB.[4]
2. *Age:* Usually, young people are involved, and 66% of the affected are in their 2nd to 4th decades of their life.[5]
3. *Sex:* Males are more commonly affected.[6]
4. *Work:* Hammering is the most common cause and constitutes 60–80% of the cause.[7]
5. *Nature of the foreign body:* 80–90% are metallic foreign bodies followed by nonmetallic foreign bodies.[7]

Some Basic Facts Regarding Trauma by Intraocular Foreign Bodies[8]

1. Smaller the wound higher the chances of retinal injury.

2. Objects that enter through sclera cause more damage than the ones which enter through the anterior route, i.e. cornea.
3. More sharp objects cause lesser destruction.
4. More the inflammation higher is the rate of proliferative vitreoretinopathy.

Approach to a Patient with Intraocular Foreign Body and Protocol for Management

Detailed History (Specifically Regarding)

a. Circumstances of injury (How? When? loss of consciousness after the injury?).
b. Chronological sequence what did the patient do after the injury like bending, lifting heavy objects.
c. Previous history of immunization against tetanus.
d. Pretrauma eye condition.
e. Nature of the foreign body injury, i.e. whether metallic or nonmetallic.
f. Any systemic problems like intracranial aneurysms.
g. Any form of primary treatment (medical or surgical or native) taken.

Examination

Complete ocular examination with special reference to other eye status is a must.

Specific points that are to be remembered are:

a. Double eversion of the upper lid for superior fornix is to be done as foreign bodies may lodge over there.
b. Iris crypts are to be looked at carefully for any nonsurgical iridotomy.
c. If possible do a gonioscopy to look for foreign body in the angle.
d. At times, intralenticular foreign bodies may be noted.
e. Fundus examination—a fully dilated pupil is a must for detailed fundus examination. Avoid atropine and instead short acting mydriatics like tropicamide can be used so as to prevent a dilated fixed pupil secondary to posterior synechiae.
f. Avoid indentation unless wound is sealed.

Radiography

CT Scan

With the advent of CT scan this has become the investigation of choice for metallic foreign bodies. This modality has 65% sensitivity to localize the foreign body if the volume is less than 0.06 mm³ and 100% sensitivity if more than 0.06 mm³. Spiral CT scan can detect up to 0.048 mm³ size objects. Wide cuts tend to miss the IOFB, so the cuts should be smaller.

Magnetic Resonance Imaging (MRI)

MRI is very useful if the suspected foreign body is nonmetallic. MRI is contraindicated if the patient has suspected metallic foreign body, implanted cardiac pacemaker and ferromagnetic implants.

Ultrasound B-scan

B-scan is of limited value as its tends to over estimate the size of foreign body but still it comes as a handy investigation when it comes to localizing the foreign body in clinical setting (Fig. 7.3.1). The "gain" setting while localizing the foreign body should be low to clearly delineate its size and location. Care must be taken to perform B-scan gently when the open wound is large in size.

X-ray

In modern era, the X-ray imaging is used lesser as an imaging tool in management of IOFB body though at many places in a developing country this may be the only investigation available. It is an unreliable investigation for small IOFBs, more so if foreign body is nonmetallic (60% false negative). It is of use when a metallic foreign body is suspected (Figs 7.3.2 and 7.3.3) and may be used as a screening investigation for metallic foreign body when CT scan is not available or patient cannot afford the cost of a CT scan.

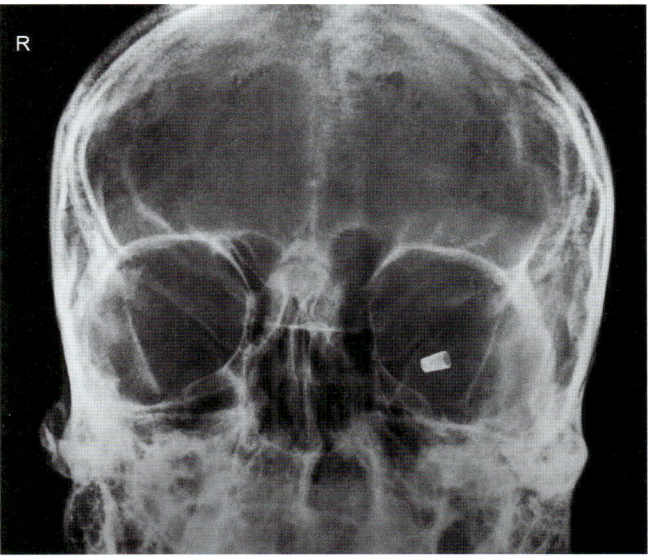

Fig. 7.3.2: Anteroposterior view of a metallic intraocular foreign body

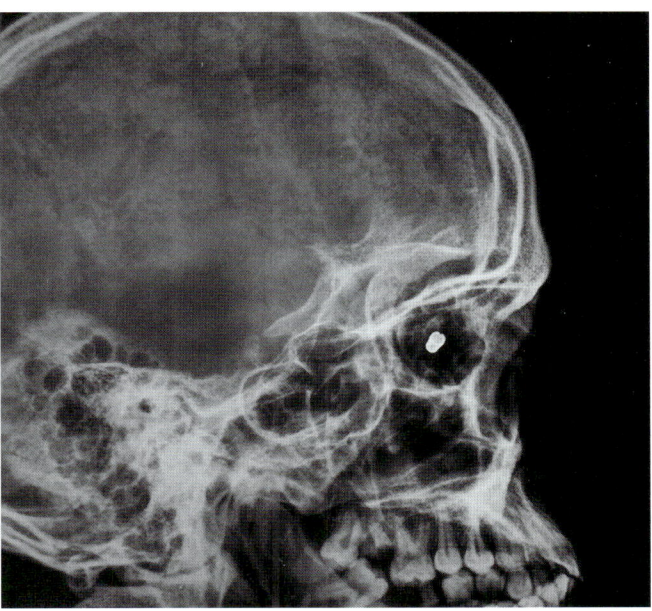

Fig. 7.3.3: Lateral view of same patient

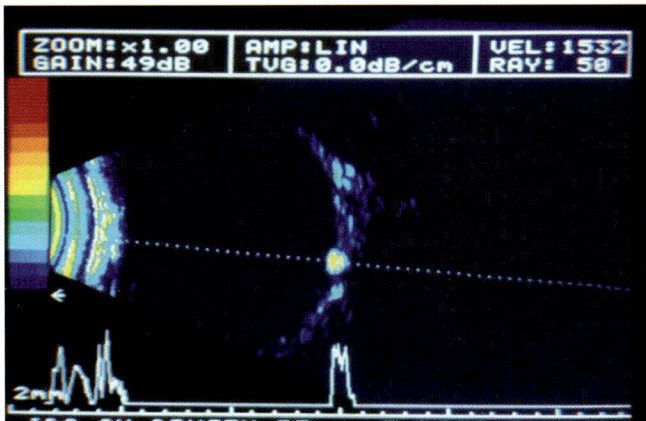

Fig. 7.3.1: Metallic foreign body delineated by B-scan (note that the gain setting is low)

Ten Points of Presurgical Work-up Protocol

1. Detailed history as described above.
2. *Physical examination:* This includes best-corrected visual acuity, pupillary reactions, wound inspection in detail, media clarity, slit lamp findings, hypopyon or signs of endophthalmitis and posterior segment findings like retinal breaks or RD.
3. Preoperative conjunctiva culture and sensitivity.
4. Patient is to be kept fasting for at least 6 hours preoperatively.
5. Systemic antibiotics as prophylaxis and prevention of infection (studies have shown a 6.8% incidence of endophthalmitis with systemic antibiotics as compared to 7.2% incidence without systemic antibiotics).[9]
6. Tetanus toxoid injection if not immunized.
7. Preoperative blood investigations to rule out any systemic infection.
8. Radiological investigations as described above.
9. Notifying anesthesia and operating room staff.
10. Detailed and informed consent is a mandatory dictum.

Principles of Intraocular Foreign Body Removal

1. Closure of all wounds in the eye.
2. Sclerotomy should be large enough for easy removal of foreign body.
3. Media to be cleared with or without lensectomy.
4. All vitreous to be removed surrounding the foreign body.
5. Removal of the foreign body should be done in the least traumatic way.
6. Associated ocular pathologies like breaks to be dealt with appropriately.
7. Foreign body to be sent for culture.
8. If endophthalimitis is present or suspected then intravitreal antibiotics should be given (vancomycin 1 mg/0.1 mL) because of its wide gram-positive coverage and also its activity against *Bacillus* species, amikacin (400 mg/0.1 mL) for gram-negative coverage. For bacilus infection *Clindamycin* 200 mg can also be injected as a substitute to vancomycin.[10,11]

Surgical Techniques for Intraocular Foreign Body Removal

The foreign body removal is a challenging task and certain minimum technical expertize is needed. The foreign body removal requires various surgical methodology as it can be lodged in various parts of the eye.

1. Foreign body in anterior segment.
2. Intralenticular foreign body.
3. Foreign body in posterior segment.
4. Intraretinal foreign body.
5. Nonmetallic IOFB.
6. Large IOFB.

Foreign Body in Anterior Segment (Fig. 7.3.4)

This is easy to deal with provided the approach is carefully planned. If foreign body is small (< 3 mm size in greatest dimension), it can be removed through the entry wound itself at the time of primary repair (Fig. 7.3.5). Nonmetallic foreign bodies like glass and plastic may be difficult to identify because of their transparency and must be visualized before grasping with a forceps so as to avoid damage to ocular tissue.

Intralenticular Foreign Body[8]

This has been dealt elsewhere.

Foreign Body in Posterior Segment

We can have two situations of intraocular foreign body in the posterior segment.
a. Foreign body is well visualized.
b. Foreign body not visualized.

Foreign Body is Well Visualized

If the foreign body is in the posterior segment and is seen well then pars plana vitrectomy and IOFB

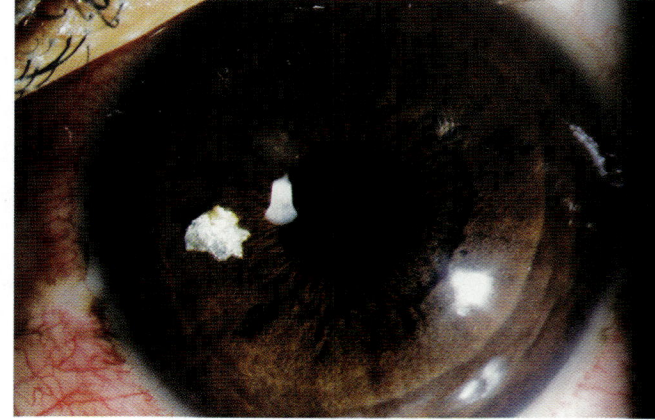

Fig. 7.3.4: Metallic foreign body in anterior chamber

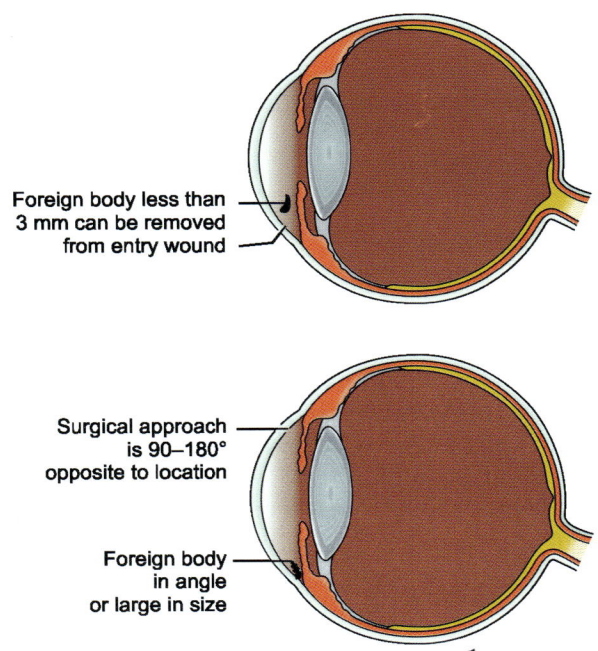

Fig. 7.3.5: Foreign body in anterior chamber

removal with or without lensectomy is a standard procedure. If planned well these patients can undergo a phacoemulsification with the insertion of an intraocular lens implant, an intraocular magnet may be of help in case of removal of metallic foreign bodies else the use of intraocular forceps is to be done if the foreign body is nonmagnetic. A drop of PFCL may be used over the macula for protection against the damage to retina in case foreign body falls back (Fig. 7.3.6).

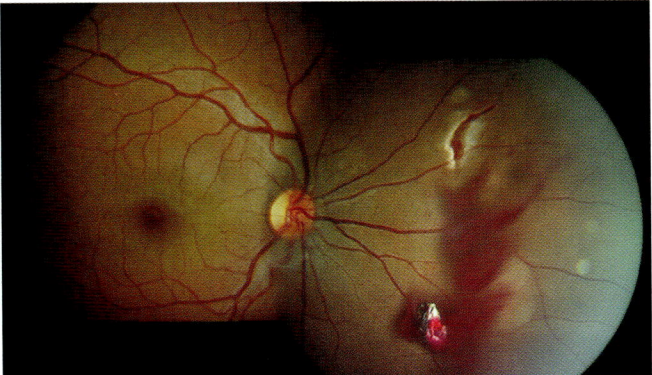

Fig. 7.3.6: Metallic foreign body in posterior segment: Note the retinal tear caused by impact of the foreign body

Foreign Body not Visualized

When the foreign body has not been visualized preoperatively then pars plana vitrectomy with or without lensectomy should be done to clear the media (Figs 7.3.7a and b). In this situation, when the IOFB is not visualized, the blind use of a magnet should be avoided as uncontrolled foreign body movement, may cause more damage. It is better to do a good vitrectomy to visualize the IOFB and then remove the IOFB using a magnet (in case of metallic foreign bodies) or forceps like Grieshaber or Wilson's vitreous foreign body forceps (for both magnetic and nonmagnetic foreign bodies) to hold the foreign body and in a more controlled manner.[12]

Magnets

These are important tools in the removal of IOFBs in the posterior segment. The action of magnet is in accordance with Coulomb's law where magnetic field (H) is dependent on strength of the magnet at each pole and inversely proportional to the distance between the poles.

$H = m \times m'/d^2$ where m and m' are strength of the magnet at each pole and d is the distance between the two poles.

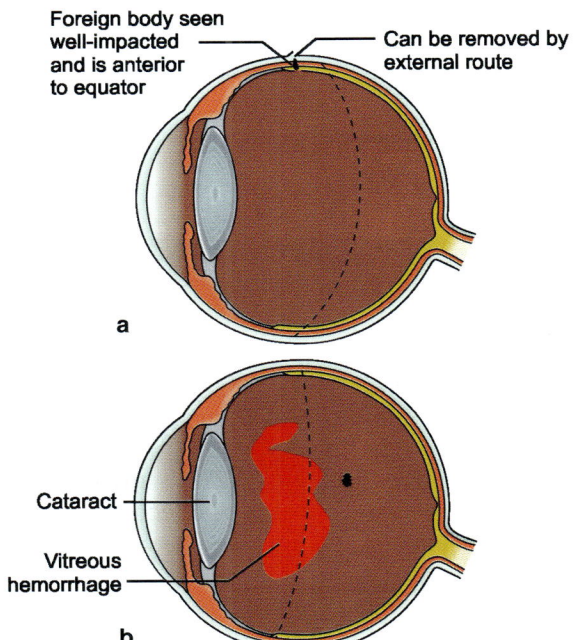

Figs 7.3.7a and b: (a) Anterior position of FB indicating choice of external route; (b) Opaque media will necessitate pars plana vitrectomy with lensectomy

Strength is inversely proportional to the cube of distance between the poles and the field decreases proportionately to distance of object from the magnet. Implication of this fact lies in that powerful magnets are needed to act at a shorter distance and objects align themselves along their long access which is facilitatory in the removal of IOFBs.

Types of Magnets

a. Rare earth magnets
b. Electromagnets.

Rare Earth Magnets (Fig. 7.3.8)

These create weak fields and work at shorter distances. They are used for contact extraction through sclerotomies.

Electromagnets

These are powerful and can be used both intraocularly and extraocularly. But, the disadvantage lies that they have to be carefully oriented otherwise damage to delicate ocular structures may occur (Fig. 7.3.9).

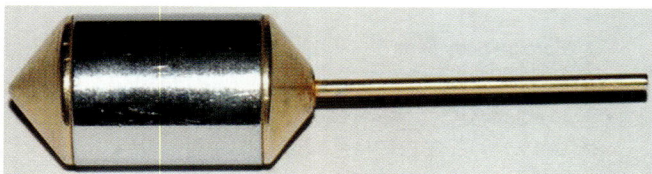

Fig. 7.3.8: Rare earth magnet

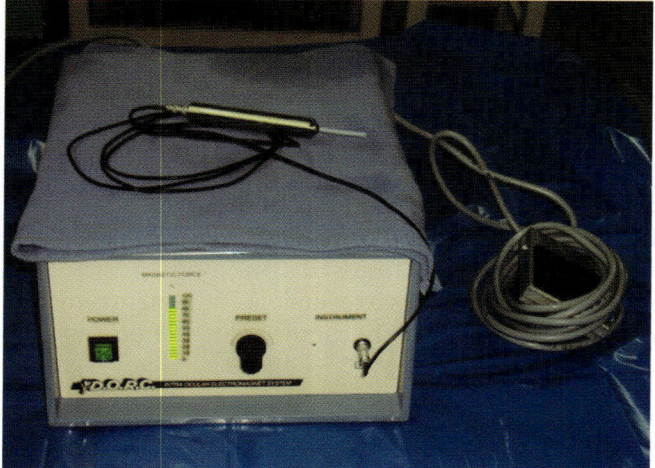

Fig. 7.3.9: Electromagnet

Intraretinal Foreign Body

Intraretinal foreign bodies are absolute indications for vitreoretinal intervention as there is a risk of RD. They can be removed via two routes.
1. Transcleral route
2. Transvitreal route.

Transcleral Route

This procedure can be undertaken only when the media is clear, the IOFB is seen well with site of impaction anterior to equator. Transcleral route is formed by the creation of "trap door scleral flap" which is followed by careful dissection of the choroidal bed and external diathermy followed by a choroidal incision and removal of the foreign body by a forceps or an external magnet.

Retinal incarceration is an unwanted complication of this procedure and prophylactic scleral buckling can be done to prevent RD.

Transvitreal Route

In this technique, pars plana vitrectomy is performed followed by laser (around the site of impaction) and if the foreign body is mobile foreign body forceps is used but if foreign body is encapsulated myringotomy blade can be used to free the foreign body. After the foreign body is released from the fibrous capsule, forceps or rare earth magnets can be used to remove it.

In this procedure, it is important to remove the vitreous around the FB, and also the complete removal of posterior hyaloid, otherwise postoperatively vitreoretinal traction or formation of macular pucker may occur. Encirclage may or may not be done depending on surgeon's choice.

The complications of this procedure are formation of a macular pucker, proliferative vitreoretinopathy and RD, if posterior hyaloid is not removed.[13]

Nonmagnetic Intraocular Foreign Bodies

The procedure for the removal of nonmagnetic IOFB is pars plana vitrectomy followed by laser around the impaction site and removal of IOFB by a forceps. Impacted inert foreign bodies can be observed.

Large Intraocular Foreign Body

These IOFBs (bomb blast pellets) can be removed by limbal incision (Figs 7.3.10a and b). If cornea is damaged then corneal grafting procedure can be combined with an open sky vitrectomy. The

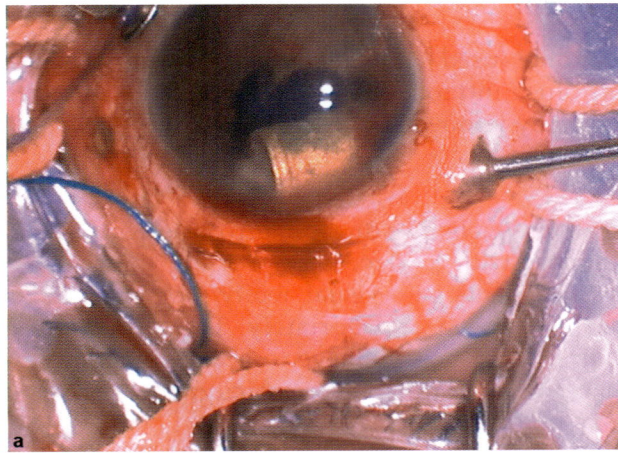

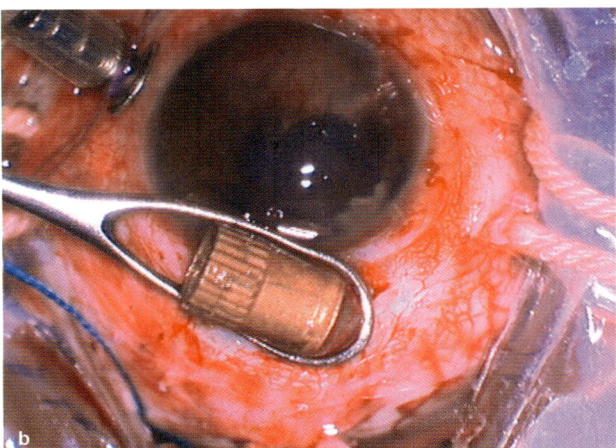

Figs 7.3.10a and b: IOFVs can be removed by limbal incision

advantages of this procedure are free instrument movement and access to peripheral structures. The disadvantages of this procedure are no IOP control, increased risk of choroidal hemorrhage or choroidal detachment, lesser control over hemotains and limited posterior dissection due to limited illumination. The resulting visual acuity after severe trauma with RD is only better than 20/200 and more often is merely perferably left (PL) to counting finger (CF) even in successful cases that may be explained by the fact that this surgery is the last resort surgery and the ocular structures are usually compromised.

Complications of the Intraocular Foreign Bodies if not Removed

1. Siderosis
2. Chalcosis
3. Effect of other metals

4. Complications associated with organic foreign bodies.
5. Complications associated with rare IOFBs.

Siderosis

This is a late occurring syndrome caused by retained IOFB of iron or steel. The initial effects are mainly due to mechanical damage and contusion and to a lesser extent secondary to a chemical reaction.

The cause of ocular siderosis is implicated to ferric iron toxicity[14] and duration of manifestation of symptoms varies from few days to years (average of 2 months to 2 years). The occurrence of siderosis depends on iron content but it does not imply that with iron foreign bodies, it is inevitable.

Clinical Features

1. Rusty discoloration of corneal endothelium.
2. Iris heterochromia.
3. "Yellow cataract" with brown deposits on the anterior capsule of the lens.
4. Dilated and nonreactive pupil.
5. Pigmentary retinal degeneration (initial complaints are of nyctalopia).
6. Constriction of visual fields.
7. Open angle glaucoma due to iron containing phagocytes and cellular debris in trabecular meshwork.
8. Attenuation of retinal vessels.
9. Optic atrophy.
10. Electroretinography shows classical increase in amplitude of the α-wave and progressive decrease in the amplitude of the β-wave subsequently.
11. Electro-oculograpy changes occur late and indicate a poor prognosis.

It is best to remove the iron foreign body early because neither encapsulation nor intralenticular location prevents development of siderosis. Even dense vitreous hemorrhage if left for a long time can cause siderotic changes in the eye.[15] However, siderosis is not always irreversible and timely removal of the iron foreign body can prevent anatomical and functional damage to the eye.

If patient has an old IOFB of iron but no siderotic changes then the management is conservative with examination of the visual acuity, slit lamp examination, indirect ophthalmolscopy, ERG and radiological investigations on regular basis.[16] If the patient cannot follow-up, then surgery should be undertaken.

Chalcosis

Copper and its alloys (e.g. bronze and brass) cause chalcosis which is a "set of chronic degenerative process in the eye". If the copper content is high in the foreign body then severe intraocular reaction inciting hypopyon and localized (sterile) abscesses within the eye develop. Corneal and scleral melting and retinal detachment may also accompany[17] the process.

These clinical features mimic pyogenic endophthalmitis or even may resemble panophthalmitis but they are refractory to antibiotics and steroids. Hence, the removal of copper containing foreign body is to be done as an emergency measure.

However, chalcosis occurs by slow diffusion with preferential deposition on basement membranes of various ocular structures (contrary to siderosis which occurs intracellularly in epithelial type cells).

Clinical Features

1. Kayser- Fleischer ring in the Descemet's membrane of cornea.
2. "Sunflower cataract" with "Greenish brown" hue on anterior lenticular capsule with spokes of copper radiating from central ring.
3. Greenish discoloration of aqueous and vitreous.
4. Copper deposits on retinal surface.

Improvement in clinical features occur soon after the removal of copper containing foreign body but chalcosis may happen due to residual copper powder in the eye.[17] As copper and its alloys are nonmagnetic it is technically more difficult to remove than iron containing foreign body.

Effect of Other Metals

They cause intraocular inflammation of varying intensity. In the decreasing order of reactivity, the metals are: mercury, aluminum, nickel, zinc and lead. Except for nickel all are nonmagnetic.

Organic Foreign Bodies

Cilia, wood and soil carry the risk of bacterial (bacillus) or fungal endophthalmitis and urgent surgery is warranted for their removal.

Rare Intraocular Foreign Bodies

Bentonite (used in dental surgeries) and pencil lead can cause intraocular inflammation and should be surgically removed.

Prognosis

Small foreign bodies due to sharp objects have a good prognosis with good recovery of visual functions (75% of the patients gain visual acuity more than 5/200) when managed appropriately. The larger foreign bodies cause more damage to ocular structures and hence the visual prognosis remains guarded even after a successful surgical removal.

Factors Having Good Visual Outcome[18,19]

1. Presenting visual acuity more than or equal to 20/40.
2. Need of a single or a maximally two surgical procedures.
3. Size of the foreign body less than 2 mm².

Factors Having Poor Visual Outcome

1. Posteriorly located entry wound.
2. Presenting visual acuity less than 5/200.
3. Wound size more than 4 mm.
4. Size of IOFB less than 10 mm.[20]
5. Blunt objects (edgeless), e.g. bomb blast pellets.[21]
6. Nonmetallic foreign body.
7. Afferent pupillary defect.
8. Endophthalmitis.
9. Multiple surgical interventions.

REFERENCES

1. Paton and Goldberg. Management of ocular injuries, 2nd Edition: 61.
2. Goldberg MF. Management of posterior segment intra ocular foreign bodies. J Miss State Med Assoc. 1970; 11:149–158.
3. Havener WH, Gloecknen SL. Atlas of diagnostic techniques and treatment of intra ocular foreign bodies. St. louis, CV Mosby Co. 1969.
4. de Juan, et al. Penetrating ocular injuries. Ophthalmology. 1983;90:1318–1322.
5. Roper Hall MJ. Review of 555 cases of intra ocular foreign bodies with special reference to prognosis. 1954; 38:65–99.
6. Punnonen E, et al. Prognosis of perforating eye injuries with intra ocular foreign bodies. Acta Ophthalmol. 1989; 66:483–491.

7. Behrens-Baumann W, et al. Intra ocular foreign bodies. Ophthalmologica. 1989;198:84–88.

8. Mester V, Kuhn F. Intra ocular foreign bodies. Ophthal. Clin of North Am. 2002; 15:235–242.

9. Thompson JT, Parver LM, et al. Infectious endophthalmitis after penetrating ocular injuries with retained intra ocular foreign bodies. Ophthalmology. 1993; 100: 1468–1474.

10. Parrish CM, O' day DM. Traumatic Endophthalmitis. Int. Ophthalmol Clin. 1987;27:112–119.

11. Schemmer GB, et al. Post traumatic *bacillus cereus* endophthalmitis. Arch. Ophthalmol. 1987;105:342–344.

12. Khani SC, Mulai S. Posterior segment intra ocular foreign bodies. Int Ophthalmol Clin. 1995;35:151–161.

13. Slusher MM, Sarin LK, et al. Management of intraretinal foreign bodies. Ophthalmology. 1982;89:369–373.

14. Davidson M, Siderosis Bulbi. Am J Oph. 1933;16:331–335.

15. Cibis P, Yamashita T, et al. Clinical aspects of ocular siderosis and hemosiderosis. Arch Ophthalmol. 1959; 62:46–53.

16. Neumann R, Belkin M, et al. A long term follow up of metallic intra ocular foreign bodies employing diagnostic X-ray spectrometry. Arch Ophthalmol. 1992;110:1269–1272.

17. Duke-Elder S. System of Ophthalmology. Vol. XIV London: Henry Kimpton; 1972:451–649.

18. Brinton GS, Aaberg TM. Surgical results in ocular trauma involving the posterior segment. Am J Ophthal. 1982; 94:271–278.

19. Hutton WL, Fuller DG. Factors influencing final visual results in severely injured eyes. Am J oph. 1984; 102:712–722.

20. Delori F, Pomerantzoff O, et al. deformation of the globe under high speed impact: its relation to contusion injuries. Invest Ophth. 1964; 8:290–301.

21. Brown GC, Tasman WS, et al. BB gun injuries to the eye. Ophthal Surg. 1985; 16:505–508.

7.4 DOUBLE PERFORATIONS MANAGEMENT STRATEGIES

• R Kim • Manish Tandon

PERFORATING INJURIES (Fig. 7.4.1)

These are the small subgroup of open globe injuries comprising of 4.4% of the total ocular trauma.[1] The mode of injury most commonly is a missile, e.g. bomb blast pellets or shot gun pellet. This subgroup had a poor visual prognosis earlier but in the modern era with sophisticated techniques the prognosis has improved considerably.

Pathogenesis

At the posterior exit wound fibrovascular proliferation occurs that on contraction causes tractional RD. Experimental evidence suggests that maximal proliferation occurs after 7 days of injury.

Management

The management is primarily the closure of the entry wound and posterior exit wound if located anterior to equator. If it is difficult to close the posterior rupture site, if the location is posterior then the attempted closure of posterior wound may cause excess pressure on the globe and optic nerve and may lead to extrusion of intraocular contents. The scleral wound seals by the 7th day of the injury and vitrectomy can be delayed up to 7 days. The surgical procedure consists of standard three port pars plana vitrectomy with or without encirclage. The PVD if not present should be induced and the vitreous stump if incarcerated in the posterior exit wound should be trimmed and not completely removed as it may reopen the posterior wound. Surgery is completed by laser barrage of the exit wound and introducing the tamponade after fluid air exchange.

Prognosis

Prognosis has improved with the modern surgical equipment. Martin et al had anatomical success in 41 of 51 cases and functional success in 32 cases (63%).[2]

Factors Affecting the Prognosis

1. If macula and optic nerve is damaged, the visual outcome is poor.
2. Removal of the posterior hyaloid increases the chance of successful surgery and hence an exit site posterior to vitreous base can have a better surgical prognosis.

Prevention

2.2 mm polycarbonate lenses can prevent small pellets from penetration of the eye and hence they should be worn in high risk group like military personnel and hunters.[3]

REFERENCES

1. Muller-Jensen K. Doppelt Perforierende Augenveletzungen. Klin. Monastbl Augenheikld. 1964; 145:754–758.
2. Martin DF, Meredith TA, et al. Perforating (Through and through) injuries of the globe: surgical results with vitrectomy. Arch Ophthal. 1991; 109:951–956.
3. Simmon S.T., Knohel GP et al. Prevention of ocular gun shot injuries using polycarbonate lenses. Ophthalmology. 1984;91:977–983.

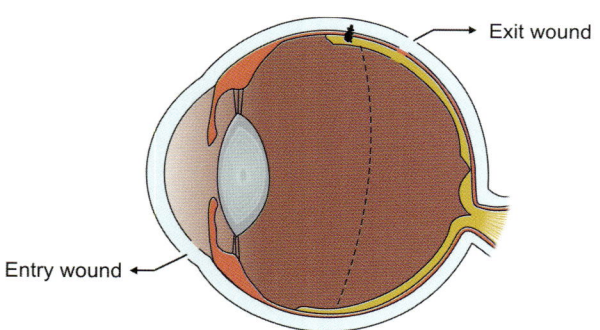

Fig. 7.4.1: Double perforation (penetrating injury) with entry and exit wound

Exit wound

Entry wound

7.5 POST-TRAUMATIC ENDOPHTHALMITIS

• DK Mehta • Deepali Garg Mathur

INTRODUCTION

Endophthalmitis is one of the most devastating diagnoses in ophthalmology. With any breach of the ocular bulbus, potential exists to introduce an infectious inoculum large enough to produce endophthalmitis leading to blindness in potentially salvageable eyes. About 25% of endophthalmitis cases occur following trauma and are sadly associated with a poorer visual outcome than otherwise similar globe injuries with only 22–42% of patients obtaining a final visual acuity of 20/400 or better.[1-3]

Studies reveal that between 2.4% and 7.4% eyes with penetrating ocular trauma develop endophthalmitis.[4] The type of injury and the nature of infecting organism greatly influence the prognosis in these eyes.[4] Increasing risk factors include dirty wound, breach of the lens capsule, delay more than 24 hours in primary repair, older age and presence of retained intraocular foreign body.[5,6] Early diagnosis and treatment with antimicrobial therapy are fundamental to optimize visual outcome.

ETIOPATHOGENESIS

The overall profile of organisms isolated from post-traumatic endophthalmitis shows *Staphylococcus epidermidis* to be the most common. With a retained IOFB, *Bacillus cereus* and *Streptococcus* are common species isolated. *Bacillus* is especially associated with more aggressive infections and with organic foreign bodies. Other species implicated include *Propionibacterium acnes, Pseudomonas, Gram-negative organisms*, fungi and mixed pathogens. Polymicrobial infections are common. There is a reported relative absence of infection caused by yeast like fungi. Most fungal infections are caused by filamentous fungi with greater virulence, e.g *Fusarium solanae*. The spectrum differs in pediatric postoperative endophthalmitis with 55% being caused by *Streptococcus* and *Staphylococcus* and *Bacillus* in only 12.5% eyes. Positive cultures do not always correlate with infection.

CLINICAL PRESENTATION

Post-traumatic endophthalmitis may occur within hours after trauma up to several weeks following it, depending on the virulence of the infecting organism. It may also result from contagious spread from an infected corneal, scleral or adjacent wound. Presentation may be masked by distortion of the normal anatomy of the eye due to trauma. Clinical symptoms typically include reduced or blurred vision, redness, pain and lid swelling. Progressive vitritis and a hypopyon are commonly seen.

Progression of the disease may lead to panophthalmitis, corneal infiltration and perforation and ultimately phthisis bulbi.

INVESTIGATIONS

Initial evaluation must exclude occult or retained foreign bodies. If the fundus view is inadequate, CT or in eyes with self-sealing or previously sutured wounds, USG B-scan may be helpful. MRI must be avoided because a retained foreign body might be magnetic. Routine intraocular culture does not play a significant role in diagnosing post-traumatic endophthalmitis. Ariyasu et al found that 33% of open globe injuries were culture positive, but none developed endophthalmitis. In contrast, the prevalence of culture negative cases of post-traumatic endophthalmitis has been in the range of 17–42%.[7]

Role of vitreous tap and vitreous biopsy has been stressed from time to time. Although vitreous culture may not be positive in more than half the cases it is worth while to take the samples before starting the antibiotics or even during the treatment for better sensitivity options.

MANAGEMENT

Endophthalmitis is one of the most challenging complication of ocular trauma. The risk of infection in trauma is significantly high as bacteria inadvertently gain entry into the eye at the time of injury. After appropriate investigation to rule out a retained IOFB (indirect ophthalmoscopy, CT scan, USG B-scan), primary repair should be performed as soon as possible after open globe injury. Delayed surgery has been associated with infection both in the presence and the absence of retained IOFB. During primary repair, it is prudent to document the extent of the wound in terms of zone, type and grade of injury. The injury if caused by an object contaminated by soil or vegetable matter is termed a "dirty wound". Any lens disruption, vitreous in wound and posterior segment complications can increase the chances of contracting endophthalmitis.[8]

Antibiotic prophylaxis, refers to antibiotics given before any evidence of clinical infection is not yet established. In high risk cases (classified as those with two out of three factors, (delay in primary repair, ruptured lens capsule and dirty wound)[8] prophylactic intravitreal antibiotics would be prudent at the time of primary repair. Most studies advocate intravitreal vancomycin 1 mg and ceftazidime 2.25 mg which is effective against most gram-positive and gram-negative organisms including *Bacillus cereus*. The susceptibility of pathogens in post-traumatic endophthalmitis to vancomycin is reported as between 80% and 100%.

The role of pars plana vitrectomy in the management of post-traumatic endophthalmitis is undetermined. Retrospective studies do not document vitrectomy with intravitreal antibiotics to be superior to intravitreal antibiotics alone. In severe forms of postoperative endophthalmitis, however, vitrectomy may allow the surgeon to obtain a larger sample of vitreous for microbiological analysis and clear the vitreous cavity of harmful inflammatory cells and bacteria.[5]

Prophylactic intravenous antibiotics are not supported by any human clinical studies though some authors recommend it on the basis of experimental trials which show adequate intravitreal concentration in traumatized eyes. Tetanus immunization must be done if immunization record is not current.

SYMPATHETIC OPHTHALMIA (Table 7.5.1)

Sympathetic ophthalmia (SO) is a diffuse bilateral granulomatous panuveitis occurring as a potential complication of penetrating ocular trauma or surgery. Accidental trauma to uvea that incites an autoimmune inflammatory response is one of the major presumed reasons of SO. It is postulated that the trauma may play a role in the breakdown of the tolerance to uveitogenic intraocular antigens by providing their exposure to extraocular located lymphatics.[9] Injury to one eye (exciting eye) possibly leads to impairment of visual acuity or even blindness in both eyes. The innocently affected eye is called the sympathizing eye. The interval between the ocular injury and the onset of SO reported can vary from 5 days to 60 years with 90% occurring within the first year.

The incidence of SO after penetrating trauma varies between 0.14% and 0.5% and that after ocular surgery is estimated at 0.01%. However, these figures are based on retrospective studies, with clinical data more than 10 years old and may not reflect the benefits of modern microsurgical techniques and immunosuppression.[11] In a study conducted in Ireland in 2000, the incidence of SO was estimated to be as low as 0.03/100,000 of the general UK population. Formerly, accidental trauma was the main cause but ocular surgery especially retinal surgery has now become the main risk factor for SO.[10] The current SO risk of vitectomy is now more than twice the previously reported 0.06%. Immunogenic risks of pars plana vitrectomy are likely to be due to increased retinal manipulation and the breakdown of blood retinal barrier with release of previously sequestered retinal antigens and possibly subclinical uveal incarceration at wound sites, a known immunogenic risk.[11]

The clinical spectrum can range from mild bilateral posterior uveitis to severe bilateral granulomatous panuveitis. It was formerly believed that purulent eye infection with penetrating trauma destroys the uveal tissue and antigens to such an extent that such eyes do not incite SO. However, recent reports show that purulent infection may not offer protection against development of SO but may potentiate its development. The incidence of coexistent SO with post-traumatic endophthalmitis is reported as between 1% and 11%.[12]

Symptoms range from minimal to severe and include problems in near vision, photophobia, floaters and decreased vision. Anterior segment findings include mutton fat keratic precipitatis (KP's) posterior synechiae and uveitic glaucoma. Posterior segment findings may host vitritis, Dalen Fuch's nodules (yellowish white mid-equatorial choroidal lesions), peripapillary choroidal lesions and exudative RD. Chronic SO can lead to cataract formation, chronic cystoid macular edema (CME), choroidal neovascularization and optic atrophy. Extraocular findings include sensorineural deafness, alopecia, poliosis and vitiligo.

Table 7.5.1: Changing trends in sympathetic ophthalmia

Parameter	Historical	Current
Etiology	Post-trauma	Postsurgery (especially vitreoretinal)
Patient profile	More common in males and children (reflecting trauma peaks)	No gender preference (positive impact of injury prevention programs) and increasing in elderly and female patients (reflects impact of ocular surgery)
Incidence[13]	0.2–0.5% following trauma, 0.01% following ocular surgery	0.3/100,000 in prospective studies 1 in 800 following vitrectomy[15]
Onset	65% within 2–8 weeks, 90%, 1 year	Many delayed presentations as well
Clinical presentation	Granulomatous panuveitis	Any clinical uveitis to be viewed with suspicion
Role of enucleation	Enucleation within 2 weeks of trauma for prevention of sympathetic ophthalmia	Enucleation only if injured eye has no visual potential
Visual prognosis	Poor (one-third patients become legally blind)[3]	Reasonable due to modern immuno-suppressives

Since Mac Kenzie and Fuch's description of SO approximately one century ago, enucleation of the inciting eye to influence the course of SO, remains controversial. In some cases, the vision in the inciting eye may be better than the sympathizing eye making the decision to enuleate even more tough. As of recent times, prophylactic enucleation of a severely injured eye should be considered within 2 weeks of vision loss to minimize the risk of SO only when the injured eye has no vision potential.

Medical treatment typically involves immuno-modulation initially with systemic corticosteroids in conjunction with a long-term noncorticosteroid immunosuppressive therapy (azathioprine, metho-trexate, mycophenolate, mofetil, cyclosporine A, chlorambucil and cyclophosphamide). Topical corticosteroids together with cycloplegic/mydriatic agents are essential in treatment of acute anterior uveitis and periocular steroids are used for CME. In a recent trial conducted in 2009, fluocinolone acetonide implant (Retisert) has been used to reduce dependence on systemic immunosuppression in patients with SO.[14] Though the treatment options are many, *early diagnosis and prompt treatment* is the key to better visual outcomes.[14]

Sympathetic ophthalmia is a sight-threatening disease with a high rate of vision loss: earlier studies have reported that approximately half of the patients experience 20 of 40 or worse vision and one-third become legally blind. The relapsing nature and potential treatment toxicity warrants long-term follow-up. Left untreated it can lead to loss of vision with cataract, secondary glaucoma and chronic maculopathy being the main causes. The use of corticosteroid and other immunosuppressive therapy along with advancements in microsurgical techniques of wound repair have markedly improved the prognosis of SO. In a recent study 12 of 16 patients achieved a final visual acuity of 6 of 12 or better atleast in one eye.[15]

PHACOANAPHYLACTIC ENDOPHTHALMITIS

Phacoanaphylactic endophthalmitis is a chronic zonal granulomatous inflammation centerd around the ruptured lens. It is mostly unilateral although bilateral cases have been reported and often misdiagnosed as SO. Histologic examination confirming a ruptured lens capsule and regional involvement is confir-matory.

REFERENCES

1. Essex RW, Yi Q, Charles PG, Allen PJ. Post-traumatic endophthalmitis. Ophthalmology. 2004;111(11):2015–2022.
2. Affeldt JC, Flynn HW, Jr, Forster RK, Mandelbaum S, Clarkson JG, Jarus GD. Microbial endophthalmitis resulting from ocular trauma. Ophthalmology 1987;94:407–13.
3. Ariyasu RG, Kumar S, LaBree LD, Wagner DG, Smith RE. Microorganisms cultured from the anterior chamber of ruptured globes at the time of repair. Am J Ophthalmol. 1995;119(2):181–188.
4. Kresloff MS, Castellarin AA, Zarbin MA. Endo-phthalmitis. Surv Ophthalmol. 1998;43(3):193–224.

5. Alfaro DV, Roth D, Liggett PE. Posttraumatic endophthalmitis. Causative organisms, treatment and prevention. Retina 1994;14:206–11.

6. Thompson WS, Rubsamen PE, Flynn HW Jr, Schiffman J, Cousins SW. Endophthalmitis after penetrating trauma. Risk factors and visual acuity outcomes. Ophthalmology. 1995;102(11):1696–1701.

7. Brinton GS, Topping TM, Hyndiuk RA, Aaberg TM, Reeser FH, Abrams GW. Posttraumatic endophthalmitis. Arch Ophthalmol 1984;102:547–50.

8. Thompson JT, Parver LM, Enger CL, Mieler WF, Liggett PE. Infectious endophthalmitis after penetrating injuries with retained intraocular foreign bodies. National Eye Trauma System. Ophthalmology. 1993;100(10):1468–74.

9. Sen HN, Nussenblatt RB. Sympathetic Ophthalmia: What have we learned? Am J Ophthlmol.2009;148:632–3.

10. Rathinam SR, Rao NA. Sympathetic Ophthalmia following post operative Bacterial endophthalmitis: A Clinico-pathollogic study. Am J Ophthalmol. 2006:141: 498–507.

11. Kilmartin D, Dick A, Forrester J. Prospective surveillance of sympathetic ophthalmia in the UK and Republic of Ireland . Br J Ophthalmology 2000;84:259–63.

12. Kilmartin D, Dick A, Forrester J. Sympathetic ophthalmia risk following vitrectomy: should we counsel patients? Br J Ophthalmology 2000;84:448–9.

13. Chan CC, Roberge RG, et al. Thirty two cases of Sympathetic Ophthalmia. Arch Ophthalmol. 1995;113: 597–601.

14. Mahajan VB, Getrs KM, et al. Management of Sympathetic Ophthalmia with the Fluocinolone Acetonide implant. Ophthalmology 2009;116(3):552–7.

15. Vote BJ, Hall A. Changing trends in Sympathetic Ophthalmia. Clinical Experiment Ophthalmol. 2004; 32(5):542–5.

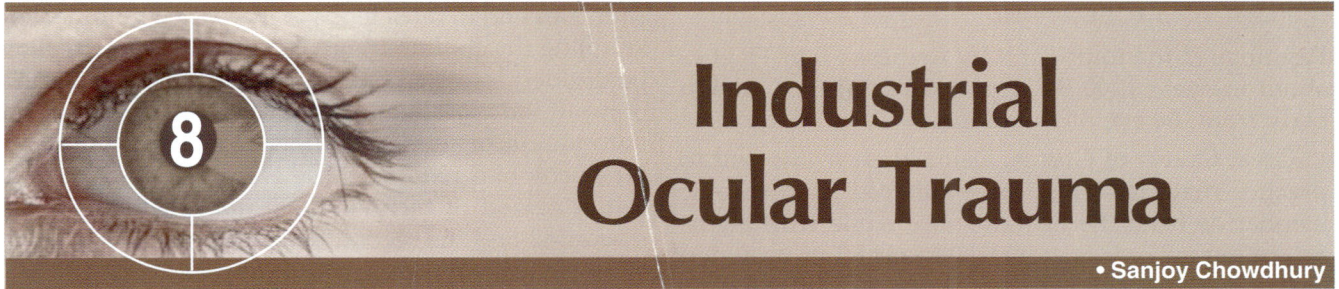

Industrial Ocular Trauma

• Sanjoy Chowdhury

"To produce and to avoid waste through errors and inaccuracies, one must see, have eyes and use them efficiently and to have two eyes or even one eye, one must guard them by suitable physical protective devices."   Dr Mrs HS Kuhn[6]

INTRODUCTION

Industrialization is the marker of development. An industrialized nation is considered as more developed nation. But life in industry is exposed to many dangers which include accidents and exposure to hazards. A healthy workforce is vital for sustainable social and economic development at global, national and local level. WHO study shows that 8% of yearly 160 million new cases of work-related illness are due to injuries,[1] ocular trauma account for substantial proportion of work-related injuries and around 50% of all eye injuries are considered to be industry related (Figs 8.1 and 8.2).[2-4] Earlier days, industries were labor oriented and produced varied types of injuries. Automation has changed the nature and profile of ocular trauma sustained by the people working there. Still the lifetime prevalence of work-related eye injuries among United States (US) workers is 4.4%.[3]

Many features, investigations and line of management are common to all types of eye injuries. Like the real need for consideration lies in that immediate treatment is of great value than that which can be given after lapse of golden period. Still another reason for special attention is the appalling danger that blindness of both eyes may be the result of injury to one of them (sympathetic ophthalmia) and like other types this is also mostly preventable more so in an industrial setup.

Therapeutics of trauma may not be very different in relation to cause and effect to specifics and but mode damage of initial care and treatment definitely affect the outcome. Besides this the real problems of

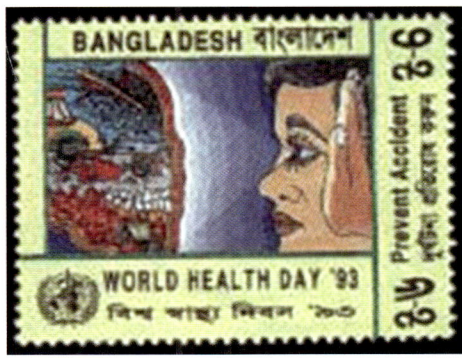

Fig. 8.1: Accidental eye injury: WHO day in a postage stamp from Bangladesh

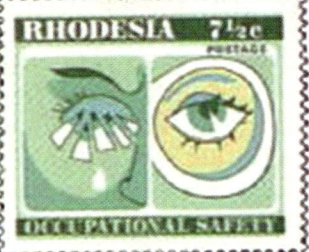
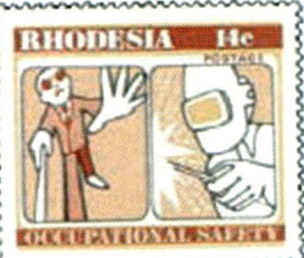

Fig. 8.2: Awareness of occupational eye disease: stamps from Rhodesia

Courtesy: Both the stamps are from collection of Royal Society of Ophthalmology, UK.

industrial eye injuries lies in prevention thereof, loss of man-hours, compensation and need for notification in many cases as per factory rules.

HISTORICAL BACKGROUND

Paintings at the tomb built by Rameses II at Thiebes about the year 1200 BC depicted removal of foreign body from the eye of a workman.[5]

Great Orator of Greece, Demosthenes was sent to practice rhetoric as his father suffered from chronic blepharitis from the heat of forge while working as an armourer.[5] Fear of industrial hazard thus provided Greece with her greatest orator.

Bernardo Ramazzani (1653–1714 AD), known as the father of industrial medicine, described ocular injuries due to occupational hazards after he came across many cases of keratoconjunctivitis among the lavatory cleaners of Paris city[5] in his book "De morbis artificum diatriba"(1700 AD).

During the first half of twentieth century, the name associated with the pioneering work in occupational eye safety was that of Hedwig Kuhn, MD.[6] Her work, "Industrial Ophthalmology" published in 1944 was the state of art in eye safety. Kuhn stressed the importance of visual need of the worker and then matches those needs with the ophthalmic evaluation report of the worker, like stereoacuity for crane operators. She summarizes the key points: adequate pre-employment tests, periodic rechecks of specific groups, practical visual survey of the plant. At the same time, emphasis was placed on the development of thorough eye protection program.

In India, industrial ocular trauma reports were initially published by Dr Venkatswamy,[7] Dr Laxminarayan[8,9] and others. Later on industrial trauma statistics were included in the Andhra Pradesh eye disease study.[10] All India ophthalmological society tried to make trauma registry but there is no such effort from Governmental agencies. Occupational eye trauma studies are mostly institutional and not population based. However, prevalence of intraocular trauma (IOT) in India is found to be similar to those of western countries of first half of twentieth century.

Although started so early under auspices so good, it must be said that practical applications of industrial ophthalmology—progressed very slowly.[11]

EPIDEMIOLOGY

The general prevalence of IOT varies greatly with the industrial development of the region involved: their occurrence, therefore, differs widely in different countries and in most tends to increase with time. For studying the epidemiology, twenty-first century may be divided into two halves: (1) depicting the period of rapid industrialization and (2) depicting period of automation or modernization. However, India and other colonial nations these two periods could be: initial period of technological import, many times discarded and the second half showing the period of self-reliance—depicting a shift in paradigm.

Approx one-third of all eye injuries are work related. Hospital based studies show that half the ocular emergencies are due to injuries and half of them are work related.

From different published data, global prevalence of ocular trauma is found to be around 5–10%, with slightly higher rate in rural population of India as compared to urban; reverse is seen in developed countries.[10,13] Annual incidence of eye injury is around 8–10 per 1,000 population, 3–4% of whom are work related. 80–90% of IOT cases are male with a mean age of 25–45 years.

Almost 70% of the injuries result from flying objects or sparks striking the eye and contact with chemicals cause one-fifth of all eye injuries. Others are by objects swinging from a fixed or attached position, such as tree limbs, ropes, chains or tools that were pulled into the eyes while working with them. But probably, the most common cause is non-wearing of eye protection. Almost all studies indicate that three out of every five workers who suffered eye injuries were not wearing eye protection at the time of incident. Others wore the wrong kind of protection.

Potential eye hazards can be found in nearly every industry, but more than 40% of the injuries occurred among craft workers such as mechanics, carpenter and plumbers. Over a third of injured workers were assemblers, sanders and grinding machine operators. Laborer suffers s one-fifth of all eye injuries. Almost half of injured workers were employed in manufacturing while slightly more than 20% were in construction job.[12]

Chemical injuries: Three to four percentage of all eye injuries are due to chemical splashing into eyes, the half of which are occupational in origin and mostly without any visual morbidity. But, severe chemical injury is common amongst painters, cleaners and assault.[16]

Table 8.1: Occupational trauma and related factors

	Human: host	*Vector*	*Physical environment*	*Socioeconomic*
Pre-event	Substance misuse	Faulty protective gear Poor vision	Work load, unaccustomed area	Shift duties
Event	Not using protective gear	Improperly maintained machinery	Unhealthy workplace	Poorly enforced factory, labor rules and woking under influence of alcohol
Post-event	Coexisting eye disorders systemic diseases like hypertension, diabetes, color blindness		Slow emergency response, poor rehabilitation program	Little help for reintegrating rehabilitated visually handi-cap people in the society

TIMING OF INJURY

Eight to ten percentage of all IOT occurs during first hour of work; in contrast half occurs after 6 hours of work which may be explained by the occupational fatigue or monotony (Table 8.1 and Fig. 8.3).[14]

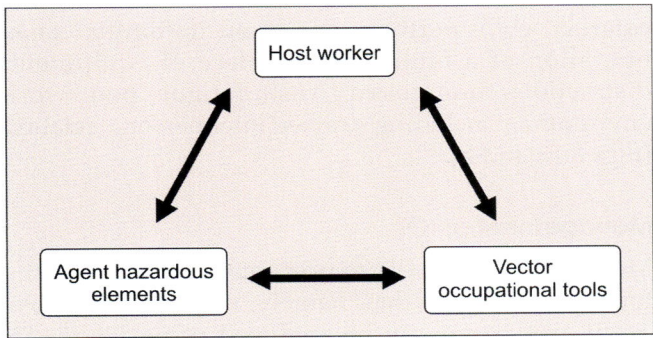

Fig. 8.3: Equation in industrial train

Wearing effective protection saves eyes. About 94% injuries to workers wearing protection resulted from objects or chemicals going around or under the protector. Only small percentage of workers who were injured while wearing protection report breakage of the equipment. Face shields or welding helmets further reduces incidence of injury as one-fifth of injured had shield or helmets on top of eye protection. Workers injured while not wearing protection often says they believed it was not required by the situation. Even though the vast majority of the employers provide eye protection at no extra-cost, about 40% of the workers received no information on where and what kind of eyewear should be used. Eye protection devices should be properly maintained as scratched and dirty devices reduce vision, cause glare and may contribute to accidents.[15]

Nature of ocular injuries occurring in the coal mines:[8,9]

1. "Blast injuries", caused by blasting in mines, the whole body of the miner is studded with coal particles including the eyes, apart from serious and fatal injuries. Along with the coal, sulphur particles in the explosives can be seen inextricably embedded in the ocular surface. The eyes are also exposed to concussion and compression injuries. Such injuries range from complete loss of both the eyeballs to loss of vision of different degrees in one or both the eyes. The associated fractures of the orbit or facial bones are invariably present depending upon the severity of the blast.

2. Retained foreign bodies (coal) entering the eyeball through anterior or posterior route is difficult to localize by X-ray, being radio-transparent and difficult to remove being nonmagnetic. Those which are big enough to be visible can be taken out with the inevitable result of loss of the contents of the eyeball and consequently complete loss of vision.

3. Metallic foreign bodies in the eyeball and its adnexa are common, as working tools are mostly metallic which get chipped off while cutting coal or stone, causing injuries of varying severity.

4. Infection caused by the varied bacterial flora found in coal mines.

5. These contaminated foreign bodies causing ulcers of the cornea seem to be highly infected. Such ulcers are not ordinarily amenable to the routine treatment and take a fulminating course. In all probability, these foreign bodies possibly are contaminated with fungi as well.

6. Foreign bodies of cornea met with in the coal mines, at times, cause corneal lesions simulating superficial punctate keratitis both nummular and macular

type. Such corneal lesions persist for a long time and undergo the usual cycle of remissions and exacerbations. Quite probably, these are contaminated with virus. Such corneal lesions lead to different type of sequallae like degenerative changes of the cornea and atheromatous ulcers with consequential end results.

7. During the fall of roof in an underground mine, the flying and fleeing coal particles catch the miners unaware causing penetrating and non-penetrating, concussion and compression injuries of the eyeball.

8. The type of perforating ocular injuries commonly met with in the coal industry can be described as in between civil and war injuries. The causative agents were metal chips of working tools, broken coal pieces and stones. Blast injuries were like the gun powder injury commonly found in war. In modern hydraulic mining eyes have been injured and even perforated by forceful jet of water (Fig. 8.4).

Etiopathologically, miner's eye injury is either due to mechanical trauma or burns out of which 75–80% minor, 15–20% severe and 2–5% ensued a permanent incapacity to work underground.[17]

In recent years ocular injuries in the coal mining industry has been lowered down relatively due to better safety measures and health education of the miners.[8] Improved surgical technique and control of infection by drugs have further reduced ocular mortality. Use of protective goggles underground could not be enforced due to fogging and restriction of field of vision. Improved mining methods and better lighting underground have eliminated miner's nystagmus and saved from many accidents.[8, 18]

Welding related IOT: Delayed presentation with severe photophobia and foreign body sensation with a history of exposure to welding arc is the diagnostic hallmark of this type of injury which constitutes 5–10% of all IOT cases.[19]

The most common welding-related eye injuries are foreign body or burns. Frequent work activities at the time of injury include welding, grinding, cleaning, brushing, or observing a welder. Workers performing welding tasks or working near welders should be trained to recognize potential hazards and the effective use of proper safety equipment to prevent ocular injury.

RISK FACTORS IOT

Comorbid ocular conditions (refractive errors, cataract, etc.), performance of an unfamiliar task, operation of a faulty tool or piece of equipment, distractions, unnecessary rush, fatigue, poor work environment including strained inter personal relation (Figs 8.5a and b).[20]

Management of IOT

Most of the IOT cases are preventable because all the four interacting factors, namely, environment, host, agent and vector can be analyzed using Haddon's matrix (Figs 8.5 to 8.9).[21]

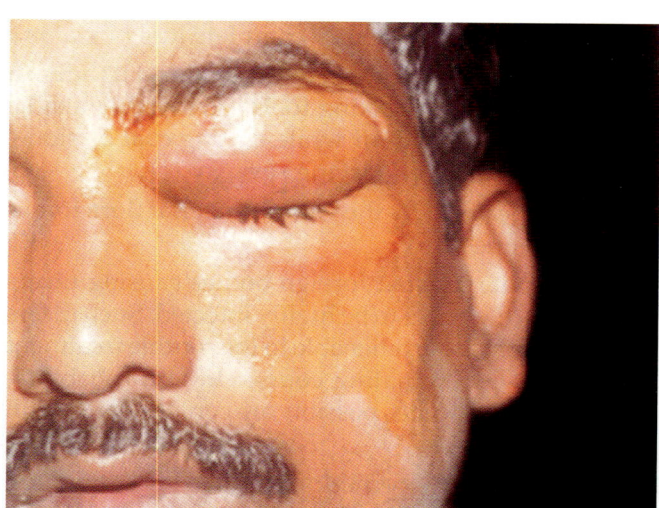

Fig. 8.4: Acute blast injury

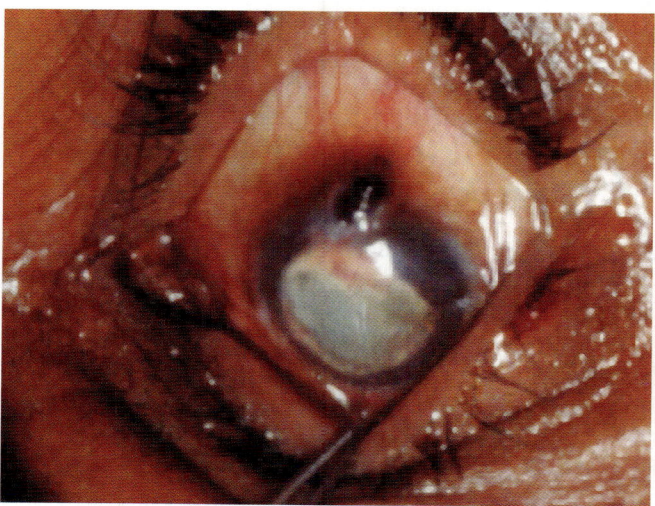

Fig. 8.5a: Risk factor in IOT comorbidity: cataract

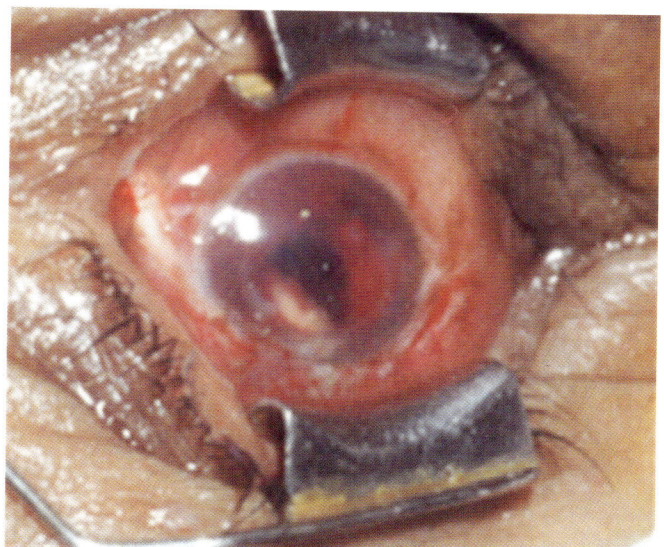

Fig. 8.5b: Risk factor in IOT: comorbidity: complicated pseudo-phakia

Appropriate interventions to prevent such accidents from occurring in future might be:

Primary prevention strategies:

- Campaigns against drinking before coming to duties
- Increased enforcement of working under the influence of alcohol (DUI) laws

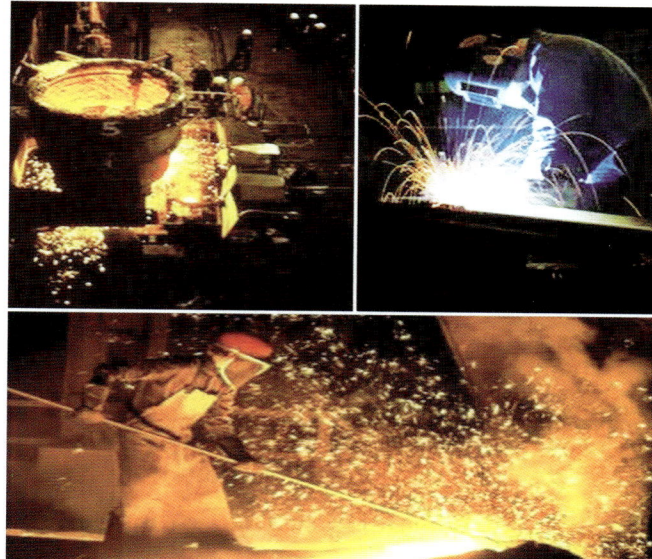

Fig. 8.6: Risk factors: unfamiliar environment

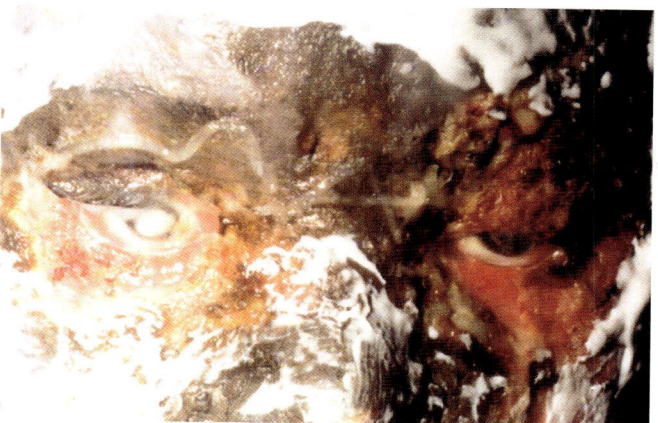

Fig. 8.7: Chemical injury: assault at workplace

- Random inspections of machine tools to ensure that they are in good condition and safe
- Laws requiring that all workers use protective gears
- Shop floor training
- Rotation of shifts.

Secondary prevention strategy:

Improved emergency response services in the form of occupational health services at factory premises.

Tertiary prevention strategy:

Better rehabilitation programs.

The above example clearly demonstrates that use of Haddon's Matrix can help to clarify which interventions might work at any or all phases of an event and which might be targeted toward any or all of the factors.

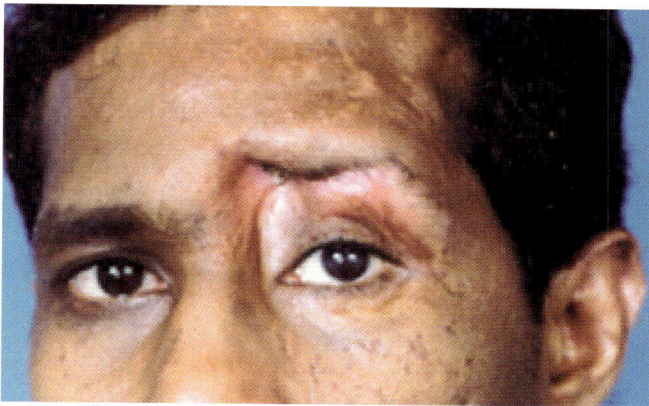

Fig. 8.8: Blast injury mines: disfigurement, traumatic cataract

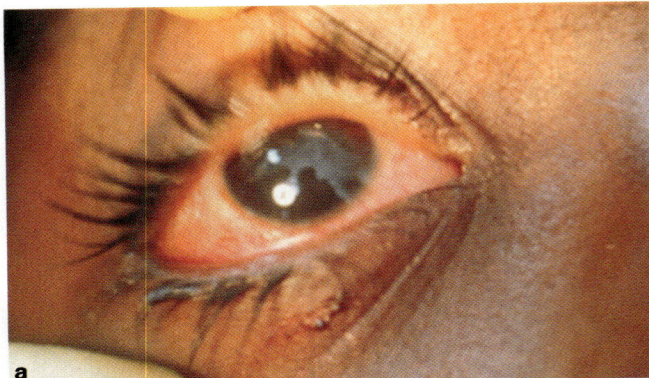

Pretreatment

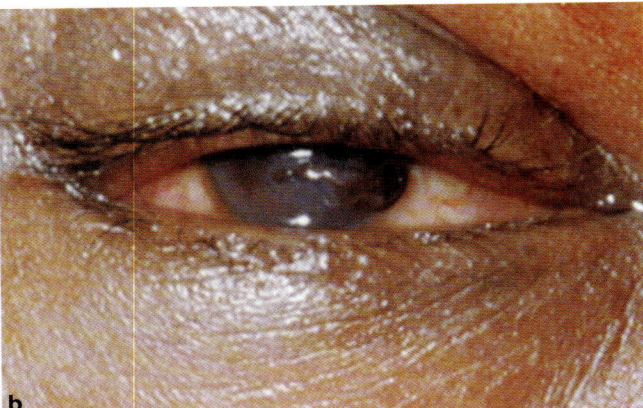

Post-treatment

Figs 8.9a and b: Chemical injury both pretreatment and post-treatment

SHOP FLOOR TRAININGS

- Do not interfere with eye injuries except minor cases. Refer the case to hospital immediately
- Symptoms of serious eye injuries are:
  1. Blurred vision that does not clear with blinking
  2. Loss of all or part of the visual field of an eye
  3. Sharp stabbing or deep throbbing pain
  4. Double vision
- Signs of eye injuries that require ophthalmologist's opinion are:
  1. Black eye
  2. Red eye
  3. An object on the cornea
  4. One eye that does not move as completely as the other eye

5. One eye protruding more than the other
6. One eye with an abnormal pupil size, shape or reaction to light
7. A layer of blood between the cornea and the iris (hyphema)
8. Laceration of eyelid specially if involves the lid margin
9. Laceration or perforation of the eye

- Crucial steps:
  1. Any chemical splashed in the eye(s) should be considered as a vision-threatening emergency. Forcibly keep the patient's eyelids open while irrigating at least for 5 minutes. then refer the patient to the ophthalmologist. Inform the ophthalmologist about the nature of the chemical contaminant.
  2. Patch the eye lightly with dry, sterile eye pad. If laceration of the eye is suspected, add a protective shield over the sterile eye pad. Instruct the patient not to squeeze the eye tightly shut because it greatly elevates the IOP. Calmly transport the patient to the ophthalmologist.
  3. Conjunctivitis, with normal vision and clear cornea, may be treated with antibiotic eye ointment for several days. If there is no improvement, referral to the ophthalmologist is indicated.
  4. Never put ointment in an eye about to be seen by the ophthalmologist. The ointment makes clear visualization of retina very difficult.
  5. Never give a patient topical anesthetic to relieve pain, such as from flash burn. The prolonged use of topical anesthetic can result in blindness from corneal breakdown.
  6. Never treat a patient with topical steroid unless directed by the ophthalmologist. Topical steroids can make several conditions much worse such as herpes simplex, keratitis, fungal infections and some bacterial infections.
  7. If in doubt as to how severe an ocular symptom sign is, always err on the side of caution and refer the worker to an ophthalmologist for diagnosis and treatment.

For making proper prevention strategy, potential sources of data on occupational injuries are very important listed below:
- Workplace records
- Labor inspector or national occupational safety records

- National insurance schemes/workers' compensation bureau
- Rehabilitation centers.

TREATMENT

Treatment of all industrial ocular injuries is provided along the standard line of other eye injuries which are dealt in detail in other chapters of this book.

REHABILITATION

The most important part of industrial ocular trauma is rehabilitation vis-a-vis compensation which is guided by the following statutory provisions:

a. Workmen's Compensation Act
b. Employee's State (ESI) Act
c. Motor Vehicle Inspection (MVI) Act
d. Railways Act
e. Civil Aviation Act
f. Quantum Damage Act.

Some of these are outdated and need revision.

The Workmen's Compensation Act, 1923 Act No. 8 of 1923 1* (5th March, 1923)

An act to provide for the payment by certain classes of employers to their workmen of compensation for injury by accident. Three types of eye injury has been described to result permanent total disablement and grouped under the heading of other injuries.

Part I List of Injuries Deemed to Result in Permanent Total Disablement (Table 8.2)

Table 8.2: Type and injury

Description of injury	Percentage of loss of earning capacity
Loss of one eye, without complications, the other being normal	40
Loss of vision of one eye, without complications or disfigurement of eyeball, the other being normal	30
Loss of partial vision of one eye	10

Two types of eye diseases, described in the Sch III of this act are infrared cataract, snow blindness.

List of Occupational Eye Diseases as per Workmen's Compensation Act (Table 8.3)

Table 8.3: Occupational diseases

Occupational disease	Employment
Occupational cataract due to infrared radiations	All work involving exposure to the risk concerned
Snow blindness in snow bound areas	All work involving exposure to the risk concerned

According to this act, serious bodily injury includes eye and reporting has to be done to appropriate authority. "Serious bodily injury" means an injury which involves, or in all probability will involve, the permanent loss of the use of, or permanent injury to, —or the permanent loss of or injury to the sight.

Reports of Fatal Accidents and Serious Bodily Injuries

Where, by any law for the time being in force, notice is required to be given to any authority, by or on behalf of an employer, of any accident occurring on his or her premises which results in death, or serious bodily injury, the person required to give the notice shall, within 7 days of the death or serious bodily injury, send a report to the commissioner giving the circumstances attending the death or serious bodily injury.

Under the statutes or Workman's Compensation, disability may be divided into three periods which are:

1. *Temporary total disability* is that period in which the injured person is totally unable to work. During this time he or she received orthopedic or other medical treatment.

2. *Temporary partial disability* is that period when recovery has reached the stage of improvement so that the person may begin some kind of gainful occupation.

3. *Permanent disability* applies to permanent damage or to loss of use of some part of the body after the stage of maximum improvement, from orthopedic or other medical treatment has been reached and the condition is stationary.

THE DOCTOR AND THE EVALUATION

The doctor may be called upon to testify as an expert witness in the court of justice. The expert witness is legally bound to declare his knowledge of the case and express his or her opinions. Effects of disability are physical, social, psychological and vocational, since the total disability is not purely a medical condition, medical man should evaluate the permanent physical impairment rather than total disability. Physical impairment evaluation certificate is to be issued only by medical doctors who are registered under "The 1st schedule of Medical Council of India (MCI) Act, 1956". Aggregate of permanent physical impairment should not exceed more than 100%. Most compensation laws today are interpreted to indicate that if any injury is inciting to the recurrence or occurrence of a pre-existing condition, then compensation must be considered from the standpoint of the injury being totally responsible for the visual loss. This has resulted in many unusual award. Some of the conditions in which the injury has been held responsible for all the visual damage produced by a condition already existing may be grouped as follows: actinomycosis, blastomycosis, herpes simplex, herpes zoster ophthalmicus, dendritic ulcers of the cornea, Reiter's syndrome (which includes inflammation of the conjunctiva of the eye along with arthritis, nonspecific urethritis and sometimes by other symptoms), Stevens-Johnson syndrome (a severe form of erythema multiforme characterized by constitutional symptoms and marked involvement of the conjunctive and oral mucosa), toxoplasmosis when accompanied by an infection of the eye, foreign body in the eye believed to be the inciting agent in an eye condition due to hypertension which has caused ill effects to the vision, foreign bodies in another part of the eye being held responsible for a malignant growth of the iris of the eye; and, diseases of the central nervous system producing optic atrophy attributed to a minor eye injury when a systemic condition was responsible (Figs 8.10 and 8.11).

GUIDELINES FOR EVALUATION OF PHYSICAL IMPAIRMENT IN EYE INJURY

The head and neck has been divided into eight equitable components. The following scoring system based on anatomical functional and esthetic factors is to be used.

Ten-point Formula for Evaluating Post-Burn (Table 8.4)

Table 8.4: Ten-point formula			
Disfigurements and deformities of head and neck			
Eyebrows	Right and left	5 + 5	10
Eyelids	Right upper	6	
	Lower	4	10
	Left upper	6	
	Lower	4	10
Split up of ten point formula for each component			
Eyebrows	Part of one or both	2.5	Lt
			Rt
	Total loss of one or both	10	Lt
			Rt
Eyelids	Upper-skin-disfigurement alone	1.5	Lt
			Rt
	Deformity or full thickness loss	6	Lt
			Rt
	Lower skin-disfigurement alone	1	Lt
			Rt
	Deformity or full thickness loss	4	Lt
			Rt

Categories of Visual Disability (Table 8.5)

Table 8.5: Categories with visual correction			
Category	Better eye	Worse eye	Age impairment (%)
Category 0	6/9 to 6/18	6/24 to 6/36	20
Category I	6/18 to 6/36	6/20 to Nil	40
Category II	6/40 to 4/60 or field of vision 10–20°	3/60 to Nil	75
Category III	3/60 to 1/60 or field of vision 10°	FC at 1 feet to Nil	100
Category IV	FC at 1 feet to Nil or field of vision 10°	FC at feet to Nil	100
One eyed persons	FC at 1 feet to Nil or field of vision 10°	6/6	30

FC = Finger count

PROCESS OF CERTIFICATION

A disability certificate shall be issued by a Medical Board duly constituted by the Central/State Government having, at least three members. Out of

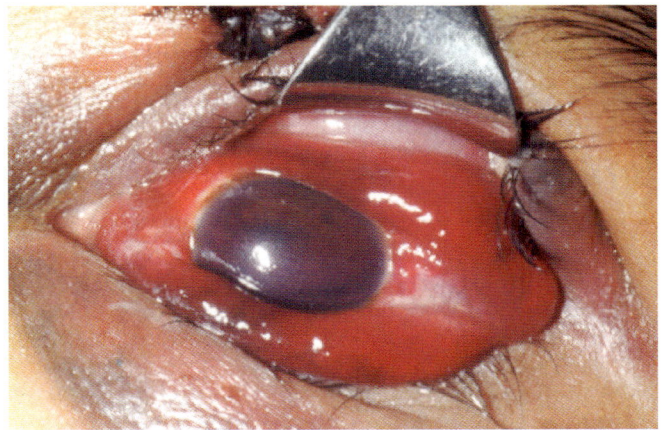

Fig. 8.10: Ruptured globe: flying object from a tyre of a truck moving inside plant. Traumatic hyphema with conjunctival chemosis leading to phthisis

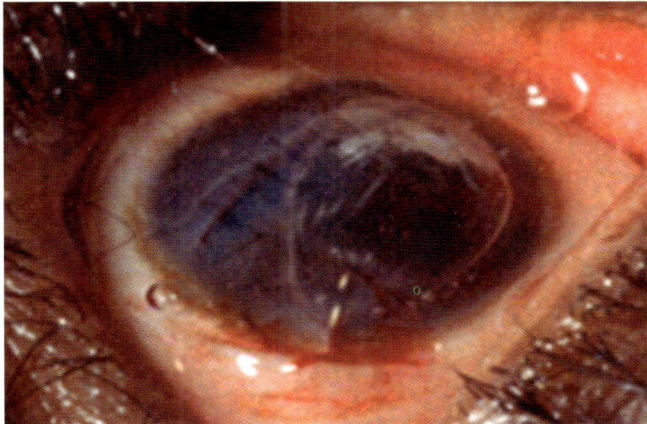

Fig. 8.11: Open globe IOT: repaired

Certificate for the Persons with Disabilities

This is to certify that Shri/Smt/Kum/wife/daughter of Shri .... Age .... old male/female, Registration No. .... is a case of physically disabled/visual disabled/speech and hearing disabled and has .... % (.........................) permanent (physical impairment/visual impairment/speech and hearing impairment) in relation to his/her ....

Note:
1. This condition is progressive/non-progressive/likely to improve/not likely to improve.*
2. Re-assessment is not recommended/is recommended after a period of .... months/years.

*Strike out which is not applicable.

Sd/-   Sd/-   Sd/-
(DOCTOR)   (DOCTOR)   (DOCTOR)
Seal   Seal   Seal

Signature/Thumb impression
of the patient

Countersigned by the Medical Superintendent/
CMO/Head of Hospital (with seal)

Recent attested
photograph showing the
disability affixed here.

which, at least one member shall be a specialist in ophthalmology. Impairment 20–40% or less may only be entitled to aids and appliances.

Classification of Severity of Visual Impairment Recommended by WHO (Table 8.6)

Category of visual impairment	Visual acuity with both eyes using best possible correction	
	Maximum less than	Minimum equal to or better than
1	6/18 3/10 (0.3) 20/70	6/60 1/10 (0.1) 20/200
2	6/60 1/10 (0.1) 20/200 3/60	3/60 1/20 (0.05) 20/400 1/60 (finger counting at 1 meter)
3	1/20 (0.05) 20/400 1/60 (finger counting at 1 meter)	1/50 (0.02) 5/300 (20/1200)
4	1/50 (0.02)5/300	Light perception
5	No light perception	
6	Undetermined or unspecified	

Table 8.6: Visual impairment

a: If the extent of the visual field is to be considered also, patients with a field of less than 10 but more than 5° around central fixation should be placed in category 3 and patients with a field less than 5° around central fixation should be placed in category 4, even if the central acuity is not impaired.

b: These categories are intended to correspond with the fourth digit of the numbering system used in the International Classification Diseases. In this system, the digit 6 customarily signifies "unspecified".

CONCLUSION

Current information regarding the total cost of eye injuries is limited to the specific types and regions. In the US, the National Safety Council estimates that occupational eye trauma (approximately one-third of all eye injuries) costs amount to $ 300 million annually. This includes medical and hospital bills, workmen's compensation and lost production time. But less than 3% of eye research budget is spent for ocular trauma, despite huge costs incurred due to eye injury. Hence injury research should be considered as an investment that will more than pay for itself by reducing the economic burden of injury and disability. Both eye trauma victims and society bear a large, potentially preventable burden.

REFERENCES

1. Dr Maria Neira. Healthy work places: a model for action. WHO Publication. 2004
2. Islam SS, Doyle EJ, Velilla A, et al. Epidemiology of compensable work-related ocular injuries and illnesses: Incidence and risk factors. J Occup Environ Med 2000; 42:575–81.
3. Justin M Kanoff, Angela V Turalba,Michael, et al. Characteristics and Outcomes of Work-Related Open Globe Injuries. Am J Ophthalmol 2010;150:265–269.
4. Welch LS, Hunting KL, Mawudeku A. Injury surveillance in construction: Eye injuries. Appl Occup Environ Hyg 2001; 16:775–62.
5. Sir Stewart Duke Elder, PA Macfaul.System of ophthalmology, Vol 14 part I, Henry Kimpton,1972
6. Kuhn HS: Industrial ophthalmology. St Louis, Mosby, 1944
7. Venkataswamy G. Industrial injuries of the eye. Indian J Ophthalmol 1968;16:169–71
8. Narain L. Perforating injuries in coal mining area. Indian J Ophthalmol 1984;32:273–6
9. Laxminarayan. Ocular injuries in coal mines. Indian J Ophthalmol 1968;16:186–91.
10. Dondona L, Dondona R, Srinivas M, et al. Ocular Trauma in an urban population in South India: the Andhrapradesh Eye Disease study. Clin Experiment Ophthalmol 2000;28:350–6
11. Pizzarello Louis D. Eye Safety and Economic impact of Eye injuries during the last century in the United States: a historical perspective.Ophthalmol Clin N Am 1999;12(3):297–301.
12. F Kuhn, R Morris, et al. Epidemiology and Socio-economics. Ophthalmol Clin N Am 15 (2002)145–151.
13. Nirmalan PK, Katz J, Tielsch J M, et al. Ocular trauma in rural south Indian population: The Arvind comprehensive eye survey. Ophthalmology 2004;111: 1778–81.
14. Nicaeus T, Erb C, Rohrbach M, Thiel HJ. An analysis of 148 outpatient treated occupational accidents. Klin Monbl Augenheilkd. 1996: 209(4):A7–11.
15. De la Hunty D. Sprivulis P. Safety goggles should be worn by Australian workers. AustN Z J Ophthalol 1994: 22(1):49–52.
16. Macdonald ECA, Cauchi PA, A Azuara-Blanco, B Foot. Surveillance of severe chemical injuries in the UK. Br J Ophthalmol 2009;93:1177–80.
17. Koraszewska-Matuszewska B, Kamińska-Olechnowicz B, Kozie o T, Formińska-Kapuœcikowa M. Causes and types

of eye injuries in miners and employees of coal mines. Klin Oczna. 1989;91(2-3):60–2

18. Desai P, MacEwen CJ, Baines P, Minassian DC. Epidemiology and implications of ocular trauma admitted to hospital in Scotland. J Epidemiol Community Health 1996; 50:436–41.

19. DA Lombardi, R Pannala, GS Sorock, H Wellman, TK Courtney, S Verma, GS Smith. Welding related occupa-tional eye injuries: a narrative analysis Inj Prev 2005;11: 174–179.

20. Chen SY, Fong PC, Lin SF, Chang CH, Chan CC. A case-crossover study on transient   risk factors of work-related eye injuries. Occup Environ Med. 2009 Aug; 66(8):517–22.

21. Injury surveillance guidelines/edited by: Y. Holder, et al. World Health Organization 2004.

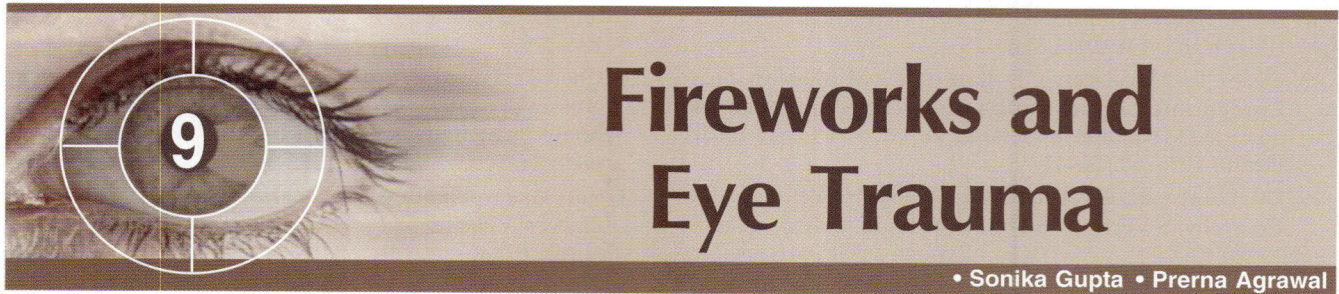

Fireworks and Eye Trauma

• Sonika Gupta • Prerna Agrawal

INTRODUCTION

Fireworks which have been a traditional form of celebration for centuries, are increasing at an alarming rate. India, China, Malaysia, are said to use fireworks in celebrations. They are used during many functions across the world, from American independence day, 4 July to Chinese lunar year. Unfortunately, the number of injuries from fireworks are also increasing. The fireworks used as lunar new year celebrations in 2009 set ablaze a newly built Mandarin Oriental Hotel at Beijing, China and reduced it to ashes. More fireworks are ignited in the United States (US) each 4th July than any other national celebration in the world. This may account for the fact that more than 2 of 3 of fireworks related ocular injuries (FROIs) occur between 16th June to 16 July in US. Netherland and Canada and even in UK, firecrackers are used to mark the national celebrations and welcome new year.

Legislation has made a little impact an incidence of these injuries. The incidence of injuries was less on Deepawali days but the incidence rose in first. Three days after the festival, Netherland has no laws against the firecrackers and a number of eyes have been lost due to firecrackers.

An estimated 16% of fireworks-related injuries affect eyes. Though bottle rocket, firecrackers and sparklers are the main source of injuries requiring hospitalization all types of legally available fireworks have caused serious injuries and even death. Fireworks are most commonly used during festival of Deepawali and Gurupurva in India. Nowadays, there is increasing trend of using firecrackers during wedding and other happy occasions also.

Firework-related ocular injuries can be devastating, with total loss of vision possible. These injuries constitute an important cause of preventable[5] blindness worldwide, and in India, such injuries are very common among children.[1,2] Eye trauma contributes to an estimated 18% of the total number of firework injuries.[3]

EPIDEMIOLOGY

Of all the reported injuries to eye, 1.6–2% are due to injury by firecrackers.[1] FROIs are common all over the world. In India, FROIs are most common during Deepawali (Diwali) and Gurupurva.[1,2] They are common in New Year's eve in China, the Prophet's birthday in Libya and 4th July in USA.[3]

Incidence of ocular damage varies globally. Sundelin (2000) reported an annual incidence in Western Sweden of 1.0/1,000,000.[4] Lee (1966) a 6-year average of 1.3/100,000 in Hong Kong.[5] Wilson (1982) a 2.6/1,000,000 on an annual basis in the USA.[6] Faber (2009) a 4.8/100,000[1] incidence around Dutch New

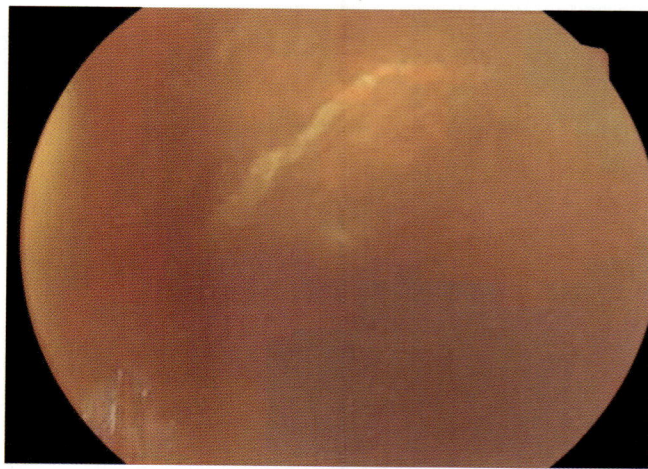

Fig. 9.1: Severe retinal concussion injury with peripheral choroidal tear due to "HAWAI" a metallic flying cracker hitting the eye with severe impact

208

Year's eve.[7] Malaysia adil Fitri figures are said to be 9.7/100,000.[8] Vernon (1988)[9] a 2.5/100,000 incidence covering a 2 week period around Guy Fawkes day in the Trent region of the UK.[10] Kuhn (2000) compared US and Hungarian registries reporting incidences of 4.4/100,000 and 0.16/100.000 respectively.[11] The faulty ignition and improvization is a major cause of those accidents. Though the crackers belonged to class C (Sane and Safe) poor quality controls were also an important cause of these serious damage (Fig. 9.1).

DEMOGRAPHY

There is an alarmingly high proportion of those injured to be children. Children make-up more than 50% of those injured in all studies. Seventy percent of the patients were 12 years old and below.[11] Lack of adult supervision was the major contributing factor. They are usually more common in boys.[1,2,7] Of 30 patients, 29 were male in a study by Rashid, et al.[8] In their review on literature of ocular firework trauma, Wisse, et al.[11] showed 75% victims were males and 67% were between age group 14 years and 30 years. By standers also were also injured in these accidents (47%).

According to one study in India[1] most common cause of ocular injuries are cracker bombs (37%) followed by sparklers (19%). Most serious ocular injuries are due to bottle rockets and bombs. The distribution of severe eye injury (hand movement-PL negative) was nearly equal in bystanders and actively involved individuals.[12,13]

In 8,600 fireworks-related injuries were treated in US hospital emergency room in 2010 and more than 1,800 of these accidents (21%) were eye injuries according to US Consumer Product Safety Commission (CPSC).

Other findings of CPSC 2010 fireworks annual report include:

1. About 6,300 firework-related injuries (73%) occurred within 30 days period that include the 4th July weekend in 2010.
2. Males sustained 65% of firework-related injuries, females accounted for 35%.
3. An estimated 265 of injuries occurred in children age 9 and younger, 53% occurred in people under 20 year of age.
4. Almost all types of fireworks caused eye injuries including sparklers.
5. For children under 5 year old, sparklers accounted for the largest number of injuries (43% of total for that age group).

6. Apart from cosmesis ocular injury cause significant visual morbidity. Eyes (21%) are involved in ocular injuries due to fireworks, other parts of body injured by fireworks were—hands and fingers (30%) legs, head (22%), face and ears (16%).

A retrospective analysis of all patients with firework-related ocular injuries attending the department of ophthalmology was done in Rennin Hospital of Wuhan University from January 20 to February 10, 2009. 25 eyes in 24 patients were enrolled in the study. It was observed that injuries were more frequent in children (under 10, 41.7%), males (79.2%), as open globe injury (62.5%).[14,15] The most common pyrotechnical products causing accidents were firecrackers (12.50%). Rural residents had significantly higher rates of injury compared to urban residents. Of 25 eyes, the most common injuries were corneal/scleral/corneoscleral open globe trauma (60%),[16] traumatic cataract (56%), vitreous hemorrhage (28%) and retinal detachment (28%). Most eyes received surgical intervention. It was therefore concluded that FROIs are common in, males children, in rural settings, are frequently severe and visually devastating. So FROI preventive measures should be strengthened including public education and legal registration on use and sale of fireworks. Removal of the legislative ban on fireworks in 1996 had a significant effect on incidence of eye. Netherland does not have any legislation and firecrackers are used to celebrate the new year. Netherland Society of Ophthalmology in their survey 2009 reported that 60% of the injured were minor 30% of them suffered a permanent eye damage and 8% eyes lead to be removed.[8] These injuries are potentially preventable with stricter control on availability of fireworks and a greater awareness of the ocular risks they pose.

TYPES OF FIREWORK INJURIES

Various types of fireworks include bombs, cone fountains, sparklers, bottle rockets, combination fireworks. Firework injuries by type of device as reported by the US-CPSC in the data collected for the year 1997 and reported bottle rockets accounted for 15% of the injuries. Sparklers accounted for 10% of the injuries. Sparklers which are often dismissed as having minimal risk, burn at 1800° which is hot enough to melt gold. This can lead to corneal burns and corneal scars (Figs 9.2 and 9.3).

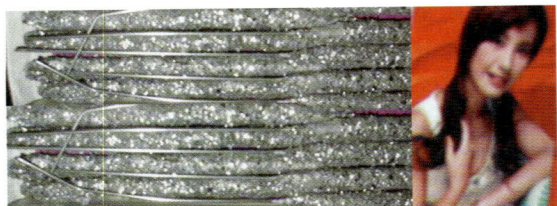

Fig. 9.2: Sparklers often thought as comparatively safer but actually are not. They cause burn at 1,800°F, can lead to corneal burns and scars, affect bystanders as well

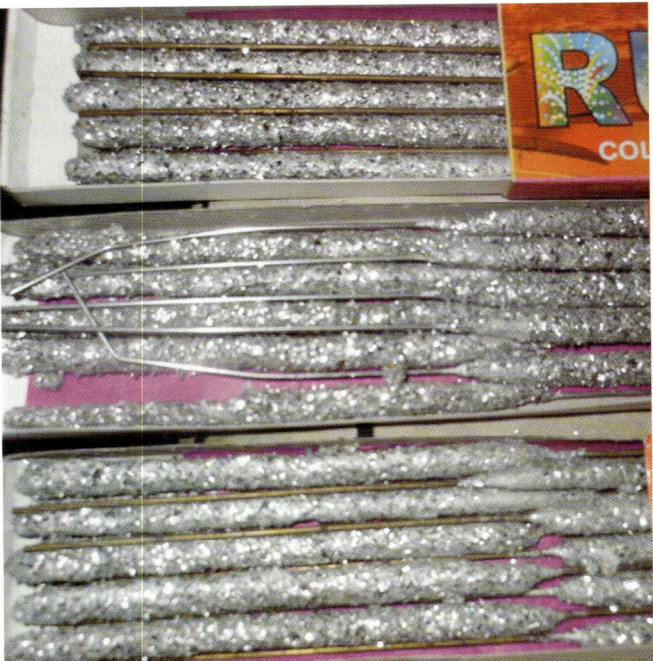

Fig. 9.3: Colored sparklers are still more dangerous, cause burn at higher temperature than simple sparklers

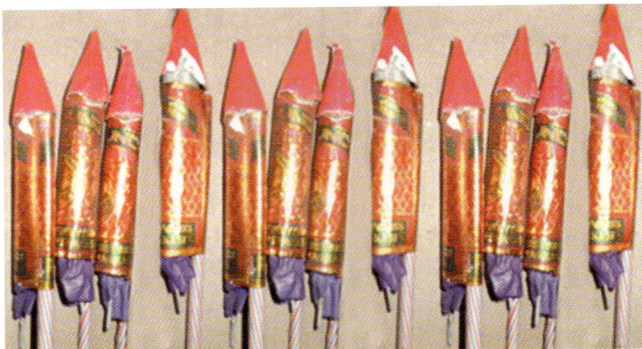

Fig. 9.4: Bottle rocket—very dangerous, flies erratically sometimes tangentially, potentially injuring bystanders, can explode showering fragments of glass or metal in all directions

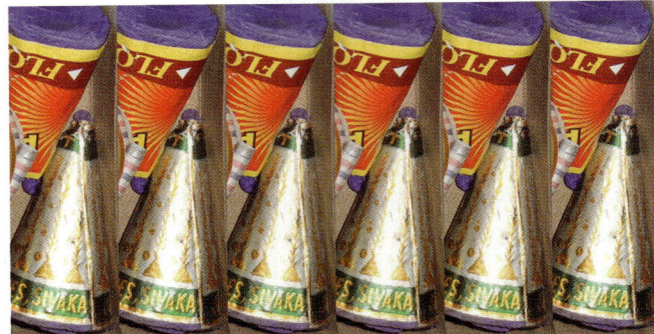

Fig. 9.5: ANAAR—one of the dangerous firecrackers, as the sparkling material attain some height above ground level, can affect bystanders also

In a prospective study of FROI,[14] over three consecutive years during Indian festival of Deepawali, bombs and cone fountains were the main cause of injury affecting 83.3% patients, followed by bottle rockets 9.52%, and sparklers 7.14% (Fig. 9.4).

An analysis of accidents involving fireworks shows that most occur because of uncertainty in the timing of explosion. Poor quality of fuse lead is responsible for these accidents. Combination fireworks (cone fountain with a bomb) (Fig. 9.5) are more dangerous than individual fireworks. The individual fireworks are in the safe category, classified as class C or "safe and sane" fireworks which includes bottle rockets, sparklers, cone fountains and bombs 1.5 inch or less in size. In combination, they are dangerous.

Many of the injuries were caused as a result of negligence of those igniting the firecrackers. Some of the severely injured patients reported device malfunction as the cause of their injury. In three cases (out of 51 patients enrolled in study) approximately 6%, the attempt to reignite or recover a failed device was the cause of injury. One (out of 51) patient suffered severe facial and bilateral ocular injuries when he attempted to ignite a homemade device made up of unburnt firecracker powder (Fig. 9.6).

CLINICAL PRESENTATION

Firecracker damage to the eye can result in mechanical, thermal and chemical injury. Most firecrackers are made of flash-powder, a mixture of oxidizer and metallic fuel that burns quickly and, if confined,

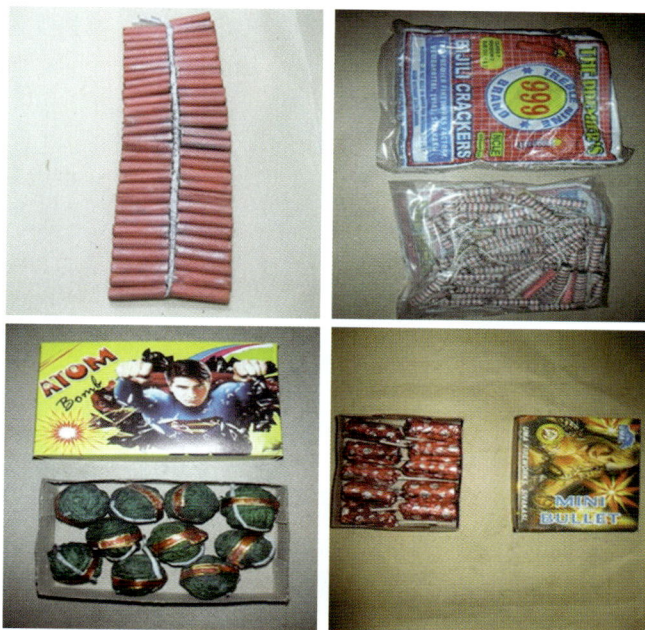

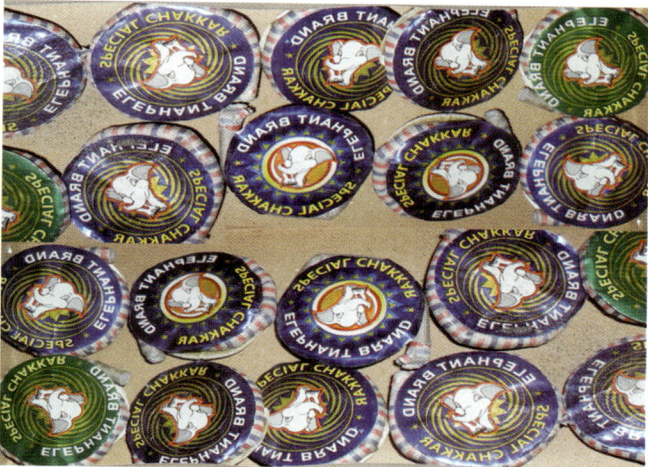

Fig. 9.7: "FIRKI"—comparatively safe for eye as they crack and rotate at ground surface and fire cracker particles do not reach at some height

Fig. 9.6: BOMBS—most common cause of FROI (37%), dangerous, big fuse lead are relatively safer

produces a loud noise.[14] Metallic particles, such as aluminum, may be found in firecrackers, and they can appear radio-opaque on computed tomography (CT) scans.

Extent of ocular trauma due to fireworks ranges from mild conjunctivitis to complete loss of vision in the eye (Fig. 9.7). Clinical features may include:

- Lid burns
- Lid lacerations
- Conjunctival burns
- Corneoscleral tears
- Corneal abrasions
- Multiple corneal foreign bodies
- Hyphema
- Cataract
- Glaucoma
- Vitreous hemorrhage
- Optic nerve injury
- Retinal detachment
- Intraocular foreign body (IOFB)
- Globe rupture.

The most common injuries reported in firecrackers are burns on lids and cornea which may be mild and resolve without much morbidity.[9,15,16] However, more severe injuries have been reported to damage the vision and cosmetic blemish. Sparkles produced only conjunctival or corneal burn or corneal abrasions (closed globe injury) without affecting the visual recovery, while rockets, cone fountain bombs and bombs caused lid laceration, open globe injury, iridodialysis, angle recession, vitreous hemorrhage and multiple corneal foreign bodies, all of which led to poor visual outcome. Corneal/scleral/corneoscleral and open globe trauma (60%).[16] Besides the initial impact of FROIs these injuries have long-term impact few studies have appropriately addressed their potential long-term impact. A 6 years retrospective survey in USA showed that 62% of such injuries involved anterior segment of which hyphema and angle recession are commonly observed. Twenty-six patients with unilateral hyphema due to FROI during celebration of Wednesday eve festival in Iran were included in the study. Their median age was 18 years (range 7–50 years) and 21 patiens (81%) were men. Two examiners independently performed gonioscopy on both eyes of these patiens 4–6 weeks after injury. It was observed that 16 patiens (62%) had angle recession with a mean extension of 180° (45–360°). Ten (63%) of these patients had an average recession of more than 180°. All cases of angle recession were associated with injuries caused by Narenjak, an illegal homemade grenade. Patients injured by Narenjak were older and teenagers and children tended to be closer to the focus of fireworks. It was concluded from the study that angle recession proved to be very common and extensive among patients with hyphema who were injured by fireworks at the time of Wednesday eve festival. The use of illegal homemade grenade was the most important risk factor for occurrence of angle recession.

PREVENTION

The most tragic aspect of blindness from fireworks is that it is completely preventable. In fact over 90% of all eye injuries can be prevented. According to one study nearly one-half of all FROIs are inflicted upon innocent bystanders.[13] A bottle rocket can hit an eye over 100 yards away and still inflict substantial damage.

Do not shake sparklers at others—sparklers are often thought of as a safe firework, but they are actually responsible for the greatest total number of injuries due to fireworks. Most of these injuries are minor burns but sparklers burn at 1,800°F. This temperature is high and can cause third degree burn. The most dangerous type of firework is bottle rocket. It flies erratically, potentially injuring bystanders. Bottle rocket can explode showering fragments of glass or metal in all direction.

PREPARATION FOR CRACKING FIREWORKS

1. Do not wear loose clothes like big-gown or duppata/stolles.
2. Aduts should supervise their children at all times (Figs 9.8a and b).
3. Fireworks should be lighted in open space with high open sky clearance.
4. Substandard or unauthorized fireworks should not be used.
5. Onlookers should maintain a safe distance and use protective eye wear.
6. Never place fireworks in tin cans or glass bottles as these can explode and pierce the eye or cause severe impact.
7. Do not attempt to make fireworks at home.
8. If a firework does not go off stay away from it and douse it with water from bucket. Cover it with wooden barrel and call the police to come and dispose it properly.

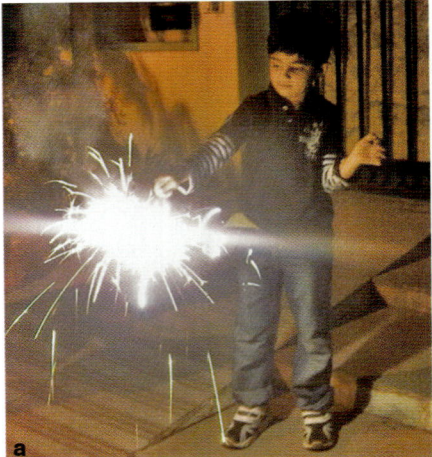

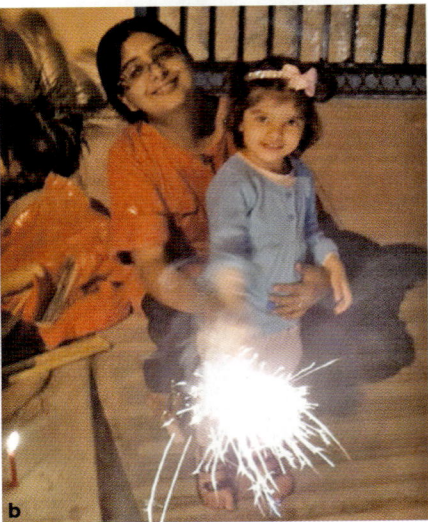

Figs 9.8a and b: (a) Safe mode—child wearing jeans, full sleeve shirt, shoes and holding firecrackers at arm's length distance; (b) Unsafe mode—child cracking fireworks without shoes, near mother's lap, with other fire crackers lying nearby

Prevention of Firework-related Ocular Injury at Manufacture's Level

1. Combination fireworks should be banned.
2. Improve the quality of fuse lead.
3. The packaging must exhibit instructions for safe use.

MANAGEMENT

If injury has occurred due to firework it should be treated as emergency and immediate measures be taken.

Immediate care: In case of a firework injury, the following measures should be taken by the patient right away at home to minimize the damage to the eye.

- Medical attention should not be delayed even for seemingly mild injuries. "Mildly" damaged areas can worsen and end in serious vision loss, even blindness, that might not have happened if treatment had occurred immediately.
- Eye should not be rubbed. If any eye tissue is torn, rubbing might push out the eye's contents and cause more damage.
- Shield the eye from pressure.
- Avoid giving aspirin or ibuprofen or other non-steroidal anti-inflammatory drugs to try to reduce the pain. They thin the blood and might increase bleeding. It is better to by-pass the drug store or medicine cabinet and get to the emergency room right away.
- Do not apply ointment or any medication. It is probably not sterile. Also, ointments make the eye area slippery. This could slow the doctor's examination at a time when every second counts.

Each patient with firework injury to eye should be subjected to detailed ocular examination, i.e. initial visual acuity, anterior segment examination by slit lamp biomicroscopy, intraocular pressure (IOP) measurement by applanation tonometer, gonioscopy, (not to be carried out in globe rupture/penetrating eye injury) direct/indirect ophthalmoscopy. Ultrasonography (A + B) scan should be carried out to assess posterior segment status, particularly, retinal detachment, vitreous hemorrhage and to rule out retained IOFB in patients with hazy media. X-ray of the orbit should be done to rule out retained IOFB.

The treatment for chemical injury to the eye from a firecracker includes copious irrigation of the eye as soon as the injury is detected. Any remaining particles in the fornices should be removed because they can cause tissue necrosis. Cycloplegics and steroid drops or ointments should be started as soon as possible to decrease inflammation. Amniotic membranes grafting can be carried out as it is known to deliver anti-inflammatory factors to the ocular surface, thus reducing scarring and providing a protective structure where the epithelial cells could replicate. Steroids must be decreased after 1 week of treatment because they can inhibit wound healing and promote infection.

Treatment for the 4 grades of corneal burns must be adjusted according to the severity of injury. In a grade I corneal burn, only corneal epithelial loss is present and no conjunctival ischemia is found. The prognosis is very good. Grade II is associated with some corneal edema and corneal haze; conjunctival ischemia affects less than one-third of the limbus and some permanent scarring may occur. Grade III is associated with significant haziness of the cornea, and limbal ischemia is less than one and half of the limbus. Prognosis is variable and vision is usually impaired. Finally, a corneal burn is grade IV. The cornea is opaque, and limbal ischemia affects greater than one and half of the limbus. Grade IV burns may be associated with globe perforation and prognosis is poor.

CONCLUSION

Fireworks cause serious preventable ocular burns and related injuries especially in children who are the most affected age group. It affects mainly eyelid and anterior segment structures which result in moderate visual loss on presentation. Health education, public awareness and tighter legislation are essential preventive measures to limit the effect of fireworks to the public. The single most effective measure may be to restrict the fireworks to public open spaces (such as parks or playgrounds). Regulating the quality of firecrackers and promoting safe use via schools and media will also have a positive impact.[13]

REFERENCES

1. Mohan K, Dhir SP, Munjal VP, Jain IS. Ocular fireworks injuries in children. Afro-Asian J Ophthalmol 1984;2:162–65.
2. Dhir SP, Shishko MN, Krewi A, Mabruka S. Ocular fireworks in children. J Paediatric Ophthalmol Strabismus 1991; 28:1–2.
3. Newell FW. Fireworks blindness. Am J Ophhalmol 1972;74:167–8.
4. Sundelin K, Norsell K. Eye injuries from fireworks in Western Sweden. Acta Ophthalmol Scand 2000;78:61–4.
5. Lee RT. Fire-cracker injury to the eyes in Hong Kong. Brit. J. Ophthalmol 1966;50:666–9.
6. Wilson RS. Ocular firework injuries. Am J Ophthalmol 1975;79:449–51.
7. de Faber JT. Firework injuries treated by Dutch ophthalmologists New Year 2008/09. Ned Tijdschr Geneeskd. 2009;153:A507. Dutch.
8. Rashid RA, Heidary F, Hussein A, Hitam WH, Rashid RA, Ghani ZA, Omar NA, Mustari Z, Shatriah I.Ocular

burns and related injuries due to fireworks during the Aidil Fitri celebration on the East Coast of the Peninsular Malaysia.Burns. 2011;37(1):170–3.

9. Vernon S. Fireworks and the eye. J R Soc Med 1988; 81(10):569–71.

10. Kuhn FC, Morris RC, Witherspoon DC, et al. Serious fireworks-related eye injuries. Ophthalmic Epidemiol 2000;7;139–48.

11. Ocular firework trauma: a systematic review on incidence, severity , outcome and prevention. Wisse RPL, Bijlsma WR, Stilma JS. Br J Ophthalmolo 2010;94:1586–1591.

12. Jing Y, Yi-qiao X, Yan-ning Y, Ming A, An-huai Y, Lian-hong Z. Clinical analysis of firework–related ocular injuries during Spring Festival 2009. Graefes Arch Clin Exp Ophthalmol. 2010;248(3):333–8.

13. Arya SK, Malhotra S, Dhir SP, SoodS. Ocular firework injuries. Clinical features and visual outcome. Indian J Ophthalmol 2001;49:189–90.

14. Green MA, Joholske J. 2006 Fireworks Annual Report: Fireworks-Related Deaths, Emergency Department Treated Injuries, and Enforcement Activities During 2006. Washington (DC): US Consumer Product Safety Commission; 2007.

15. Ravi Kumar, Manohar Puttanna, K S Sriprakash, BL Sujatha Rathod, Venkatesh C Prabhakaran Indian Firecracker Eye Injuries during Deepavali Festival: A Case Series J Ophthalmol. 2010 Mar-Apr; 58(2): 157–159. doi: 10.4103/0301–4738.60095.

16. US Consumer Product Safety Commission. Estimated firework trauma. National Electronic Injury Surveillance System.

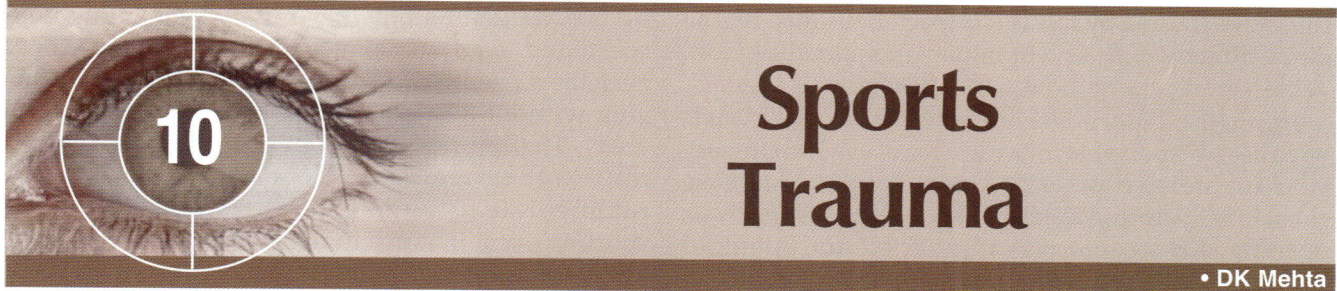

Sports Trauma

• DK Mehta

INTRODUCTION

Recreation and sports has been important for all aspects of life even the animals indulge into some playful activities for mental and physical fitness. Injuries are bi-products of all recreational activities. From bow and arrow to fun shooting or simple ball games also have been responsible for the eye injuries. While facial injuries attract attention quickly ocular injuries are often neglected with far reaching results due its position and delicate status.

Facial and eye trauma has become more intensive in present era of speed and increased mechanization of sports. The figures are alarming even from developed countries where as the figures are not easily available from developing and developed countries. It is noted that every 4 hours a sports-related injury is registered in emergency in American Hospitals. And 40,000 eyes are injured every year where every 8th eye injury due to sports is serious.[1]

Sports-related injuries have a prevalence rate of 2.4%, incidence 14.75% and 24% of "injury blindness" is due to sports in north India.[2] Anterior segment trauma is more common due to sports injuries and pure posterior segment injury is seen in 8–11% with 40–43% injuries have combined damage.

Younger population is greatly affected leading to substantial loss of man hours and economic loss in the long run. It is reported that 37% of total sports injury in USA are in under 16 years of age. In India average age is 24.2 years[3] and in Pakistan most injuries are below 25 years.[4] Similar figures are available from Portugal and New Zealand.[2-8] World over 50% of the severe sports eye injuries are below 25 years of age. It may be noted that 80–90% admissions under 14 years are due to severe ocular trauma. According to a 1989 report from India,[7] only 47% of the ocular sports injury achieve final visual acquity of 20/200 or better.[3]

The eye may be involved in isolation or with other facial injuries. While isolated eye trauma is less severe it takes a toll due to relative delay and more often missed posterior globe damage. Baseball, Soccer, Football, Handball, Hockey and Rugby are more severe on the orbit and adenexa, and small balls and missile games may injure the globe directly. Anterior segment involvement alone is seen in 40–48% of the cases in various studies and 30–40% cases show combined involvement of anterior and posterior segment. Where as pure post-segment damage is seen in one-tenth of the sports injury.

It is difficult to classify as the different types of sports are available, some in conventional sense while others may be improvised games and sports:

1. Conventional (with set norms)
2. Improvised (with no set norms). These sometimes are more damaging due to uncontrolled/improvised shrapnel and erratic actions/behavior of the components (bow and arrow, gulel, cracker bombs, twigs used as bat and hockey).

American Medical Association has divided different sports activities into three categories depending on the anticipated eye damage while indulging in them.

a. *Low risk:* Games with no ball, no body contact like cycling swimming, track events.
b. *High risk:* Ball and racquet games and body contacts
c. *Very high risk:* Strenuous body contact like boxing Wrestling and Martial arts.

Collision being the main factor in eye damage in Wrestling, Kabbadi and Khokho in Indian scenario. Football, Hockey, Rugby and Lacrosse rule the western world in eye injuries. Whereas rough contact in basketball, Baseball and Soccer may lead to orbital injuries, track and cross country events and swimming

215

cause eye trauma by fall and impact. Balls may hit the globe directly with severe impact in sports like Golf, Table Tennis, Badminton and Cricket.

Improvised sports like Bow and Arrow, *Gulli Danda* have been responsible for a number of eye losses every year in India. Bow and Arrow injuries increase substantially during Dashehra and Deepawali festivals in India. Arrow that was responsible for killing of Ravana the demon, in Ramayana is used symbolically by children games. In fact improvized arrows prepared out of Broom sticks end up with severe endophthalmitis with open globe injury (Figs 10.1 and 10.2). *Gulli Danda* a game that is inexpensive is played with a wooden stick hitting a small spindle like chiseled wood piece measuring 2–4 inches. The game is played by two or more people and the *Gulli* (spindle) kept on the ground is hit and lofted by hitting it hard

by the wooden Baton. The "missile" thus flown has speed and mass, sometimes hits the other players or even the passerby since the game is played in any open area without any boundaries more so in the rural areas. The injuries caused by a flying "Gulli" may result into severe closed globe injury or even globe rupture. Kite flying in India is taken as an exciting sporting event in north India. Incidence of significant eye trauma by kite flying directly is reported to be 016%[3] whereas fall from the roof and electrocution may have major polytrauma including serious eye damage (Fig. 10.3).

Rugby football combines speed and direct physical contact and one of the common causes of facial and eye injuries. Famous Rugby player Gavin Quinine in 2010 was injured and operated upon for eye injury and finally lost the eye (Fig. 10.4). This Game is dangerous due to it speed and impact. While open globe injuries are very common along with polytrauma, closed globe injuries are also known to have been responsible for giant retinal tears.

Racquet games often have two distinct types of injuries. Injuries sustained by Racquets in a doubles game, and accidentally being hit with a racquet whiling sitting in the stand or while walking across close to the arena. The injuries have been caused by a broken racquet flying like a missile. Unusual incident caused in the field resulted into the loss of vision in eye of international hockey player of India Balbir

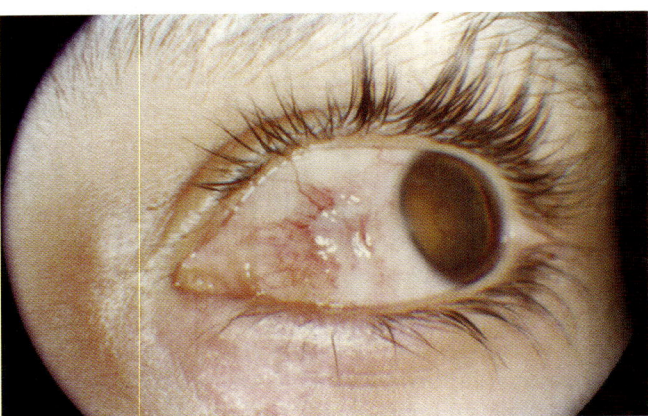

Fig. 10.1: Arrow injury localized conjunctival tear with vossius ring due to severe impact of blunted arrow tip

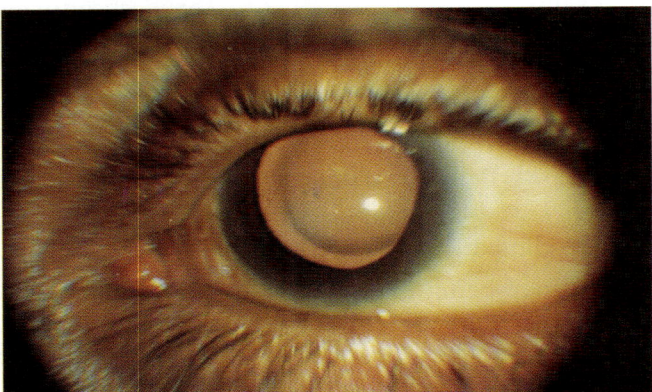

Fig. 10.2: Closed globe injury stone hitting the eye with a Katty (gulel)

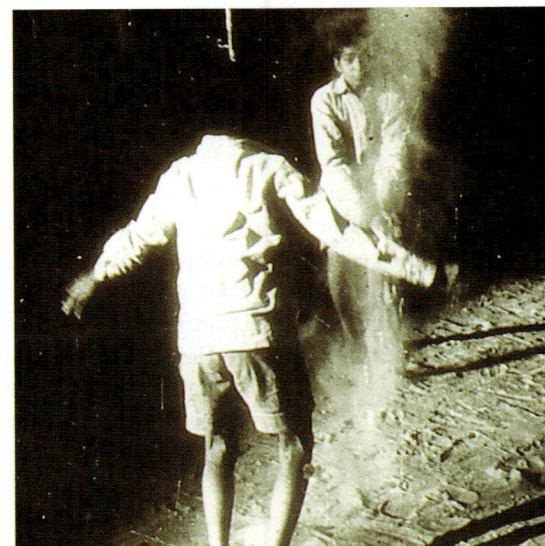

Fig. 10.3: Fun play and foreign body in the eye

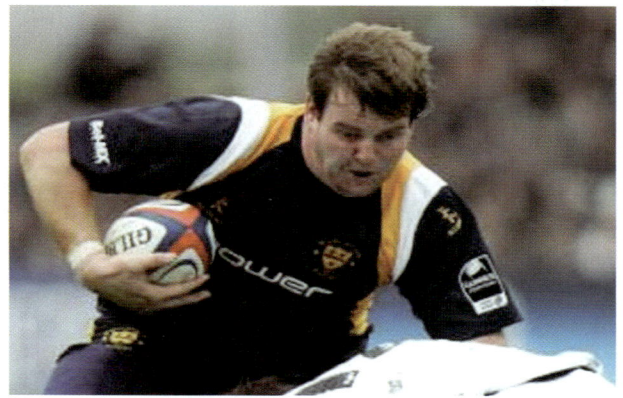

Fig. 10.4: Famous Rugby player Gavin Quinine lost the eye in a Rugby game 2010

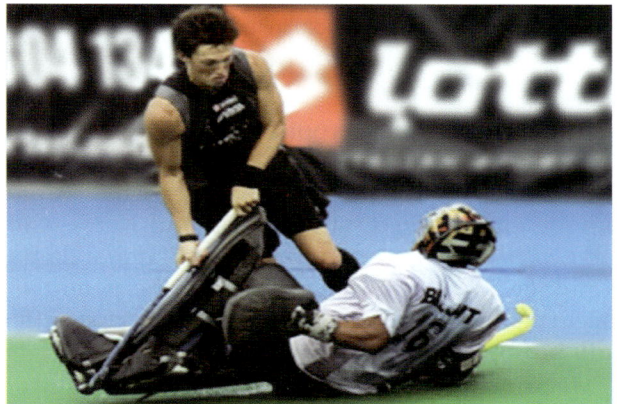

Fig. 10.5: India hockey goal keeper injured the eye with golf ball while practicing in 2010

Singh (Fig. 10.5). The goal keeper was practicing with a golf ball unprotected. Smaller balls have been responsible for orbital trauma and closed globe injury due accidental puncture and bursting. Bigger balls have resulted into eye injuries in weight lifters zone by falls and hits on the ground. Swiss ball a soft inflatable ball measuring 18–30 inches has seen its increasing use since 1960 in a number of sports arena and gyms apart from physio-armamentarium.

Balls and injury caused by racquets is responsible for one-third of all eye injuries. Golf, Tennis, Cricket, Badminton, Baseball, Soccer, Football, Table tennis and now new Paintball games are responsible for closed globe injuries of the eye and resulting into high visual morbidity. Table tennis balls and Badminton shuttle cocks are known to hit the globe end on due to its size smaller than orbital rim and cause anterior chamber damage like hyphema and angle dehiscence,

iris dialysis and sphincter tears and even lens subluxation. With the preference for fast games, Lacrosse and Paintball have become very popular in USA and 20.8% of sports injury are due to Paint ball and 89% of the these injuries are seen in under 14 years of age[9] (Figs 10.6 and 10.7). It is interesting to note that the injury with smaller balls is more severe on the globe as compared to big diameter balls. Balls less than 2.5 cm work like a end on missile on the anterior part of the globe directly or over the lids transmitting all the force to the globe and result in sudden expansion of the scleral coats creating a shearing force at sclerochoroidal and uveoretinal attachments. The structures going under stress suddenly are (angle of anterior chamber, zonules, iris diaphragm and vitreoretinal fixations). This type injury does not appear very severe compared to big balls and they damage the vision more. Baseball, Soccer, Hand ball,

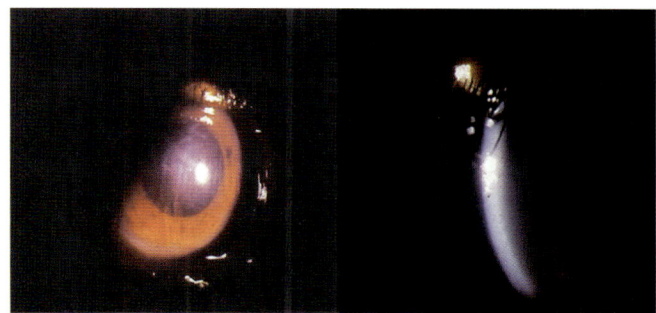

Fig. 10.6: Descemet's rupture with a cricket ball

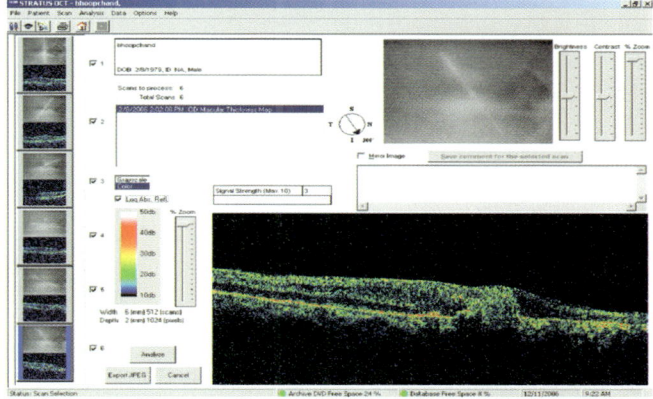

Fig. 10.7: OCT in injury a young man reported to be hit with a tennis ball couple of months ago. OCT reveals pigment proliferation, occult SRNVM, patchy RPE breaks, neurosensory lift

Volleyball, Hockey and Cricket ball may damage the orbit and adenexa and the globe at same time. Thus speed, size and trajectory with which these missiles hit the eye decide the extent of visual deficit and the outcome because of it direct uninhibited impact with great velocity. Stone pelting, Katty (*Gulel*) *Gulli Danda* and other improvized toys also cause a lot of ocular injury and ocular morbidity in the same manner.

Cricket ball injuries are very common in India and other cricket playing countries. Cricket ball injuries showed a magical rise (46% of all injuries) in Mumbai during Indian Premium League 2008. The vision-threatening injuries are often related to combine orbital and closed globe injury. A month long cricket competition and 20% of them were not playing themselves. Interestingly, soft tennis ball and smaller plastic ball used in street cricket causes more globe injury and visual deficit than regular hard cricket ball because of latter's nonelastic nature getting orbital rim support in dampening the chances of globe damage in contrast to resilient smaller balls taking conical shape to protrude in the orbit. Similar reports from Pakistan in 2003[5] indicated that 27% cases of severe sports njuries were caused by tennis ball (soft) used as cricket ball (Figs 10.6 and 10.7).[5]

Shuttle cock and table tennis balls are often responsible for traumatic mydriasis, hyphema (Fig. 10.8) and angle recession hitting directly on the cornea (Fig. 10.9), due to relative firm limbus compared to stretchable cornea and scleral coats and

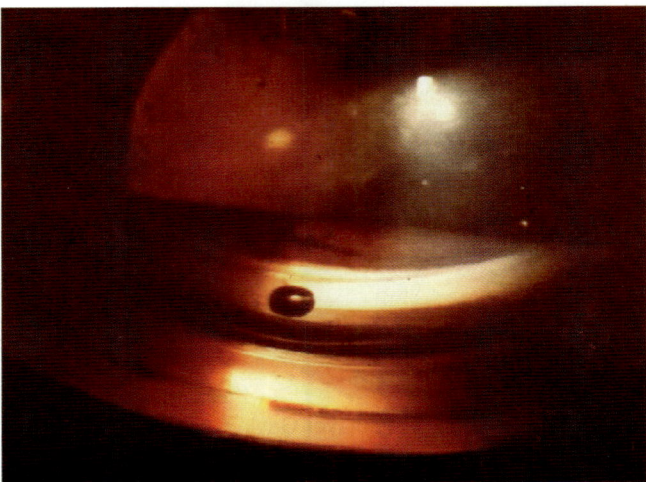

Fig. 10.9: Angle recession old injury caused by cricket ball

contracoupe impact on root of the iris from the post-segment. In more severe cases of impact subluxation of the lens, vitreous herniation and capsular rupture may be encountered. Small stone and Katty (*Gulel*) and *Gulli danda* injuries may also have similar damage in milder impact but have the have the potential of rupturing the globe (picture of ruptured globe after a gulli hitting the eye) (Figs 10.10a and b).

Macular hemorrhage choroidal infarction and choroidal tears can be seen in golf ball hitting the globe directly with severe impact. Atypical choroidal rupture have been noted in follow-up cases of golf ball injury hitting the eye with an impact without visual deficit (picture of atypical choroidal rupture) (Figs 10.11 and 10.12).

A number of factors contribute to the extensive ocular damage with direct messile effect of smaller objects on the globe, viz.

a. Variable scleral thickness and elasticity allowing differential impact in different areas.

b. Inelastic vascular choroidal tissue giving way while elastic retina escaping the hurt and scleral coat resisting the shearing force.

c. Potential space between photoreceptors and neurosensory retina filling up with fluid in altered permeability and initiation of inflammatory response.

d. Globe fixity at optic nerve, muscle attachments making them more vulnerable to retina in severe rotatory ocular movements.

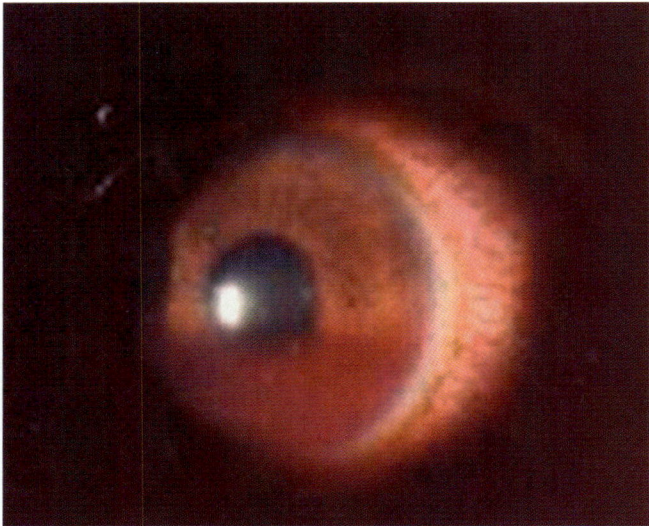

Fig. 10.8: Hyphema due to shuttle cock injury

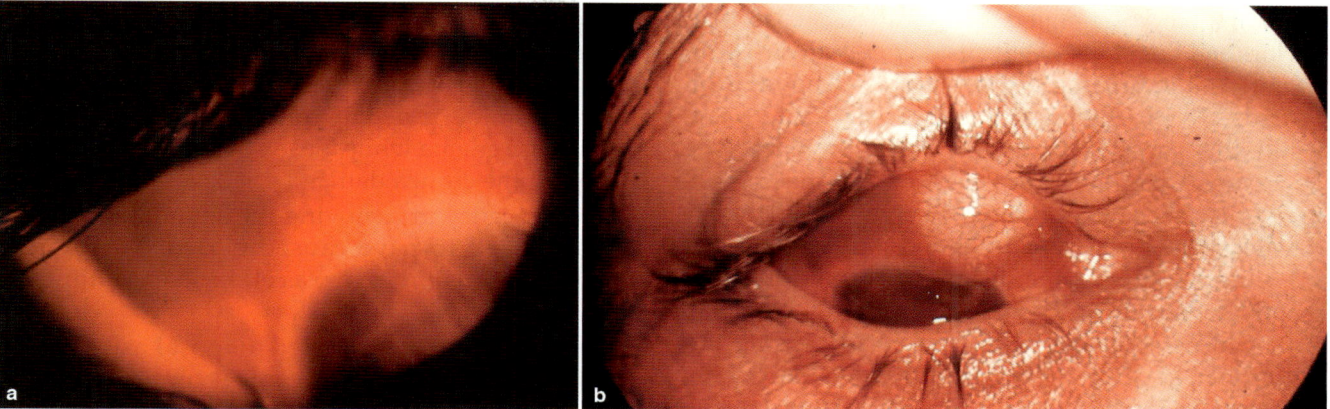

Figs 10.10a and b: (a) A stone missile released by a Katty (*Gulel*) and (b) Wooden missile (*Gulli*) injury—scleral rupture at the limbal area in two separate cases 'Gulel' injury

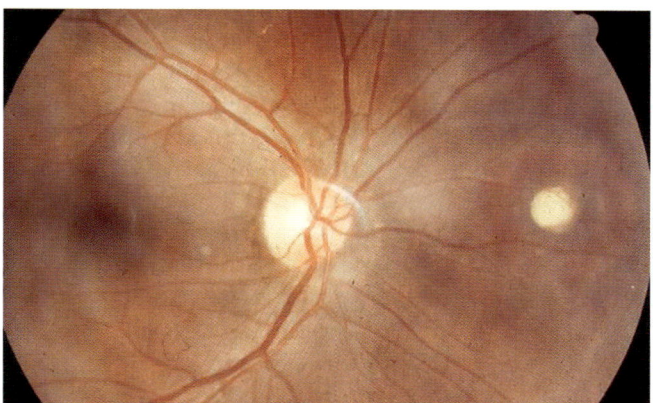

Fig. 10.11: Atypical choroidal tear caused by squash ball injury

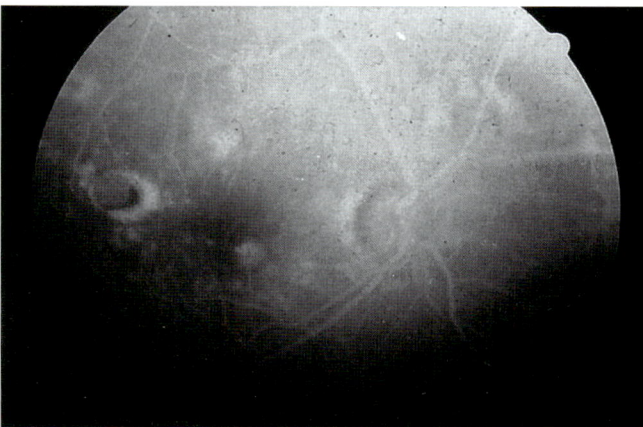

Fig. 10.12: Late film FFA with a golf ball injury (old injury) atypical choroidal rupture

e. Nonexpansile nature of limbus and crucial tissue relationship of root of iris, attachment of zonules and angle configuration at limbus and resultant contracoupe effect is responsible for angle and iris and zonular damage.

f. Independent choroidal and retinal circulation.

Golf club, hockey stick, tennis, squash and badminton racquets though not common cause very severe facial and orbital injuries with soft-tissue damage and bony fractures. Archery and Bow and Arrow may be responsible for open globe injury and may have a disappointing outcome.

Bungee jumping may have retinal hemorrhages due to sudden pressure changes in vertibrobasilar circulation aggravated by sympathetic stimulation. Wills Eye Hospital recorded 67 cases of Bungee cord injury in 1994–1999. Sixty-three percent had hyphema and 5.5% Commotio retinae. Thirty-one percent of these cases required some surgery and 6% needed anti-glaucoma surgery. Ten percent landed up with open globe and 4% needed enucleation.[9] Valsalva maneuver recommended in *Yoga* also result into Valsalva retinopathy characterized by hemorrhages in inner retina.

Paint ball/trademark game/survival game (invented by Charles Nelson to mark the trees, etc.) has been extremely popular as group and team game in children and adults as an entertainment and past time and now even as competitive sport. There are more than 50 clubs with regular teams playing paint ball in USA. The game is also being used in Army training. The game is played in variety of situations some of them unregulated environment like icecream parlors and bus stops. Seeing its vulnerability to ocular trauma minimum age for this game is kept as 16 in Canada, 18 in USA, and South Australia 12 years. While this game is banned in Tasmania since 1996, UK issues a paintball gun license if the speed of the marker exceeds 300 feet/sec. Whereas this game has developed into a million dollar industry it is catching up in India as team game and corporate entertainment mainly in Bengaluru, Chennai and Mumbai. The game is played using a soft water/dye filled capsule shot with the help of an air shot gun. The standard game has accessories like CO_2 cartridges and protective glasses. The injuries caused by this game are closed globe injuries sustained due to direct impact of the cartridges hitting the globe and cartridge taking the shape within the orbital wall due to its soft elastic nature. The cartridge hitting the spectacles may shatter the lens that may be responsible for open globe injuries.[10]

Games with extensive physical contact like wrestling, baseball and sumo are prone to orbital and adenexal injury boxing may have serious globe injury due to high speed and impact. Speed combined with reverse motion has resulted into retinal breaks, retinal detachments, and vitreous hemorrhage. It is estimated that 18.7% of all Wrestlers sustain injury around the eye during their carrier.[11] But unfortunately no protective gears have been possible in this game since these gears are going to be injurious to the opponent accidentally or intentionally. Karate judo, Taekwondo and other Martial arts-related sports are relatively less dangerous. 4.5/eye injuries have been reported in Taekwondo championship at Canada in 2004.

Snow sports, Skiing and other snow-related activities are very fast and dynamic. They require extra-protection and they are often having a restrictive mobility due to sports gear and clothing they wear. Hypoxia due to high altitude and increase in circulation may cause retinal hemorrhages. Skiing sticks have been known to cause the loss of eyes when the stick got stuck between face and protector. Skiis are dangerous to the co-player in event of a fall of the player ahead of others.

Swimming yachting, fishing, scuba diving and water sports like Water polo are common sports from decades and still very popular. Certain common factors need extra-caution in these activities.

1. Prolonged exposure to chorine is not healthy for cornea for all water indulgence.
2. Ill-fitting swimming goggles some time are responsible for ocular trauma. Tight bands may cause lid edema while loose goggles may suddenly slip on the cornea damaging it severely.
3. Complacency in removing the swimming goggles is reported to have caused closed globe injury (subluxation of the lens) as elastic band hitting the globe severely.
4. Diving is not recommended for post Lasik patients for the additional risk of corneal ruptures.
5. Scuba diving has been responsible for periorbital Baro trauma due to sudden environmental pressure changes.

Water polo is a sport that combines swimming, throwing and martial arts in one and is very popular in Euorope. It was initiated in 19th century with an imported Pulu (inflatable ball) imported from India. Direct impact injury on the face collision and hit from the ball on the face can damage the eye. Injury with finger nails may be responsible for mild corneal aberrations to penetrating injures. Hyphema and more severe closed globe injuries may be encountered with the ball or collision adenexal and orbital injuries have been seen to cause periorbital hematomas proptosis and blowout fractures.

Fishing is a very tranquil sport meant for people having lot of patience. But, fishhook penetrating injuries are not uncommon and loss of the eye in few cases.[12,13]

Corneal penetration and laceration are common with fish hook injury and entangled fish hook removal needs a special mention where the hook has to be moved through forward or tip to be cut before the removal of the fish hook followed by restoration of edges and suturing (Figs 10.13a to c).

MANAGEMENT

The management of the injuries caused have been discussed elsewhere in appropriate chapters.

Since outcome of the sports injuries caused is not a very favorable one in high percentage, the sports trauma must be taken seriously and avoid dangerous games and observe all precautions to safeguard vision and provide guidelines to the sportsmen and design suitable protective gears and make them available at affordable cost.[14-16]

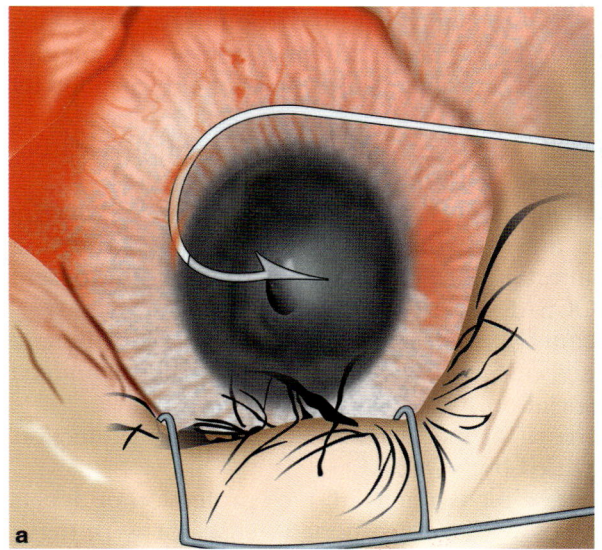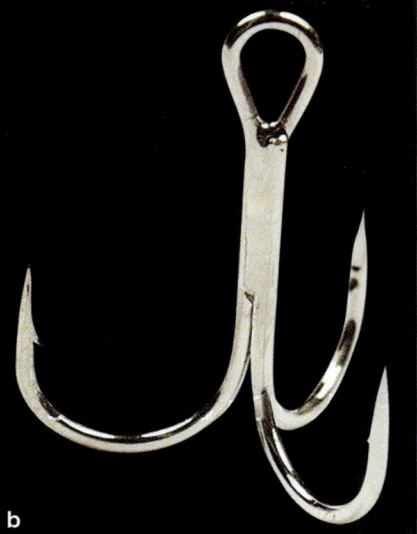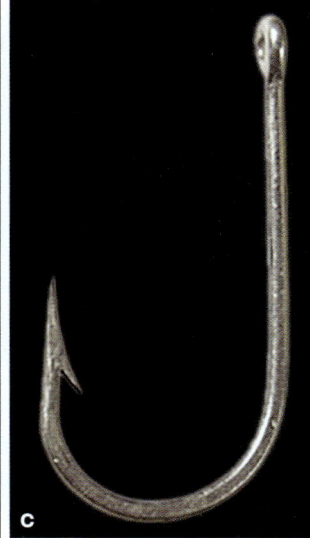

Figs 10.13a to c: Fish hook

PREVENTION AND PROTECTIVE GEARS[17-19]

It is very important to understand that 90% of ocular injuries are preventable and at that injuries encountered at sports should be preventable to nearly 100%. The best way to protect eyes while participating in sports is to follow the rules of the game. Avoid over indulgence and ensure appropriate sports eyewear.

STANDARD GEARS

Ordinary sunglasses do not protect any kind of mechanical trauma and instead they may be more dangerous in inflicting collateral trauma in case of racquet games. It is advisable not to use fashions eye wears to protect the eyes from anticipated mechanical trauma. It is advisable that rimless glasses and contact lenses must not be worn during high impact and children and racquet games players be asked to wear polycarbonate lenses in robust spectacle frames. Functionally one eyed athletes and those who had eye injury in the past or had an eye surgery must not play high risk games like boxing where no protection to eye has been devised and body contact games like wrestling it may not be practical.

Polycarbonate lenses are impact-resistant and lightest lenses you can buy. Polycarbonate is also the most shatter-resistant lens material and it filters 100% of ultraviolet (UV) light (which will help prevent radiation eye injuries). A 3 mm polycarbonate lens is considered adequate protection to the eye. Polycarbonate glasses are certified by Protective Eyewear Certification Council (PECC) in USA and generally affordable.

For the best sports protection, select glasses with polycarbonate lenses. Light tint with at least 75% light clearance Gray and Amber tints are nearly ideal.

Swimming and diving glasses have special features to save eyes from water and chemical onslaught. Similarly snow and water sports need protection from UV and infrared injuries to the eyes apart from protection from mechanical trauma.

The glasses used for cricket like games may be modified for additional visual enhancing filters and glare reducing and clarity enhancing filters.

Wrestling has a low incidence of eye injury. Although no standards exist, eye protectors that are firmly fixed to the head have been custom made. The wrestler who has a custom eye protector made must be aware that the protector design may be insufficient to prevent injury and also safe for the opponent.

For sports in which a facemask or helmet with an eye protector or shield must be worn, it is strongly recommended that functionally one-eyed athletes also wear sports goggles that conform to the requirements of American Society for Testing and Materials (ASTM) F803 (for any selected sport). This is to maintain some level of protection if the face guard is elevated or removed, such as for hockey or football players on the bench. The helmet must fit properly and have a chinstrap for optimal protection.

Athletes should replace sports eye protectors that are damaged or yellowed with age, because they may reduce the clarity and contrast.

Eye Safety in Boxing

The International Amateur Boxing Association (AIBA) Medical Commission has been monitoring eye safety for a number of years. An annual examination is recommended:

- To maintain a reasonable limit for boxing
- To check the state of the eye
- To detect preexisting lesions around the retina
- To advise on preventive treatment (laser photo-coagulation.

Certification

Protective eyewear certification; there is a need to develop a system for a competitive and totally safe environment for a sport. It is desired that following sectors be carefully addressed for safe sports:

- Certification of sports material
- Protective gears and their certification/Standardization designing, availability, implementation
- Host-related rules of the game—guidelines and rules of the game, minimal sports arena and trained personnel
- Agent-related equipment and accessories handling, protective gears
- Environment related a number of injuries are inflicted to the third party. Proper enclosures and availability of infrastructure and management in high density sports areas
- Arena and restricted entry in high speed missiles and ball games
- Legislation against harmful/dangerous games/toys. Manufacture of safe toys
- Got policies and implementation.

Protectors that have been tested to an appropriate standard by an independent testing laboratory are often certified and should afford reasonable protection.

Some of the sports have standardized protective gears for professional and practice game sessions in USA.

- Baseball or softball polycarbonate or wire face guards on the Batter's helmet and sports goggles with polycarbonate lenses on the field (certified by PECC).
- Basketball, soccers sports goggles with polycarbonate lenses certified by the PECC.
- Football a polycarbonate eyeshield attached to wire face mask certified by the National Operating Committee on Standards for Athletic Equipment (NOCSAE).
- Racquet sports; sport goggles with polycarbonate lenses certified by PECC and Canadian Standard Association (CSA).
- Lacrosse for men Helmet with full-face protection (certified by NOCSAE).
- Lacrosse for women full-face protection or sports goggles with polycarbonate lenses or wire mesh (certified by PECC).
- Field hockey a full face mask for the goalie and sports goggles with polycarbonate lenses on the field (certified by PECC).
- Ice hockey helmet with full-face protection. Certified by the Hockey Equipment Certification Council (HECC).
- Skiing high-impact resistant eye protection or sports goggles with polycarbonate lenses they should also filter ultraviolet (UV) and excessive sunlight (certified by PECC).
- Paintball full-face protection (certified by PECC).

The PECC has begun certifying protectors that comply with the some of the approved standards:

- ASTM F513, ice hockey
- ASTM F659, skiing
- ASTM F803, racquet sports, basketball, baseball, women's lacrosse and field hockey
- ASTM F910, youth baseball batters and base runners
- ASTM F910, The HECC certifies those for which there are standard specifications include youth baseball batters and base runners
- ASTM F1776, paintball
- ATSM Z 803–86, racquet sports, basketball, baseball, women's lacrosse and field hockey
- ASTM F2713, field hockey.
- Z 262 , ZM -7810, hockey
- CSA-CAN3, hockey
- CSA P4007, the CSA certifies products that comply with the Canadian racket sport standard (which is similar to the ASTM standard).

Other protectors with specific standards are available for different situations.

1. Street wear (fashion) spectacles that conform to the requirements of American National Standards Institute Standard Z80.3.11 but these are not recommended for sports.

2. Safety eyewear that conforms to the requirements of American National Standards Institute Z87.1, 12 which is mandated by the Occupational Safety and Health Administration for industrial and educational safety eyewear. Prescription or nonprescription (Plano) lenses may be fixed in these frames.

3. An athlete who requires prescription spectacles has three options for eye protection:
   a. Polycarbonate lenses in a sports frame that passes ASTM F803 for the specific sport
   b. Contact lenses plus an appropriate protector
   c. An over-the-glasses eye guard that conforms to the specifications of ASTM F803 for sports in which an ASTM F803 protector is sufficient.

4. Athletics: ASTM-F803-01 Frames with 2 mm polycarbonate glasses for low risk events and 3 mm thick glasses for athletes wearing contact lenses/glasses.

5. Archery, Javelin, Discus and Shot-put have a small but definite potential for injury especially to the spectators and passerby. However, good field supervision can reduce the extremely low risk injury to near negligible.

JOINT POLICY STATEMENT[19]

Protective Eyewear for Young Athletes

American Academy of Pediatrics, Committee on Sports Medicine and Fitness, American Academy of Ophthalmology, Eye Health and Public Information Task Force

American Academy of Pediatrics and the American Academy of Ophthalmology strongly recommend protective.

Eyewear for all participants in sports in which there is risk of eye injury. Protective eyewear should be mandatory for athletes who are functionally one-eyed and for athletes whose ophthalmologists recom-mend eye.

REFERENCES

1. American Academy of Ophthalmology. Of a variety of certified sports eye protectors. Ophthalmology 2004;111:600–603

2. Jaison SG, Silas SE, Daniel R, Chopra SK. A review of childhood admission with perforating ocular injuries in a hospital in North-West India. Indian J Ophthalmol. 1994; 42(4):199–201.

3. Vats S, Murthy GVS, Chandra M, Gupta SK, Vashist P, Gogoi M. Epidemiological study of ocular trauma in an urban slum population in Delhi, India, Indian J. Ophthal 2008;56:313–316.

4. McGwin G, Xie A, Owsley C. Rate of Eye Injury in the United States. Arch Ophthalmol 2005;123.

5. Jan S, Khan S, Mohammad S. Hyphaema due to blunt trauma. J Coll Physicians Surg Pak. 2003;13(7):398–401.

6. Filipe JAC, Barros H, Castro-Correia J. Sports related ocular injuries. A three year follow-up study. Ophthalmology 1997;104:313–8.

7. Michael P. Slade ,Ocular Trauma, ANZ J.of Surgery , 2002; 69,582–83.

8. MacEwen CJ. Sport associated eye injury: a casualty department survey. *Br J Ophthalmol.* 1987;71(9):701–705.

9. Babar TF[1], Khan MT, Marwat MZ, Shah SA, Murad Y, Khan MD. Patterns of ocular trauma. J Coll Physicians Surg Pak. 2007 Mar;17(3):148–53.

10. Aldave AJ, Gertner GS, Davis GH, Regillo CD, Jeffers JB. Bungee cord-associated ocular trauma. Ophthalmology. 2001;108(4):788–92.

11. Fineman MS, Fischer DH, Jeffers JB, Buerger DG, Repke C: Changing trends in paintball sport-related ocular injuries. Arch Ophthalmol 2000;118:60–64.

12. Mohican Kazemi and Willy Pieters, Canadian Taekwondo. Atheletic injuries at a Canadian National Taewondo Championships—A prospective Study, BMC Musculoskeletal disorders 2004;5(22):1471–2475.

13. Seiff SR. Ophthalmic complications of water sports. Clin Sports Med. 1987;6(3):685–93.

14. Rodriques JO, Lavina AM, Agrawal A, Prevention and Treatment of Common eye injuries in sports. American Family Physician 2003;67;1481–8.

15. Barr A, Baines PS. Desai P, MacEwen C J. Ocular Sports Injury The Current Picture, Brit J. Sports medicine 2000;34:456–8.

16. Pardhan S, Shacklock P, Weatherill J. Sport-related eye trauma: a survey of the presentation of eye injuries to a casualty clinic and the use of protective eye-wear. Eye. 1995; 9 (Pt 6) Suppl:50–3.

17. Capão Filipe J A, A Rocha-Sousa, Falcão-Reis, F , Castro-Correia J-Modern sports eye injuries Br. J Ophthalmol 2003;87:1336–1339.

18. Vinger PF. A practical guide for sports eye protection. Physicians Sports med 2000; 28(b).

19. American Academy of Pediatrics, Committee on Sports Medicine and Fitness, American Academy of Ophthalmology, Eye Health and Public Information Task Force Joint Policy Statement Protective Eyewear for Young Athletes Ophthalmology 2004;111: © 2004 by the American Academy of Ophthalmology.

Ocular Trauma in War and Insurgency

• RP Gupta • VK Baranwal

INTRODUCTION

The injuries sustained in wars are extremely varied and differ in various wars as the technique of combat changes. In first World War, the pattern of casualties was due to machine gun fire and blast effect of artillery. In second world war and recent wars the extensive use of mines, tanks and aerial bombing has changed the pattern of injuries.[1] Nonconventional combat is present all around the world. In recent years, there has been an increase in insurgents using improvized explosive devices (IED), hand mines, rocket-propelled grenades (RPG) and explosive formed projectiles. Although the exposed part of the eyes constitute only 1 of 375 part of body surface, the incidence of ocular injuries is comparatively much higher.[2]

Ocular injury is a frequent cause of morbidity in blast victims in war or insurgency. It occurs in 28% of survivors.[3]

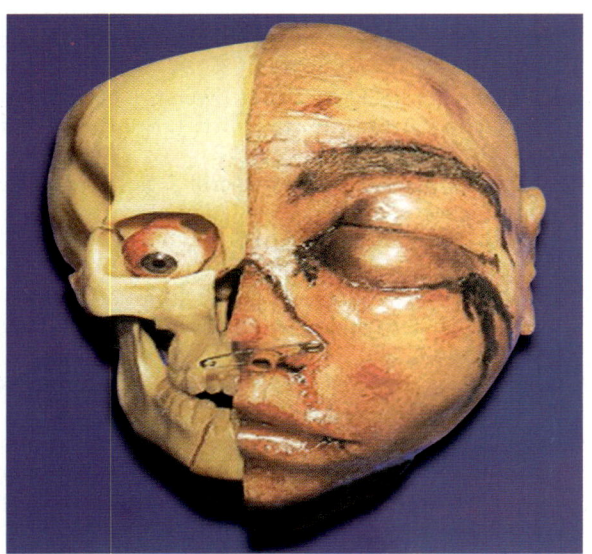

Fig. 11.1: Reconstruction face in blast injury

Secondary blast injury caused by flying fragments or debris is a peculiar threat to the eye. Such injuries are usually bilateral, varying from minor corneal abrasions and foreign bodies (FBs) to extensive eyelid lacerations, open globe injuries, intraocular foreign bodies or orbital fractures.Glass is a major source of lacerations and FBs affecting the eye. Explosive devices tend to accelerate metallic fragments and also propel soil and organic matter (Fig. 11.1).

MECHANISM OF BLAST INJURIES

Eyes

Weapons depend on high and low explosive potentials. All weapons change potential energy to kinetic energy in a very short period of time, resulting in a blast wave. The spherical front of the blast wave exhibits increase in pressure, density and temperature, known as shock front. This blast wave can inflict several types of injuries and eye is commonly prone to such injuries.

The primary blast wave impacts on eye wall, facilitate rupture of the eye ball. Partial or full thickness laceration of cornea/sclera weakens the eye wall and increases the possibility of rupture by lower primary blast wave stress impact.[4]

The secondary blast effect plays a major role in ocular injuries. Penetrating fragments made of different kinds and shapes ranging from conventional shell fragments to vehicle fragments, ground particles, and and pebbles or other components may cause devastating damage to the eye.

In conventional war, the most common weapons responsible for ocular injuries are shell fragments from rockets, grenades, mines and other nonmagnetic particles. Combat eye penetrating FBs are approximately 55% nonmagnetic, reflecting the nonferrous composition of mines and secondary missiles. In places having buildings, glass fragments from windows are notorious for causing ocular injures. Since the explosively propelled fragments of glass travel at high speed, there is no time for blink reflex to operate.[5]

Tertiary blast effect is by flames from toxic burnt materials. These fumes cause high thermal explosive effects on the cornea.

Orbit

Primary blast wave impact on nasoorbital ethmoidal skeleton leads to compression of orbit and ocular region. This is followed by expansion phase which brings it back to its original shape. The implosion and miniature re-explosion leads to crush injury to this region. The primary blast effect shock wave propagates through the globe and related orbital anatomical tissues causing concussion-contusion to organs and tissues in this region. It may also affect brain tissue by transverse wave propagation through orbital roof, damaging the cribriform plate and olfactory plate causing frontal and ethmoidal sinus fracture.

MINES EYE BLAST INJURIES

Mines continue to injure civilians and soldiers during conflict and long after a ceasefire. Bilaterality of damage is seen in 78.4% patients. The prevalence of blindness caused by mine blast injuries is quite high.[6]

ROCKET PROPELLED GRENADE (RPG-7 AND 29) BLAST INJURIES

RPG-7 is available worldwide and is cheap. Many soldiers loose their vision from this weapon explosion. Its blast wave is followed by second explosion blast which melts spall metal, which is main cause of penetrating injury by small metal fragments, blast wave and thermal effects. RPG-29 is capable of destroying even a modern tank. Antitank weapons contain more explosive material and provide a greater primary blast effect. This may cause catastrophic wounds to the soldiers who are hit, especially eye injuries because of the effect of large secondary fragments and the primary blast wave. Metal spall are small fragments from the melted metal from external armor plate. It produces a shower of small, irregularly shaped, very hot, metallic fragments at metal melting

point. The victims are very close to explosive and are therefore exposed to high thermal burns. Primary blast front wave and small metallic spalling particles of 2–3 mm size penetrate or rupture the eyeball and many a times shower the exposed face.[7]

CLINICAL PRESENTATION

Ocular Injuries

Blast eye injuries may present with a wide range of symptoms varying from minimal discomfort to severe pain or loss of vision. It is important to appreciate that significant eye damage may be present with normal vision and minimal symptoms which include eye irritation, FB sensation, bleeding and bruising. Minor blast injuries include:
- Eyelid lacerations (Fig. 11.2)
- Superficial FBs
- Conjunctivitis
- Corneal abrasions

Serious blast related eye injuries commonly include open globe injuries, i.e. penetrating or perforating injuries to the cornea or sclera with retained IOFB (Fig. 11.3). Signs of globe rupture include hyphema, a peaked tear drop-shaped or otherwise irregularly shaped pupil, exposed uveal tissue (Fig. 11.4) and extraocular movement restriction. Subtle signs of globe rupture include localized conjunctival chemosis, subconjunctival hemorrhage, conjunctival laceration or enophthalmos.

Globe rupture if not treated can lead to endophthalmitis (Fig. 11.5) or panophthalmitis. Serious nonpenetrating eye injuries include:

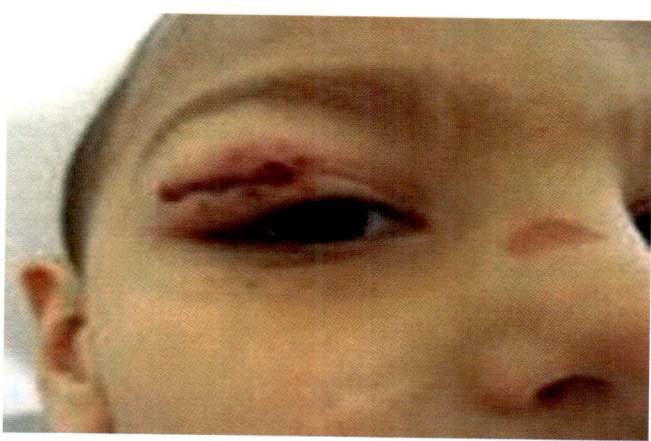

Fig. 11.2: Eyelid lacerations

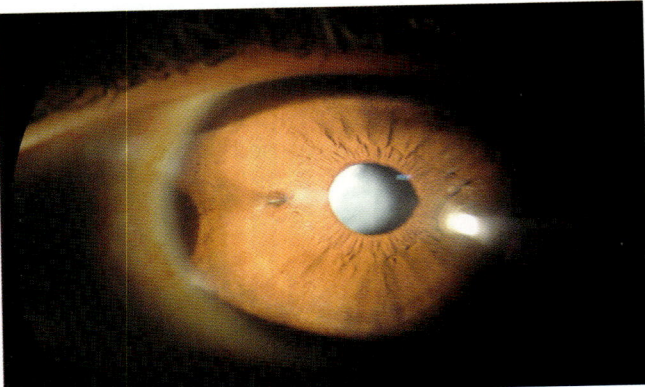

Fig. 11.3: Penetrating injury with retained IOFB

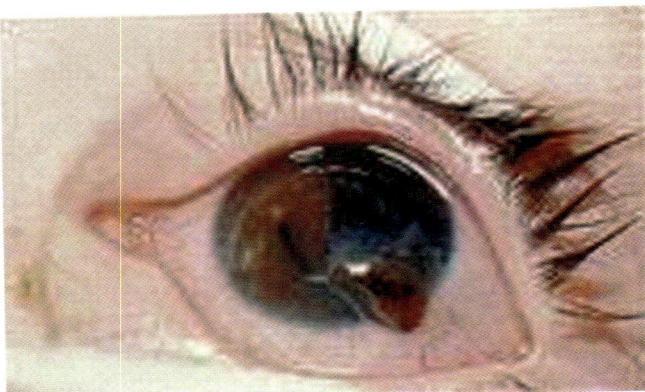

Fig. 11.4: Corneal tear with iris prolapse

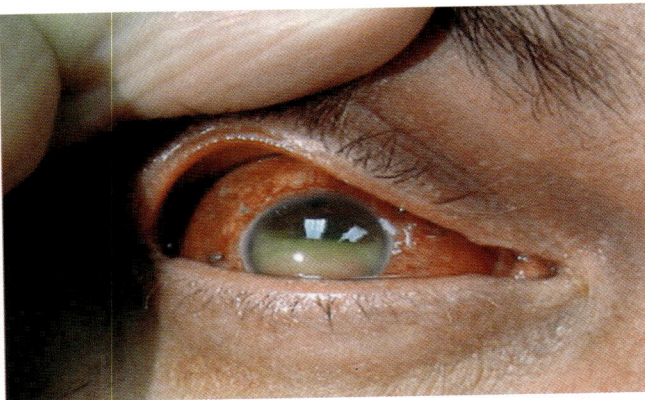

Fig. 11.5: Open globe injury with hypopyon (endophthalmitis)

- Hyphema
- Traumatic cataract
- Vitreous hemorrhage
- Retinal detachment
- Choroidal rupture.

Orbital Injuries

- Bomb blast commonly leads to penetrating orbital injuries which may effect superior orbit, involving anterior cranial fossa and deep orbital injury involving middle cranial fossa.

- Anatomic structure of orbit often allows large pieces of metal or organic matter to be embedded without significant signs and symptoms. Chronic structural compression effects and secondary infection can also occur. Composition of FB contributes to severity of injury. Metals such as iron, steel, aluminum and lead are inert. Copper alloys such as brass and bronze causes chronic, less destructive reaction. Stone and glass are well tolerated unless they cause infection. Copper causes purulent inflammation. Organic FBs like wood causes granulomatous reaction. Most common sequelae of orbital FB is diplopia following injury to muscle or nerve.

- Blow out orbital fracture occurs typically if orbit is struck by an object greater than 5 cm in diameter such as stone. Most common fracture occurs along floor of orbit. Orbital injury may lead to proptosis of the globe, elevation of intraorbital and intraocular pressure causing vascular insufficiency of optic nerve and retina. When the pressure within the orbit exceeds central retinal artery (CRA) pressure, ischemia results from insufficient blood supply. It is more serious in retrobulbar hematoma as pressure effect of fluid is higher than air. Retrobulbar hematoma (Fig. 11.6) may result in blindness if not decompressed by drainage. Optic nerve injury may lead to visual dysfunction.

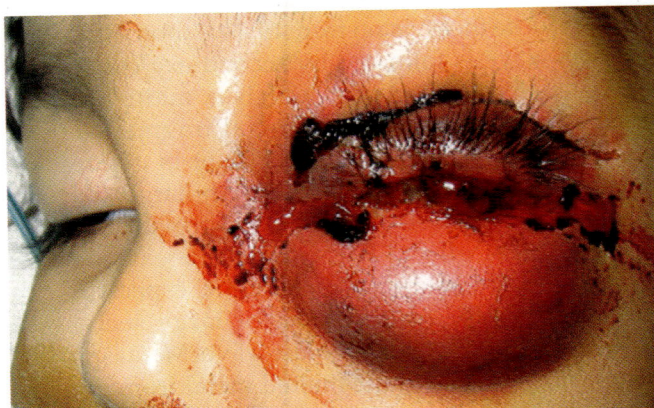

Fig. 11.6: Retrobulbar hematoma

TRIAGE

- On the battle field or at the site of detonation, all casualties are priortized in three groups depending upon severity of injuries. Group 1 includes most severe injuries requiring immediate life and limb saving measures. Group 2 include moderate injuries and Group 3 includes other minor injuries and walking wounded patients. But during this time of handling mass casualties, in severe injuries basic and advanced life support is the primary objective until the patient is stabilized. If neurosurgical concern prevents pupillary dilatation, comprehensive evaluation of retina, choroid and optic nerve head may be deferred.[8]
- But, at this critical time during handling of mass casualties and multisystem major injuries, primary or secondary eye/orbital injuries may unfortunately remain untreated because of life-saving priorities. In the case of continuous flow of new casualties in longstanding front line battle, severe eye injuries should not be missed. Patient should be examined and primary diagnosis determined. First responders at all levels should be trained to screen for eye injuries.
- The eyes are promptly checked for gross deformities, extraocular movements, globe perforations, hyphema, chemosis, enophthalmos or exophthalmos. The visual evaluation compares sight in the injured eye to uninjured eye. Severe vision loss in the non-ruptured eye is a strong indicator of serious injury. Most of the eye injuries should be covered immediately by a convex plastic or metal shield for protection. No pressure should be applied on the open globe.
- The eyes should be re-examined when the surgeon screens the blast injury patient from head to toe prior to anesthesia.

Detailed Evaluation

- Obtain visual acuity of each eye-test for light perception (PL), hand movements (HM) and counting fingers (CF).
- Check for relative afferent pupillary defects.
- Lids should be checked for subtle canalicular laceration or evidence of occult injury (Fig. 11.7).
- Evaluate globe for occult injury: Many a times underneath conjunctival swelling or ecchymosis, we find large scleral tear or perforation.

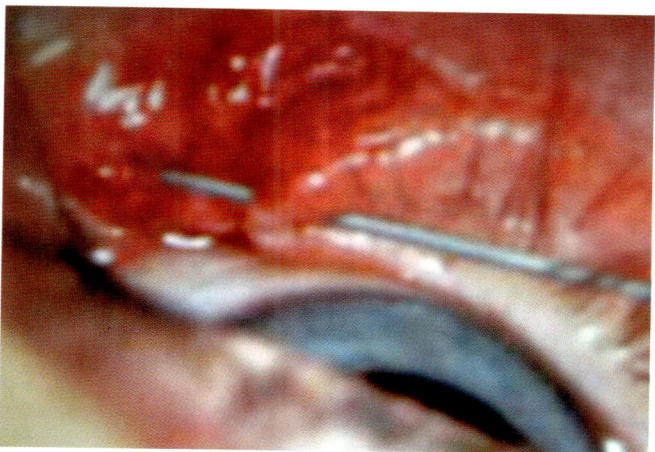

Fig. 11.7: Canalicular laceration

- Fundus evaluation to rule out occult perforation or contusive injury.
- Intraocular pressure
- Extraocular motility
- Look for periocular signs in blow out fractures, i.e. ecchymosis, edema and subcutaneous emphysema. Infraorbital nerve anesthesia, diplopia and enophthalmos.
- Ultrasonography (USG) (A-B scan) is useful for evaluating the globe in opaque media.
- Thin slice computed tomography (CT) scan is useful in evaluating bony orbit, globe and retrobulbar area (Fig. 11.8). In addition involvement of intracranial extension can also be seen.

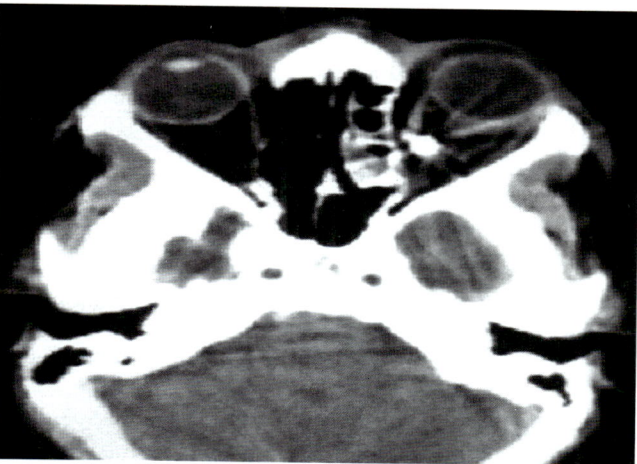

Fig. 11.8: Computed tomography (CT) scan revealing intraorbital foreign body traumatizing left optic nerve

- Magnetic resonance imaging (MRI) is contra-indicated in metallic FBs. It is useful in non-metallic FBs and soft-tissue injuries.

MANAGEMENT

Ocular Injuries

Management of ocular injuries is usually in three phases:

    i. Initial management at forward medical center
   ii. Management in an eye center
  iii. Definitive treatment at advanced ophthalmic center.

Management at Forward Medical Center

In war, casualities reach forward medical establish-ments with in few hours of the injury. At this forward treatment center, following norms are followed:

      i. Do not force the lids open to examine the eye. Defer examining eye if there is massive swelling or hematoma of the lids.
     ii. Assume all eye injuries harbor a ruptured globe. Do not put any pressure on an eye that may cause rupture or increase the already existing corneoscleral tear.
    iii. Do not apply a patch or bandage to the eye. Use a convex plastic or metal shield and tape it properly to surrounding bones to protect the eyes.
     iv. Administer tetanus toxoid.
      v. Administer intravenous broad spectrum antibiotics (particularly if ruptured globe is suspected). Suggested antibiotics presently include vancomycin/ceftazidime. Consider IV clindamycin for dirty soil/organic material contaminated wounds.
    vi. Administer anti-emetics to reduce nausea and vomiting.
   vii. If globe is intact, sterile saline wash can be given to remove particles of dirt and start broad spectrum antibiotic eye drops—0.5% moxi-floxacin topically.
  viii. Do not put any ointment in a ruptured globe.
    ix. Do not try to remove impaled FB.
- Above management can be carried out in forward center by a medical officer, when an ophthalmologist may not be available.
- Ear, nose and throat (ENT) cross consultation with surgeon, maxillofacial surgeon, neuro-surgeon, pulmonologist and orthopedician may be required.

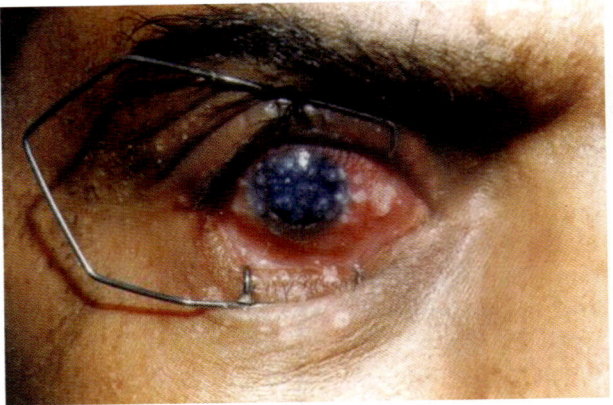

Fig. 11.9: Multiple FBs in deep corneal stroma

Management at an Eye Center of Military/Civil Hospital

      i. Lid wounds are cleaned and repaired
     ii. All conjunctival and superficial corneal FBs should be removed under slit lamp biomicro-scope to minimize damage. Multiple FBs lying in deep corneal stroma (Fig. 11.9), if removed causes lot of scarring, hence their removal should be avoided as far as possible. Cornel opacities due to multiple FBs clear remarkably in 50% cases in 6–9 months.[1] If FBs in deep stroma requires removal, these should be removed in operation theater (OT) under microscope, so that in the process of removal, if it falls in anterior chamber (AC), it can be adequately managed. Sterile glass FBs in deep stroma can be left safely without causing any opacification.
    iii. Corneal and scleral tears are repaired. If any portion of iris is prolapsing out and is dirty, it is abscissed. If it is fresh and not contaminated, it is cleaned with sterile ringer lactate and reposited. But if the prolapse is of 24 hours or more, it is better to do abscission of the iris. Any flocculent material inside AC is aspirated with Simcoe's cannula and AC is formed with balanced salt solution. In cases of scleral tear with exposed uveal tissue, lightly heated platinum tip cautery is applied to uveal tissue which stops oozing and causes its retraction. Thereafter, it may be easy to approximate the margins of scleral tear.
    iv. In badly mutilated eyes, evisceration or frill excision is done. It can be carried out simul-taneously when the patient is operated under general anesthesia for his other injuries.

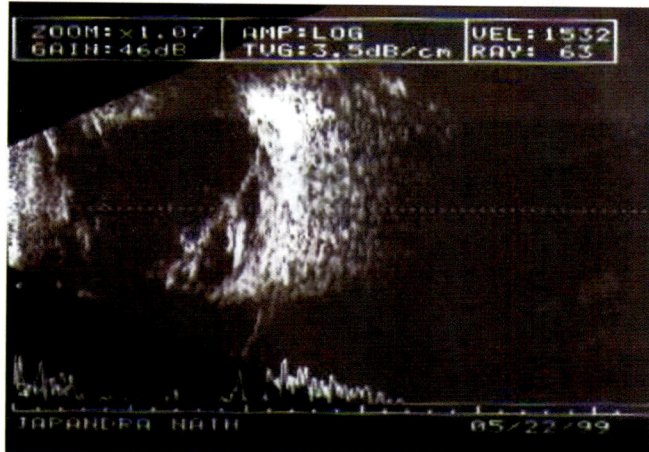

Fig. 11.10: Scan revealing retinal detachment

Definitive Management at Advanced Ophthalmic Center

i. Reconstruction of traumatic coloboma of upper or lower lid is done by oculoplastic surgeon.

ii. In all cases of closed globe injuries having hyphema, cataract or vitreous hemorrhage, USG is done to see underlying status of retina (Fig. 11.10). If retinal detachment is present, patient is taken for lensectomy/vitrectomy, endodrainge, endolaser photocoagulation and vitreous temponade as indicated. These vitreo-retinal procedures should be carried out as early as possible. Delay in performing these procedures compromise prognosis.

iii. Retained intraocular foreign body (IOFB) should be removed through pars plana route by intravitreal FB forceps or intravitreal magnet under full visualization through binocular indirect ophthalmo microscope (BIOM) or EIBOS.

Orbital Injuries

i. Blast wave leads to implosion of paranasal air cells, which allows passage of air cells into the orbit. Orbital emphysema usually deflates through fractured orbital walls. Orbital emphysema decompression can also be done by performing a small orbitotomy via lateral orbital rim by small incision on zygomaticofrontal suture region. Orbital canthotomy or inferior cantholysis could be the alternative, when the orbital pressure is high and expected to last longer.

ii. Retrobulbar hematoma may result in blindness if not decompressed by drainage. Retrobulbar decompression should be done within 90–120 minutes of developing hematoma at forward medical center. Retrobulbar emergent decompression should be done by lateral canthotomy and inferior cantholysis.[9] Canthotomy may compensate for small increase in orbital volume by forward movement of globe. Suspected globe rupture is a contraindication for lateral canthotomy.

iii. Optic nerve injury: If there is suspected optic nerve injury, no fracture in vicinity of optic canal and no hematoma, then medical decompression should be done by starting injection methyl prednisolone 1.5 g once a day for 5 days followed by oral steroids in tapering doses. In penetrating gun shot injury of orbit or splinter injury, optic nerve avulsion may occur or muscle transaction can occur. Sometimes optic nerve avulsion and transaction of muscles may occur together as revealed in (Fig. 11.11). In such situation, one has to do enucleation.

iv. Orbital FBs: Many a times, splinters from the medial or lateral side enter and lodge behind the eye. If these splinters are causing infection or compression, these should be removed via lateral orbitotomy. Many a times, these splinters may be sterile, due to velocity of splinters coming out of projectile and generation of heat around. It is better to leave such splinters inside the orbit if they are not causing any compression symptoms, because removal of these splinters itself may cause damage to eye/orbital structures around. Author has experience of leaving such splinters in orbit in 3 such cases with no untoward effects.

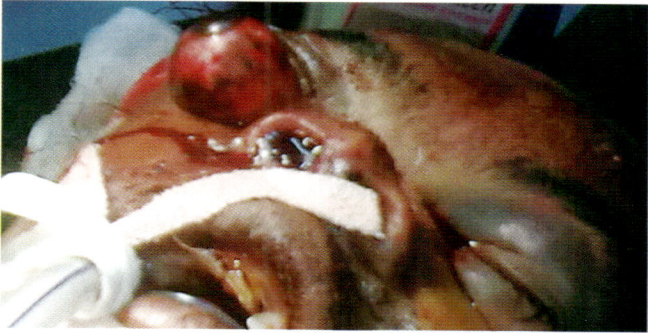

Fig. 11.11: Right eyeball having optic nerve avulsion and transaction of muscles

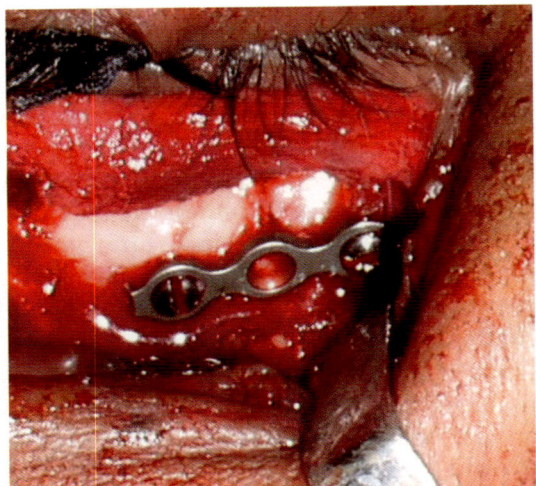

Fig. 11.12: Fixation of inferior orbital rim fracture with titanium plate

v. In orbital floor fractures presenting with diplopia or enophthalmos, reconstruction of orbital floor must be carried out in co-ordination with maxillofacial surgeon within 5–7 days. Autogenous bone graft can be harvested from iliac crest to reconstruct the floor. If there is associated inferior orbital rim fracture, it is fixed with titanium plate and screws (Fig. 11.12).

PROTECTION

In war scenario wearing helmet along with visor provides adequate ballistic protection against minor fragments/splinters and flying debris emanating from antipersonnel and antitank mines (Fig. 11.13).

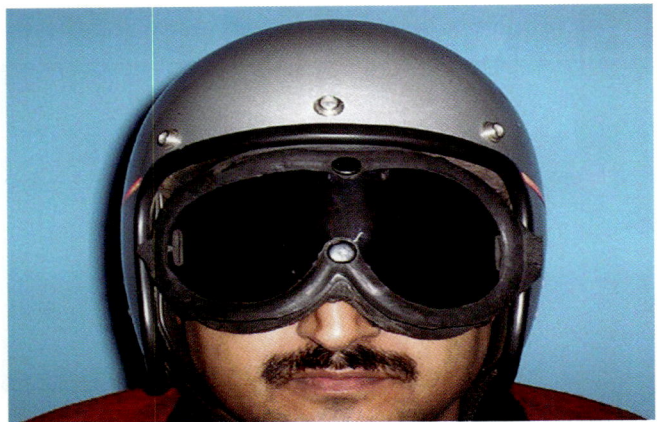

Fig. 11.13: Helmet with protective ocular goggles

It is recommended to use 4 mm thick transparent polycarbonate visor screen and suitable attachment harness which can be used with current combat helmet and turban for soldiers. The polycarbonate sheet is quite strong, highly transparent, tough and ductile. It does not shatter or spall under ballistic impact. Hence it is not only advisable for soldiers but also for civilians working in industries.[1,10]

CONCLUSION

Blast injury of eye/orbit requires special attention and interest among ophthalmologists. Thousands of people loose their vision due to penetrating, perforating and ruptured eyes because modern vitreoretinal surgeries are not being performed at appropriate time, due to lack of expertise, experience and/or equipment. The likelihood of restoring a soldier's vision has direct correlation to the immediate management of eye injury by proper antibiotics and vitreoretinal procedures performed as needed. Combination of vitrectomy and antibiotics is quite useful in managing post-traumatic endophthalmitis.

New vitreoretinal surgical techniques certainly helps in a big way in management of traumatized eyes with blast injuries in war or insurgency. Presently it is available in advanced eye centers only. It should be offered to victims all over the world. This area of ophthalmology should receive increased attention more so in developing countries where adequate facilities for performing such procedures are lacking.

Sympathetic ophthalmitis was reported in large number of cases in first and second world war. This dreaded complication has decreased markedly due to microscopic surgery, improved techniques and use of steroids. Author did not encounter a single case of sympathetic ophthalmitis while dealing with hundreds of cases of ocular injuries in wars, insurgency and terrorism in recent past. No hurried attempt should therefore be made to enucleate an eye immediately following trauma because of fear of sympathetic ophthalmitis since enucleation immediately following the injury is likely to cause additional psychological trauma to the already emotionally disturbed and wounded individual.

REFERENCES

1. Col. NB Singh, Lt. Col V K Madan, Lt. Col M Deshpande, Maj. RP Gupta, Maj. SK Srivastava, Medical Journal Armed Forces India 1990;46:3.

2. Stewart Duke Elder. System of ophthalmology, Part 1 Mechanical injuries, London, Henry kimpton, 1972; 14:50–51.

3. Thach AB. Ophthalmic Care of the Combat Casualty. Borden Institute Army Mil. Publisher Department of the Army. Washington, DC, USA, 2003;421–29.

4. Bailey A, Murray SG. The chemistry and physics of explosions. Explosives, Propellants, and Pyrotechnics, 2nd Edition. In: Bailey A, Murray SG (Eds). Land Warfare, London, UK, v;1–19.

5. Guy RJ, Kirkman E, Watkins PE, Cooper GJ. Physiologic responses to primary blast. J Trauma 1998;45(6):983–7.

6. Pillgram-Larsen J, Mellesmo S, Peck R. Injuries from mines. Tidsskrikt for Den Norske Laegeforening 1992;112:2183–87.

7. Shuker ST. Rocket-propelled grenade maxillofacial injuries and management. J Oral Maxillofac Surg. 2006; 64:503–10.

8. Kluger Y. Bomb explosions in acts of terrorism – detonation, wound ballistics, triage and medical concerns. Isr Med Assoc J (IMAJ) 2003;5:235–40.

9. Goodall KL, Brahma A, Bates A, Leatherbarrow B. Lateral canthotomy and inferior cantholysis: an effective method of urgent orbital decompression for sight threatening acute retrobulbar haemorrhage. Injury 1999;30(7):485–90.

10. Boparai MS, Sharma RC. Ocular war injuries. Ind J Ophthalmol. 1984;32:277–79.

12 Polytrauma

12.1 ROAD TRAFFIC ACCIDENTS

• Anand Verma • DK Mehta

INTRODUCTION

From prehistoric era, people wander in search of food in jungles. As civilization developed, people started travelling from one place to another place for trading and other purposes using carts and chariots but science advanced still further, leading to new inventions day by day blessing world with newer automobiles, high speed cars, bikes, buses and trains, etc. This modern high speed mode of transportation increases incidence of road traffic accidents.

The world's first road traffic death involving a motor vehicle is alleged to have occurred on 31 August 1869.[1] An Irish scientist Mary Ward died when she fell out of her cousins' steam car and was run over by it.

Many different terms are commonly used to describe vehicle collisions. The World Health Organization (WHO) use the term *road traffic injury*[2] while the United States (US) Census Bureau uses the term *motor vehicle accidents (MVA)*[3] and transport Canada uses the term "motor vehicle traffic collision".[4] Other terms that are commonly used include *auto accident, car accident, car crash, car smash, car wreck, motor vehicle collision (MVC), personal injury collision (PIC), road accident, road traffic accident (RTA), road traffic collision (RTC), road traffic incident (RTI), RTA* and later *RTC*, as well as more unofficial terms including *smash-up* and *fender bender*.

Some organizations have begun to avoid the term "accident". Although auto collisions are rare in terms of the number of vehicles on the road and the distance they travel, addressing the contributing factors can reduce their likelihood. For example, proper signage can decrease driver error and thereby reduce crash frequency by a third or more.[5] That is why these organizations prefer the term "collision" rather than "accident".

Road accidents have earned India a dubious distinction. With over 130,000 deaths annually, the country has overtaken China and now has the worst road traffic accident rate worldwide.

Every hour, 40 people under the age of 25 die in road accidents around the globe. According to the WHO, this is the second most important cause of death for 5–29 years old.

In India alone, the death toll rose to 14 per hour in 2009 as opposed to 13 the previous year. The total number of deaths every year due to road accidents has now passed the 135,000 mark, according to the latest report of National Crime Records Bureau (NCRB).

While trucks and two-wheelers were responsible for over 40% of deaths, peak traffic during the afternoon and evening rush hours is the most dangerous time to be on the roads.

While death surely cannot be passed off lightly. It is the morbidity and ocular morbidity that keeps the victim as under previlaged and the government that has to support its handicapped population for a preventable cause. Each year more than 2.5 million eye injuries occur and 50,000 people permanently lose part or all of their vision.[6]

Worldwide, there are approximately 1.6 million people blind from eye injuries, 2.3 million bilaterally vision impaired and 19 million with unilateral vision loss;[1] this being one of the most common cause of unilateral blindness today.[7]

Developing countries like India, carry the largest burden, yet are the least able to afford the costs. Though majority of these injuries leave the final vision unaffected and only 2–3% require hospitalization.[8,9] Noteworthy is the fact that of the patients hospitalized, over 10% will lose useful vision in the injured eye.

As per information available from the Healthcare Cost and Utilization Project (HCUP) on emergency department (ED) (the HCUP Nationwide Emergency Department Sample (NEDS) is a unique and powerful database that yields national estimates of ED in US visits related to eye injuries in 2008. Across all ED visits related to eye injuries, among the top five causes of eye injuries, MVA (3.3%) ranks fourth. Ocular injuries by motor vehicle accident involving collision with parked vehicle (E812.0) accounts 0.8%. Among all the patients attending ED for ocular injuries, patients requiring in-patient care were the most commonly due to fall (36.1%), followed by motor vehicle traffic accident (19.1%).[10]

Eye injuries that occur during motor vehicle crashes have increased progressively since 1998, according to a study published in a 2005 issue of Archives of Ophthalmology. Statistics from the American Society of Ocular Trauma show that 8.9% of ocular injuries are caused by motor vehicle crashes. Those crashes are also the leading source of bilateral eye injuries. According to a study conducted in UK, the mean age of this group of patients was 33 years (3–84) with a sex ratio female 5:1.[11]

The Eye Injury Registry of Alabama has been collecting epidemiologic, treatment, final outcome, and rehabilitation information on serious ocular trauma since 1982. By December 31, 1989, 150 motor vehicle crash-related eye injuries had been registered. This is the largest series of motor vehicle crash-related serious eye injuries reported. The mean age of those injured was 29 years; 61% were between 16 years of age and 35 years of age, and 73% were males.[12]

Road traffic accidents are a major cause of visual loss in young adult population, and Canavan et al. found that they caused 30.2% of perforating eye injuries in Northern Ireland from 1967 to 1976.[13]

In pediatric age group (11–15-year-old children), cause of eye injuries due to road traffic accidents was 11%. This study was conducted at Baltimore, USA.[14] Similar study based on pediatric ocular trauma conducted in Iran indicates that cause of eye injuries due to road traffic accident accounts 13.3%.[15]

The observations made above make RTA very important cause of ocular morbidity worldover stressing its prevention and timely management.

NATURE OF INJURIES IN CAR ACCIDENTS

Most of the accidents are due to collision of one car with another vehicle, often in head-on impact overtaking on one-way routes, or at road traffic crossings. At times, the injury is caused by a careless driver injuring a pedestrian.

Glass-splinters from the windscreen can cause cut wounds to the face, eyelids, conjunctiva and corneas. Lid lacerations, muscle disinsertions and sclera lacerations may be seen some times due to splinters hiting the eye. Sometimes rupture of the globe is also found. In some cases, the injuries may be limited to the external eye only with superficial abrasion to the cornea. In some instances, for example, pieces of glass and the frame of the spectacles pierced the eye causing a perforating injury. In a few instances, the steering wheel and dashboard were struck by the forehead, face and the eye causing severe blunt trauma. Rarely, a fracture of the orbital margin resulted. Intraocular foreign bodies (IOFBs) or extraocular foreign bodies impacted in the soft tissues of the eyes or adnexae may have to be carefully looked for. It is usually not possible to distinguish whether the glass fragments were from windscreen glass or spectacle plastic lenses however glass lenses can be identified by its weight and sharper edges.

Study depicting types and nature of injuries encountered in RTA was conducted in UK. The types of eye injuries encountered were orbital wall fractures (61%), periorbital swelling or hematoma (46%), subconjunctival hemorrhage (23%), periorbital lacerations (22%), optic nerve trauma (11%) and penetrating eye injuries (6%). Visual impairment resulted in about 67% of survivors, including loss of eye in 24%. Diplopia requiring intervention was seen in 24% of the cases.[11]

In America from 1982 to 1989, 10 individuals (7%) suffered bilateral eye injuries. The retina was injured in 47% of eyes. The initial visual acuity was 19/200 or worse (legal blindness) in 47% of eyes. Of eyes with at least 3 months of follow-up, 63% had worse than 20/200 initial visual acuity and 41% remained legally blind. Twelve percent of eyes required removal. Possibly due to the large number of blunt ruptures, motor vehicle crash-related eye trauma carries a particularly unfavorable treatment prognosis.[12]

A study conducted on RTA and ocular trauma: Libya 16 of 276 traumatized eyes of 248 patients. One hundred and eighty-six (75%) patients were male and 62 (25%) were female. The mean age was 32.5 years. Types of injuries found were:

Extraocular: Eyelid bruising 104 (37.7%), eyelid edema 98 (35.5%), eyelid laceration 49 (17.8%), avulsion of extraocular muscle 12 (4.5%), orbital rim fracture 3 (1.1%).

Anterior segment: Subconjunctival hemorrhage 117 (42.4%), corneal abrasions 84 (30.4%), corneal perforations 129 (46.7%), scleral perforation 64 (23.2%), hyphema 138 (50%), iris injury 164 (59.4%), traumatic angle recession 29 (10.5%) traumatic cataract 88 (31.9%), lens dislocation 21 (7.6%).

Posterior segment: Vitreous hemorrhage 65 (23.6%), commotio retinae 55 (19.9%)

IOFB: Intraocular foreign body: 27 (9.8%).

Globe: Ruptured globe (with prolapse of uveal tissue, lens and vitreous) 27 (9.8%).

In a study conducted in, Glasgow, midfacial fractures revealed higher association with ocular injury.

Road traffic accident was associated with the highest incidence of severe ocular disorder (9/45 = 20%) whilst assaults had the second highest incidence at 11% (20/181). One-third of all patients with comminuted malar fracture suffered a severe ocular disorder (9/27) whilst blow-out fracture came second at 16.7% (6/36).[17]

NATURE OF INJURIES IN MOTOR CYCLE/ CYCLE ACCIDENT

According to a study , conducted in Nigeria on motor cycle related ocular injuries shows most commercial motor cycle riders are mainly young men (21–30 years of age). Mostly affected eye structures were conjunctiva, eyelids and cornea. This was expected because of anterior location of structures. Involvement of the conjunctiva (24.1%) either in form of traumatic conjunctivitis, subconjuctival hemorrhage or conjuctival lacerations were the most common conditions seen. Corneal lacerations, abrasion or ulceration and lid lacerations were the next most common type of ocular injuries (22.8%) recorded. This

again is not surprising because most most motor cycle riders do not wear protective glasses.[18]

Posterior indirect traumatic optic neuropathy and visual system injury is a serious and infrequently found condition where treatment is controversial and permanent visual loss is almost evident.[19-23]

It can occur following an innocent ipsilateral injury over the superior temporal orbital rim and is characterized by vision loss without external or internal ophthalmic evidences of injury to the eye and its nerve.[24]

Posterior indirect traumatic optic neuropathy is seen in up to 5% of all the cases of closed head trauma. Superior temporal orbital rim injury, even when minor, carries a potential risk for development of blindness from indirect posterior indirect traumatic optic neuropathy in two-wheeler drivers. Presenting signs do not correlate with visual status. Only visual evoked potential (VEP) has prognostic significance and the condition is untreatable. Posterior indirect optic neuropathy is not so common as shown in a study from North-East region of India,[25] in this study out of 129 consecutive cases of cranio-orbital injury,[35] had posterior indirect traumatic optic neuropathy with minor ipsilateral superior temporal orbital rim trauma and none used any protective headwear. Presenting clinical features like relative afferent pupillary defect ($P = 0.365$), optic disc status ($P = 0.518$) and VEP ($P = 0.366$) were disproportionate to visual loss, only VEP had prognostic significance.

RISK FACTORS RESPONSIBLE FOR RTA

A 1995 study using British and American crash reports as data, found that 57% of crashes were due solely to driver factors, 27% to combined roadway and driver factors, 6% to combined vehicle and driver factors, 3% solely to roadway factors, 3% to combined roadway, driver, and vehicle factors, 2% solely to vehicle factors and 1% to combined roadway and vehicle factors.[26]

Human Factors

This includes all the factors related to drivers and other road users including driver behavior, visual and auditory acuity, decision-making ability, and reaction speed. On analysis it was found that driver error, intoxication and other human factors contribute wholly or partly to about 93% of crashes.[26]

A Rent-A-Car (RAC) survey of British drivers found that most thought they were better than average drivers; a contradictory result showing overconfidence in their abilities. Nearly all drivers who had been in a crash did not believe themselves to be at fault.[27]

In AXA survey concluded Irish drivers are very safety-conscious relative to other European drivers. However, this does not translate to significantly lower crash rates in Ireland. Eighty-three percent of Irish drivers think a 0% alcohol limit would be a good idea according to a recent survey by AXA insurance. The survey, which was carried out across Europe, shows Ireland to be one of the most ardent supporters of the idea. In contrast, the average EU support for a 0% alcohol limit stood at 68%.[28]

Age

Young people tend to have good reaction times, disproportionately more young male drivers feature in accidents,[29] with researchers observing that many exhibit behaviors and attitudes to risk that can place them in more hazardous situations than other road users.[30] This is reflected by actuaries when they set insurance rates for different age groups, partly based on their age, sex, and choice of vehicle. Older drivers with slower reactions might be expected to be involved in more accidents, but this has not been the case as they tend to drive less and, apparently, more cautiously.

Youth

Insurance statistics demonstrate a notably higher incidence of accidents and fatalities among teenage and early 20-aged drivers, with insurance rates reflecting this data. Teens and early 20-aged drivers have the highest incidence of both accidents and fatalities among all driving age groups. This was observed to be true well before the advent of mobile phones. Females in this age group suffer a somewhat lower accident and fatality rate than males but still well above the median across all age groups. Also within this group, the highest accident incidence rate occurs within the first year of licensed driving. For this reason many US have enacted a zero-tolerance policy wherein receiving a moving violation within the first 6 months to 1 year of obtaining a license results in automatic license suspension. No US allows 14 years-old to obtain drivers licenses any longer.

Old Age

With some jurisdictions requiring driver retesting for reaction speed and eyesight after a certain age.

Physical Impairment

Poor eyesight and/or physical impairments, with many jurisdictions setting simple sight tests and/or requiring appropriate vehicle modifications before being allowed to drive.

Distraction

Research suggests that distracting sounds such as conversations and operating a mobile phone while driving also divert driver's attention. Many jurisdictions now restrict or ban the use of some types of phone within the car. Recent research conducted by British scientists suggests that music can also have an effect; classical music is considered to be calming, yet too much could relax the driver to a condition of distraction. On the other hand, hard rock may encourage the driver to step on the acceleration pedal, thus creating a potentially dangerous situation on the road.

Sleep Deprivation

Fatigue and deprivation of sleep impair the reflexes of driver and worsen the performance of driver.

Alcohol and Drug Use

Consumption of alcohol causes severe effect on driving performance and similarly drugs like antihistamines, opioids and muscarinic antagonists, and illegal drugs impairs driving performance. Combining low doses of alcohol and cannabis has a more severe effect on driving performance than either cannabis or alcohol in isolation.[31]

MOTOR VEHICLE SPEED

The US Department of Transportation's Federal Highway Administration review research on traffic speed in 1998.[32] The summary states:
- That there is evidence that crash risk is lowest near the average speed of traffic and increases for vehicles traveling much faster or slower than average.
- That the risk of being injured is lowest for vehicles that travel near the median speed and it increases

exponentially with speeds much faster than the median speed.

- That the severity of a crash depends on the change in speed of at impact. International research indicates the change in injury crashes will be twice the percentage change in speed squared, and fatal crashes will be four times the percentage change in speed.
- That there is limited evidence that suggests that lower speed limits result in lower accident rate on a system wide basis and that most crashes related to speed involve speed too fast for the conditions.

VEHICULAR DESIGN

The design and safety factors must be carefully crafted to reduce the morbidity also in cases of a vehicular trauma. Handle and brake lever of the bicycle have been responsible for damage the eye resulting in ocular perforation and even cause gauging of the globes a proper designing may save a lot of such unpleasant situations.

Car should be designed to take protective and safety measures and insist of their compliance An analysis of the safety measures provided is given to highlight its usage in reference to ocular trauma.

1. Seat belt
2. Airbag
3. Windscreen
4. Bluetooth.

Seat Belt

Seat belt is safety harness designed to secure the occupant of a vehicle against harmful movement. The ocular injury caused by a RTA is usually associated with multiple facial lacerations and may affect both the eyes. The mechanism of injury comprises impact of victim head against a shattered windscreen and perforation caused by flying glass.

Seat belt wearing by front seat occupants of vehicles became compulsory in Northern Ireland from 1 February 1983. Two hundred and forty-six patients with ocular perforation were treated at the Royal Victoria Hospital, Belfast, in Northern Ireland between 1 February 1981 and 31 January 1985. RTAs were responsible for 63 injuries, all of which affected front seat occupants, and 45 occurred before implementation of the seat belt law on 1 February 1983. Following legislation there was a 60% reduction in ocular

injuries[33] and this study corresponds with the observation of Hall et al in Wessex, England who reported that the estimated annual incidence of perforating eye injuries as a result of RTAs has decreased by 73% following legislation for the compulsory wearing of seat belts by drivers and front seat passengers[34] and Vernon and Yorston found a 58% reduction during comparable 6 months periods before and after compulsory use of seat belt.[35] It recorded a decrease of 83.3% of perforating eye injuries in the year after legislation.[36]

Similarly, a review of all penetrating eye injuries was treated by the Manchester Eye Hospital over 4 years (1 February 1982–31 January 1986) was undertaken. One hundred and ninety-six penetrating eye injuries were seen, of which 16 (8.2%) were due to road traffic accidents. Eight patients (nine eyes) were seen in the 12 months prior to the introduction of the seat belt legislation on 1 February 1983. None of these patients was wearing a seat belt whereas two of the eight patients (10 eyes) seen after the seat belt legislation were. Both these patients suffered severe visual loss due to intraocular glass from shattered windscreens.[37]

Therefore, it is clear that the risk of serious ocular injury by windscreen impact is greatly reduced by seat belt use. It is again observed that injuries continue to occur which may be due to the non-use of belts, faulty belts, and injury caused by flying glass from toughened windscreens[38] emphasised the danger of flying windscreen glass as a cause of ocular perforation. According to MacKay view these injuries may be further reduced by compulsory fitting of laminated windscreens instead of toughened windscreens in all newly registered motor vehicles and rigorous enforcement of the seat belt legislation.[39]

Airbag

For years, the trusty seat belt provided the sole form of passive restraint in our cars. There were debates about their safety, especially relating to children, but over time, much of the country adopted mandatory seat belt laws. Statistics have shown that the use of seat belts has saved thousands of lives that might have been lost in collisions. Like seat belts, the concept of the airbag—a soft pillow to land against in a crash—has been around for many years. The first patent on an inflatable crash-landing device for airplane was filed during World War II. In the 1980s, the first commercial airbags appeared in automobiles.

Airbag is a flexible envelop that can inflate during automobile collision to prevent occupants from striking interior objects such as steering wheel or a window. Airbags are safety devices designed to deploy in frontal but not other types of crashes. Most airbags will deploy only in a moderate-to-severe frontal crash. They are devices of proven value that supplement the protection provided by seat belts. Air bags are connected to sensors that detect sudden deceleration. When activated, the sensor sends an electrical signal that ignites a chemical propellant, and when ignited, this propellant produces nitrogen gas, which inflates the airbag. This process occurs very quickly—in less than one-twentieth of a second— faster than the blink of an eye. Most airbags have internal tether straps that shape the fabric and limit the movement of the airbag. Vents in the rear allow the bag to deflate slowly to cushion the head as it moves forward into the deploying airbag.

With all the flying debris it is no surprise that the eyes are at risk for severe injuries. Since the introduction of air bags, injuries that are caused by windshield and other things on dashboard have been minimized but what is more surprising that many eye injuries are caused by airbags. Airbag induced eye injuries may not be as common as eye injuries cause by flying debris but they are severe enough for concern. There is proof that airbags may do more harm than good. Studies show that the risk of an extreme eye injury and other serious injuries outweigh the benefits of airbags. The eye seems to be particularly vulnerable to injury especially if spectacle are worn. Eye injuries can range in severity from bruises in the eye socket to orbital fractures, retinal detachment, lens rupture and ruptured eyeballs, which can result in blindness or other long-term injuries to eye. Front seated children are at greater risk of eye injuries.

Chemical injuries of the eye are a rare complication of airbag deployment and result from seepage of the chemical, causing inflation through vents in the airbag. Severe cases of bilateral alkali eye injury upon airbag contact in a RTA were reported.[40]

Airbag Faults—Deployment Problems

Since their introduction as safety measures, airbags have been recorded as the cause of a number of very serious accidents. These can happen when an airbag:

- Inadvertently deploys when a vehicle hits a pothole, bump or for no discernible reason.
- Deploys because of a chafing condition in the steering wheel wiring of radio/tape controls. This has been a particular problem for drivers of general motors (GM) vehicles when changing the settings.
- Explode while deploying.

Airbags were developed to be an added safety measure, but they are proving to be more of a risk than anything. Airbags were designed to work with a male of a height around 5 feet 8 inches. Since this is far from the average size of women and men, airbags have a major flaw. They are not designed to suit women drivers or those of short stature. Anyone larger than the model used is also at risk.

While there have been notices made that children under the age of 12 years should sit in the backseat to avoid the possible harms of airbags, the truth is that every passenger is still at risk from the flying debris of an airbag. So, no matter where you sit in a car with airbags, you are at risk for eye injuries caused by them.

The airbags cause injuries because they deploy late. Manufacturers have known for at least 25 years that the airbag must be fully inflated before there is an interaction with the occupant. However, because of sensor designs, location of sensors, and the wiring systems utilized by manufacturers, airbags frequently do not deploy in a timely manner. As a result, the airbag partially inflates into the occupant, causing inflation-induced injuries.

Late deployments can be proven by downloading the black box to airbags. The black box is a computer database on each car, called the Sensing Diagnostic Control Module. It records information concerning the accident. In particular, it will show when the airbag was not fully inflated when it interacted with occupant.

In an accident, ocular injuries due to airbags may have grounds for seeking compensation from car manufacturer. To prevent eye injuries from airbags, one should follow all instructions from the manufacturer about safety. This includes keeping children in the back seat and using aids to help you sit higher in your seat if you are driving and are of a short stature.

Eye injuries from a car accident may happen from any flying debris. You may be able to prevent them by using airbags carefully and being aware of the risks they pose. It cannot hurt to get information and learn how to minimize your chance of a traumatic eye injury in a car accident. Wearing eyeglasses, safety glasses or sunglasses while driving or riding in a car could also be helpful.

Smart Airbags

These devices are still in the trial phase, but are looking promising for the future. Different car occupants would be sensed, and a number of alterations automatically made to the airbag. Potential developments include adjustment of the triggering force, gas volume and inflation rate. Advanced sensing and control systems will be necessary for these to become reality.[41]

Windscreen

In a car accident, the small pieces of glass from a shattered windscreen can cause damage to the inner or outer parts of the eye.

Automotive glass is manufactured into two different types of safety glasses to protect both the structure of the vehicle and the occupants inside. The first type of glass is called laminated glass, which is for the windshield. The second type of glass is known as tempered glass, which is used for the vehicle's side and back windows.

Laminated glass is made by sandwiching a layer of polyvinyl butyral (PVB) between two pieces of glass. The glass and the PVB are sealed by a series of pressure rollers and then heated. That inserted layer of PVB is what allows the glass to absorb energy during an impact and gives the glass resistance to penetration from flying projectiles. It also deflects up to 95% of ultraviolet (UV) rays from the sun.

Laminated glass can break and be punctured. The inner strong chemical bond with the PVB the splinters from two surfaces of glass on either side do not move more than few mm in the air. Careful consideration of the thickness of the glass should be maintained for its safety and weight factor to make the vehicle fuel efficient. A glass, thickness of the glasses less than 3 mm is unsafe.

Laminated and tempered glass each have different functions, but together, they keep you inside the vehicle in an accident, shield you from flying sharp glass, retain the roof's rigidity in a rollover and allow the side airbag to protect you when it's deployed. The Federal Motor Vehicle Safety Standards (FMVSS) for automotive glass (FMVSS 219) —this standard states that no part of most passenger vehicles can penetrate the windshield more than 6 mm (0.24 inches) in a crash.

In a study 64 cases of RTAs with eye injury were seen between January, 1966 and April, 1971. Fifty-one of these cases were studied in detail. Most of the accidents involved frontal collision with another vehicle and produced eye injuries to the unbelted driver or the front seat passenger. Ninety percent of the eye injuries in this series were caused by tempered glass windscreen. Perforating injuries that are bilateral or involve the expulsion of the lens at the time of accidents have the worse visual prognosis. Most of the injuries can be prevented by wearing safety belts and installing high penetration resistant laminated glass windscreens. Paper presented at The Royal Society of Medicine, 21–22 May, 1971, Eye injuries in RTA. KG Soni West Norfolk and King's Lynn General Hospital, King's Lynn, Norfolk, UK.

BIKE DESIGN

1. *Airbag:* Fuel tank mounted airbags as well as wearable jacket airbag devices change the way we think about the risks involved with motorcycles. Accidents occur within a very short time and a rider may not be able to instinctively protect him or herself when a crash takes place. This is where an airbag device becomes useful.

2. *Helmet:* A full-face helmet provides the most protection. Thirty-five percent of all crashes show major impact on the chin-bar area.[1] However, 3 of 4 and 1 of 2 helmets also are available. Bike helmet should fit you properly. It should not be too small or too big. Never wear a hat under bike helmet. It is also necessary that it should be worn in right way so that it can protect. It should be worn level and cover the forehead.

3. *Goggles or helmet visor:* Eye protection is of utmost importance—an insect or a kicked-up pebble in the eye at speed has enough momentum to cause significant damage. Such an event could easily cause the rider to lose control and crash. Besides this danger, squeezing into the wind is unpleasant at best and watering eyes are quite distracting.

REFERENCES

1. WHO/Road Safety issue : a public health issue, 29 March 2004.

2. Margie Peden et al. WHO; World report on road traffic injury prevention 2004.

3. US Census Bureau. The 2012 Statistical Abstract, National Data Book: Motor Vehicle Accidents and Fatalities"1103, 1104,1105.

4. Statistics and Data - Road and Motor Vehicle Safety - Road Transportation - Transport Canada".

5. Desktop Reference for Crash Reduction Factors Report No. FHWA-SA-07-015, Federal Highway Administration September, 2007.

6. Eye Injuries: Recent Datas and Trends in the United States;American Academy of Ophthalmology and American Society of Ocular Trauma, United States Eye Injury Registry summary report, 1998–2002.

7. Negrel AD, Thylefors B. The global impact of eye injuries. Ophthalmic Epidemiol 1998;5(3):143–69.

8. MacEwen CJ. Eye injuries: a prospective survey of 5671 cases. Br J Ophthalmol 1989;73(11):888-94

9. Chiapella AP, Rosenthal AR. 1 year in an eye casualty clinic. Br J Ophthalmol 1985;69(11):865–70.

10. Pamela L Owens, Ryan Mutter. Emergency Department Visits Related to Eye Injuries 2008, Health carecost and utilization project;statistical brief no. 12;May 2011.

11. Georgouli T, Pontu I, Chang BYP, Glannoudis PV. European Journal of Trauma and Emergency Surgery; Volume 37 Number 2, 135–140, DOI: 10.1007/s00068-010-0029-6).

12. Ferenac Kuhn, Pat Collins, Robert Morris, C Douglas. Epidemiology of motor vehicle crash related serious eye injuries; Accident Analysis and Prevention; 1994; 26(3):385–390.

13. Canavan YM, O' Flaherty MJ, Archer DB, Elwood HJ. A ten year survey of eye injuries in Northern Ireland 1967-76; Br J Ophthalmol, 1980; 64:618–25.

14. Strahlman E, et al. Causes of pediatric eye injuries. Apopulation based study. [My paper], Br J Oral Maxillofac Surg. 1991;29(5):291–301

15. MR Shoja and AM Miratashi. Paediatric ocular trauma , Acta Medica Iranica, Vol 44, No 2(2006)127.

16. Shtewi M El, Shishko MN, and Purohit G K, Road Traffic Accidents and Ocular Trauma: Experience at Tripoli Eye Hospital at Libya; Journal of Community Eye Health. 1999; 12(29):11–12.

17. A al-Qurainy, Stassen L F, Dutton G N, Moos K F, A el-Attar. The characteristics of mid facial fractures and the association with ocular injury: aprospective injury; Ophthalmology, 2006;113(1):109–16[My paper]

18. Enock ME, et al. Motor cycle related ocular injuries in Irrua specialist teaching hospital, Irrua, Edo State,

Nigeria; JMBR Journal of Biomedical Sciences 2007 Vol. 2007;7:1,2:5–11

19. Levin LA, Beck RW, Joseph MP, Seiff S, Kraker R. The treatment of traumatic optic neuropathy. Ophthalmology. 1999;106:1268–77.

20. Kline LB, Morawetz RB, Swaid SN. Indirect injury of the optic nerve. *Neurosurgery.* 1984;14:756–44.

21. Kallera I, Hyrkas T, Paukku P, Iizuka T, Lindqvist C. Blindness after Maxillofacial blunt trauma. J Oral Maxillofac Surg. 1994;22:220–5.

22. Lessell S. Indirect optic nerve trauma. *Arch Ophthalmol.* 1989;107:382–6.

23. Steinsapir KD, Goldberg RA. Traumatic optic neuropathy. *Surv Ophthalmol.* 1994;38:487–518.

24. Walsh FB, Hoyt WF. Clinical neuro-ophthalmology. Baltimore: Williams and Wilkins; 1969. p. 2375.

25. Harsha Bhatacharjee, et al. Indirect optic nerve injury in two wheeler riders in northeast India. Indian J Ophthalmol. 2008;56(6): 475–80.

26. Harry Lum, Jerry A. Reagan. "Interactive Highway Safety Design Model: Accident Predictive Module". Public Roads MagazineWinter 1995;59(2).

27. "I'm a good driver: you're not!". Drivers.com. 2000-02-11. Date 24 January 2008 ,http://drivers.com/article/157

28. Joseph Galvin. Eight out of ten drivers favour zero tolerance on alcohol-AXA-survey; Poltico Social & Political issues; Friday 2010;17:01

29. Thew, Rosemary (2006). "Royal Society for the Prevention of Accidents Conference Proceedings" (PDF). Driving Standards Agency. http://www.rospa.com/roadsafety/conferences/congress2006/proceedings/day2/thew.pdf. "Most at risk are young males between 17 and 25 years.

30. The Good, the Bad and the Talented: Young Drivers' Perspectives on Good Driving and Learning to Drive (Road Safety Research Report No. 74 ed.). Transport Research Laboratory. January 2007.

31. Road Safety Part 1: Alcohol, drugs, ageing and fatigue (Research summary, TRL Report 543 ed.). UK Department for Transport. Spring 2003.

32. Synthesis of Safety Research Related to Speed and Speed Limits". US Department of Transportation,Publication Number: FHWA-RD-98-154; Date: July 1998.

33. Johnston PB and Armstrong MF. Eye injuries in Northern Ireland two years after seat belt legislation.Br J Ophthalmol. 1986;70(6):460–462.

34. Hall NF, Denning AM, Elkington AR, and Cooper PJ. The eye and the seatbelt in Wessex. Br J Ophthalmol. 1985; 69(5): 317–319.

35. Vernon SA, Yorston DB. Incidence of ocular injuries from road traffic accidents after introduction of seat belt

legislation, Journal of Royal Society of Medicine, 1984; 77(3): 198–200.

36. Rutherford WH, Greenfield T, Hayes HRM, Nelson JK, The medical effects of seat belt legislation in the United Kingdom, Department of Health and Social Security Office of the Chief Scientist. Research Report No. 13, London :HMSO , 1985

37. BC Patel and LH. Morgan Penetrating eye injuries in road traffic accidents. Arch Emerg Med 1988;5(1):21–25.

38. Blake J, Kelly G, Fahey C, Khan MA. Eye injuries in road traffic accidents. Ir Med J 1983;76:120–4.

39. MacKay GM. Eye injuries and the windscreen. Dublin: Irish Faculty of Ophthalmology, 1975.

40. Subash M, Manzouri B, Wilkins M. Moorfields Eye Hospital,UK. Airbag-induced chemical eye injury. Eur J Emerg Med. 2010;17 (1):22–3.

41. Wallis LA, Greaves I; Injuries associated with air bag deployment. Emerg Med J 2002;19:490–3.

12.2 POLYTRAUMA IN THE DEPARTMENT OF CASUALTY

• Anand Verma

INTRODUCTION

Polytrauma patients usually suffer from both life-threatening injuries, where early intervention is mandatory to prevent mortality. Vital maintenance, resuscitation and treating the patient for shock and uncontrollable hemorrhage—especially during the "golden hour" is necessary and secondary injuries of lower priority receive delayed referral or treatment during this golden period. Non-life-threatening injuries can sometimes be overlooked and so remain untreated until a much later stage which may leave life time morbidity to the patient.

The casuality officer should inspect for lid injuries for abrasion, full thickness lid injuries, any lid tissue loss, any skin tags, area of lacrimal sac whether it is lacerated causing damage to the canaliculi and punctum, ocular proptosis, orbital fractures, endophthalmos and integrity of ocular globe. Look for scleral and corneal injuries (laceration), prolapse of inner ocular coats, hyphema and impacted foreign body. Casuality officer if they are not ophthalmologist, should be trained enough so that they can examine and inspect above mentioned ocular injuries in cases of polytrauma. Patch the eye without pressure with or without putting antibiotic eye drops. Ophthalmologist should be called in the casuality. If not possible, these cases should be referred to ophthalmologist.

Further management of ocular trauma has been given elsewhere in this book.

RECOMMENDATIONS FOR THE PREVENTION OF OCULAR AND ORBITAL INJURIES IN ROAD TRAFFIC ACCIDENT

- Strict observation of the rules of the road shall reduce the rate and severity of ocular trauma in traffic accidents.
- Regular surveillance by CCTV cameras on high ways will not only serve as deterrent but also its footage can be used in educational and training programs.
- Road markings and display sign boards need to be appropriately placed and repainted more frequently. Paint should be fluorescent so as to be clearly visible during darkness.
- Regular renewal of driving license must be done with credit and penalty points.
- Punishment for reckless driving and dangerous overtaking to the extent of cancellation of driving license.
- There is urgent need for traffic and vehicle-related education of the public through the use of news media and television programs.
- Introduction of awareness and training related to road traffic rules should start from school level.
- Passengers sitting in the front seats more commonly sustain ocular trauma. Hence front seat occupants must be more cautious while traveling long distances.
- The practice of sitting younger children on the lap of a parent on one of the front seats should not be allowed.
- The use of safety seat belts must be made compulsory and compliance essential.
- All road vehicles must have laminated glass winds screen and certified thickness must be displayed.
- The use of unbreakable plastic spectacles (polycarbonate) should be encouraged.
- The benefit of wearing seat belts in road vehicles and protective goggles in industry and sport should receive more publicity on radio and television and via poster campaigns.
- Strict ban on use of mobile phone while driving vehicle. Marketing of the cars equipped with bluetooth should be promoted.
- The government should make law for compulsory wearing of helmet by motorcycle riders as well as passenger. In order to facilitate this, motorcycle merchant should be made to include the cost of two helmets when selling a motorcycle.
- Visors used in riding must be made of polycarbonate with appropriate thickness (2 mm or more).

12.3 EYE SIGNS IN HEAD INJURY

• Zia Chaudhuri • Rajat Chaudhary

INTRODUCTION

Head trauma is a common cause of ophthalmic disorders. Ophthalmologists encounter injuries not only to the globe and ocular adnexal structures but also to the anterior and posterior visual pathways, the pupilomotor path way, the cranial nerves, the supranuclear and internuclear pathways.[1-7]

Most patients sustaining head injury are males with a 4:1 preponderance over females.[1,2,8] The age of patients range from approximately 10 to 50 years, with peak incidence in the 20–30 year-old-age group, with MVAs associated with most of the cases. In particular communited orbitozygomatic fractures are associated with the highest incidence of ocular injuries.[6,8]

Ocular signs in head injury are important because they have immediate localizing as well as prognostic implications.[9-12] Broadly they can be divided as follows:[1-7]

Visual pathway signs
- Retina and optic disk
  - Papilledema
  - Purtscher retinopathy
- Optic nerve
  - Traumatic optic neuropathy
- Optic chiasma
  - Infrequent usually from contusion
  - Retrochiasmal.

Motor signs
3rd, 4th and 6th nerve palsies, conjugate gate palsy, internuclear ophthalmoplegia.

Pupillary signs
- Fixed dilated pupil
  - Transtentorial/uncal herniation (3rd nerve palsy)
  - Traumatic 3rd nerve palsy
  - Traumatic Mydriasis
- Small pupil
  - Horner's syndrome
  - Traumatic miosis
  - Pontine hemorrhage
  - Hutchinson's pupil (early stages of transtentorial herniation)

Late signs
- Subdural hematoma
  - Late 3rd nerve palsy (transtentorial herniation)
  - Late 6th nerve palsy [raised pressure cerebral palsy (ICP)]
- Aberrant 3rd nerve regeneration
- Carotid cavernous fistula
- Late Horner's syndrome.

INCIDENCE

Considerable variation exists in the literature regarding the incidence of ocular injuries in patients who sustain head trauma. The reported incidence ranges from 2.7 to 90%.[1,2,4-8] Most reported studies are retrospective. There is no formal estimate of the percentage of the total number of closed head injury patients who had visual symptoms or signs. An informal estimate was in the range of 30–50%.[8,9]

EVALUATION OF PATIENTS

Patients sustaining trauma a to the visual system often have concomitant neurological, orthopedic, and internal organ injuries, some of which may be life-threatening. As with all traumatized patients, initial assesment and management must emphasize airway management, control of hemorrhage, hemodynamic stabilization and neurological assessment. Proper assessment of the trauma patient necessitates a multidisciplinary approach. The cooperation of neuro, general and trauma surgery, and otolaryngology or craniofacial trauma services is imperative for optimizing prompt evaluation and treatment of patients.[10] Appropriate time for ophthalmic examination is early in the course of illness once the patient is hemodynamically stable. Because the existence of ocular injuries influences the timing of repair of craniofacial injuries, a comprehensive ophthalmologic examination should be conclded as soon as possible.[10,11]

Formal visual acuity testing may be difficult if the patient has a decrease level of consciousness or is heavily sedated. However, the presence or absence of gross visual acuity, even bare light perception, may be prognostic when it is interpreted in the context of radiologic and neuro-ophthalmological findings.[1,11,12]

TRAUMATIC VISUAL LOSS

Optic Nerve Injury

Optic nerve trauma is often associated with severe head trauma. Most cases of traumatic optic neuropathy are associated with motor vehicle accidents which produce high-energy deceleration type head trauma.[2-5]

Patients with unilateral traumatic optic neuropathy demonstrate a relative afferent pupillary defect and decrease in vision. The diagnosis of traumatic optic neuropathy should not be made in the absence of these two findings. The nerve can be injured at any point between the optic chiasma and the globe. The fundus picture may be variable with an absolutely normal looking optic nerve to one that looks visibly affected.

Injury of the Intraorbital Optic Nerve

Traumatic optic neuropathy caused by injury of the Intraorbital portion of the optic nerve may result from direct or indirect mechanisms. It may occur as a result of:

- Contusion of the nerve in penetrating orbital trauma
- Traction on the nerve caused by severe axial globe displacement
- Compression of the nerve from space occupying intraorbital hemorrhage or sequestrated air
- Avulsion from the globe with blunt orbital injuries.
- Direct trauma to the optic nerve causing hemorrhage within the sheath.

Optic disk swelling and hemorrhage, in addition to retinal whitening suggestive of central retinal artery occlusion may be observed. Immediate surgical intervention with optic nerve sheath fenestration has been reported to relieve compression of the anterior optic nerve and to improve optic nerve function.[3-5]

Injury of the Intracanalicular and Intracranial Optic Nerve

Injury to the intracanalicular portion of the optic nerve is the most common cause of traumatic optic neuropathy. This segment of the optic nerve is protected within the bone of the optic canal, within the canal, the dura of the optic nerve is tightly adherent to the bone of the canal. The intraorbital and intracranial segments of the optic nerve are less tightly held in position, hence with forceful trauma the orbital and intracranial contents shift, thus applying tractional forces on the tightly bound intracanalicular portion of the optic nerve. This may lead to both shearing of axons and interruptions of the vascular supply of the optic nerve. If a comminuted fracture is present, the displaced fragments may impinge on the optic nerve. In addition to the optic nerve ophthalmic artery enters the orbit through the optic canal within dural investments of the floor of the canal. Disruption of the pial vessels, which supply the intracanalicular portion of the optic nerve, induces optic nerve ischemia and axonal necrosis. Secondary edema of time optic nerve may ensue and create a compartment syndrome within the canal.

MANAGEMENT OF TRAUMATIC OPTIC NEUROPATHY

There is no universally agreed on management algorithm for optic neuropathy. Although cases of spontaneous visual recovery after profound visual loss have been reported these represent the exception rather than the rule.[3-5]

TREATMENT PROTOCOL

1. Establish the diagnosis at traumatic optic neuropathy based on a reduction at visual acuity and the presence of a relative afferent pupillary defect (RAPD). Quantitate the RAPD with neutral density filters.

2. Institute high-dose intravenous methylprednisolone therapy after ruling out contraindications and consulting with other physicians involved in the patient's care:
   - *Loading dose:* 30 mg/kg (infused over a minimum of 30 minutes)
   - *Maintenance dose:* 5.4 mg/kg/hours for 48 hours

3. Monitor therapeutic response closely with serial visual acuity (VA) and RAPD measurements. After 48 hours of high-dose methylprednisolone
   a. If VA or RAPD improves, change to oral predinisone therapy and taper rapidly. If VA or RAPD worsens during oral prednisone therapy, reinstitute high-dose intravenous methyl-

prednisolone and consider surgical decompression of the optic canal.

  b. If VA or RAPD fails to improve, consider surgical decompression of the optic canal.

OPTIC CHIASM INJURY

Head injury severe enough to cause chiasmal trauma is often life-threatening. Multiple cranial neuropathies, traumatic optic neuropathy and hypothalamic dysfunction may occur in association with chiasmal trauma.

Traumatic injury of the optic chiasm will result in complete bitemporal hemianopia. The mechanism of injury, may be contusion necrosis, disruption of blood supply or penetrating trauma. In addition to a bitemporal hemianopia, optic atrophy may develop approximately 6–8 weeks after the traumatic event.

POSTCHIASMAL VISUAL PATHWAY INJURY

Structures of the postchiasmal visual pathways include the optic tracts, lateral geniculate nuclei, the geniculocalcarine radiations, and the occipital cortex. Postchiasmal lesions, unless bilateral should not produce decrease in visual acuity unless they are associated injury to structures of the anterior visual system.

All postchiasmal lesions result in contralateral homonymous visual defect. Lesions more posterior in the postchiasmal pathways, nearer the occipital cortex, are usually more congruous.

Optic Tract Lesions

Incongruous homonymous hemianopia, bilateral retinal nerve fiber layer or "bow-tie optic atrophy and contralateral relative afferent pupillary defect (in the eve with temporal field loss).

Isolated lesions of the lateral geniculate nucleus are rare, and two types of visual-field loss are possible:
1. An incongruous homonymous hemianopia.
2. A congruous homonymous horizontal sectoranopia.

Fibers the inferior hemiretina course anteriorly from lateral geniculate nucleus into the temporal lobe as Meyer's loop fibers.

Fibers from the superior hemiretina course directly posteriorly into the parietal lobe on their way to occipital cortex. This superior-inferior separation of the fibers is thee basis of topographic diagnosis of posterior visual lesions.

Injury to the temporal lobe thus produce homonymous visual-field defects that are denser above, and parietal lobe lesions produce homonymous defects that are denser below.

Occipital Lobe Lesions

They produce congruous homonymous hemianopias. As a rule, lesions superior to calcrine fissure yield inferior quadrantanopic defects and those below the calcarine fissure produce superior defects, Lesions of the optic tract, temporal lobe lobe, and occipital lobe may produce a homonymous heminopia. Thus, it is not a localizing finding.

Post-traumatic Transient Cerebral Blindness

It is rare occurring in less than 1% of all cases of head trauma, patients usually have a history of migraine headache or seizure disorder. Patients are usually symptomatic for 1–24 hours. Spontaneous resolution follows in most cases. site of abnormality is proposed to be in the occipital or front temporal lobes. The mechanisms proposed are contusion edema of the brain parenchyma or cerebrovascular spasm.[12] Patients sustaining severe head trauma experience visual perception disorders. Patients may experience visual hallucinations, either formed with temporal lobe lesions, or unformed, associated with occipital lobe lesions. Patients may also demonstrate aphasia, agnosia, alexia, and hemifield neglect.[12]

PUPILLARY ABNORMALITIES[3-5,7]

For an accurate assessment of the integrity of the afferent and efferent pupillary system, the pupil size (in dim and bright light), reactivity, and presence of a RAPD must be carefully evaluated. If RAPD is present it should be quantitated with neutral density filters. It is imperative that the patient fixate on a distant object to control for pupillary changes associated with near synkinesis. Anisocoria of greater than 0.5 mm that varies in dim and bright light warrants further evaluation.

Traumatic Mydriasis

Traumatic mydriasis results from structural damage to the iris most commonly tears in the sphincter. Differentiation of traumatic mydriasis from a pupilomotor defect and pharmacologic blockade is possible with pharmacologic testing. A mydriatic pupil caused by iris sphincter tears fails to constrict after instillation of 1% pilocarpine.

Horner's Syndrome (Oculosympathetic Paresis)

The clinical signs include: Relative miosis, papillary dilatation lag, and narrowing of the palpabral fissure because of upper eyelid ptosis, and higher than normal lower eyelid position due to reverse ptosis. The miosis may be subtle, 0.5–1.0 mm, is more appreciable in dim light. Interruption of the sympathetic innervations of the Müller's muscle of the upper lid and the inferior tarsal muscle produces narrowing of the palpabral fissure.

Horner syndrome is due to a deficiency of sympathetic activity. The site of lesion to the sympathetic outflow is on the ipsilateral side of the symptoms. The following are examples of conditions that cause the clinical appearance of Horner's syndrome:

- *First-order neuron disorder:* Central lesions that involve the hypothalamospinal pathway (e.g. transaction of the cervical spinal cord).
- *Second-order neuron disorder:* Preganglionic lesions (e.g. compression of the sympathetic chain by a lung tumor).
- *Third-order neuron disorder:* Postganglionic lesions at the level of the internal carotid artery (e.g. a tumor in the cavernous sinus).

Pupil Involving Oculomotor Nerve Paresis

Traumatic injury of the 3rd nerve may result in pupillary mydriasis and accommodative paresis as a result of interruption of the parasympathetic innervation to the pupillary sphincter and the ciliary body. Compression of the 3rd nerve against the tentorium cerebelli resulting from herniation of the uncus may occur as a result form cerebral edema. Interruption may also occur as a result of direct trauma to the ciliary ganglion or avulsion of the short ciliary nerves they enter the globe.

Traumatic Miosis

The differential of this condition in a comatose patient after head trauma includes: narcotic ingestion, parasympathatomimetic ingestion or topical use, and pontine hemorrhage. Neuroimaging should detect intracerebral hemorrhage and should demonstrate the extent of brain injury. Topical naloxone, a narcotic antagonist, may be used as a diagnostic test to reverse miosis when it is caused by narcotic intoxication.

CRANIAL NERVE INJURIES[13–17]

Oculomotor Nerve Paresis

Oculomotor nerve paresis as a squeal of minor head trauma is unusual and should alert the clinician to the possibility of an occult intracranial tumor. Patients may have horizontal, vertical, or oblique diplopia; difficulty with near vision; and light sensitivity. Because of the severity of head trauma associated with oculomotor nerve paresis, the patient may have a reduced level of consciousness, prohibiting detailed assessment of ocular motility. The 3rd nerve may be injured anywhere along its course from the midbrain to the orbit. Severe head trauma may induce brainstem contusion, edema, and infarction, causing damage to the oculomotor nucleus. As the nerve exits the brain stem and travels in the subarachnoid space, it is prone to injury as it courses near the tentorium cerebelli. Cerebral edema secondary to contusion or intracerebral hemorrhage may lead to downward displacement of uncal portion of the temporal lobe. Here, the nerve is prone to compression on the edge of tentorium cerebelli. As the nerve travels in the lateral wall of cavernous sinuous it is vulnerable to compression by aneurysms of the carotid artery, cavernous sinus thrombosis, and carotid cavernous fistulas. The nerve may also be injured as it enters the orbit through superior orbital fissure in cases of comminuted orbital apex fractures.

Trochlear Nerve Paresis

The trochlear nerve nuclei, located in the ventral midbrain at the level of inferior colliculi, innervate the contralateral superior oblique muscles. Head trauma is the most common cause of trochlear nerve paresis in adults. As many as third cases are bilateral. With blunt head trauma, rapid deceleration causes displacement of the brain and brainstem within the cranium. The subarachnoid segment of the nerve is vulnerable to injury from the free edge of the tentorium cerebelli near the point where the nerve pierces the dura to enter the cavernous sinus. In bilateral cases, the site of injury is likely in the anterior medullary velum, where the fascicles decussate before exiting the midbrain. Patients with paresis of one or both trochlear nerve may have vertical binocular diplopia and tilting of images. The findings of unilateral trochlear nerve paresis include: diminished depression of the eye in adduction, vertical tropia in primary gaze that increases in gaze to ipsilateral side and head tilt to the contralateral side, and excyclotorsion of less than 10°.

Abducens Nerve Paresis

The abducens nerve nuclei are located in the pontine tegmentum, near the midline and ventral to the fourth nerve ventricle. Abducens nerve paresis is most commonly caused by infarction due to microvascular disease. However, it is commonly a squeal of head trauma. Injury to the nerve may occur at several locations. The subarachnoid portion is the most prone to the injury. The nerve is tethered to the skull base as it passes beneath the petroclinoid ligament. Head trauma cause rapid displacement of the brain within the cranium, which may induce shearing forces on the nerve. Downward displacement of the brainstem, occurring due to raised intracranial pressure, may stretch or avulse the delicate nerve fibers. The nerve may also be injured within the cavernous sinus as a result of traumatic carotid aneurysms and carotid-cavernous fistulas. The combination of an abducens paresis and ipsilateral Horner's syndrome localizes the site of injury to the cavernous sinus. Patients will have horizontal diplopia, often more bothersome with distant viewing than with reading. An abduction deficit and a manifest esodeviation are apparent.

DISORDERS OF SUPRANUCLEAR AND INTERNUCLEAR GAZE PATHWAYS[18,19]

Horizontal Gaze Palsy

The neural pathways mediating horizontal gaze are located in the pons. The abducens nucleus functions as the horizontal gaze center. It connects to the ipsilateral lateral rectus and contralateral medial rectus though the medial longitudinal facsiculus (MLF). The abducens nucleus is in turn under the control of ipsilateral parapontine reticular formation (PPRF). The frontal eye fields stimulate the contralateral PPRF causing saccadic eye movements to the opposite side. Thus frontal lobe injury may produce contralateral horizontal gaze palsy. Gaze in the direction away from the side of the lesion is not possible. In some cases, tonic deviation of the eyes

toward the side of the frontal lobe injury may result due to unopposed action of the intact contralateral frontal lobe. Lesions of at the level of pons affecting 6th nerve nucleus, PPRF also produce ipsilateral horizontal gaze palsy. Lesions of the MLF, which is composed of the interneurons from the abducens nucleus to the contralateral oculomotor nucleus result in an internuclear ophthalmoplegia (INO). The hallmark of INO is a slowed adducting saccade of the ipsilateral eye in conjugate gaze movement toward the side opposite the lesion. Traumatic INO may spontaneously resolve within months after the traumatic event.

Vertical Gaze Palsy

The neural pathways for the control of vertical and torsional eye movements are located in the midbrain and are associated with the occulomotor and trochlear nuclei. The paired rostral interstitial nuclei of the MLF receive afferent input from the frontal eye fields, the vestibular nuclei, and the PPRF. The rostral interstitial nuclei of the MLF project bilaterally to the 3rd nerve nuclei and to the ipsilateral trochlear nucleus. The interstitial nucleus of Cajal has been proposed as the neural integrator of the vertical gaze and is responsible for vertical gaze holding.

Thus injury to the midbrain may affect the rostral interstitial nuclei of the MLF and may lead to vertical gaze paresis.

Skew Deviation

Skew deviation is a uniocular vertical deviation not due to extraocular muscle restriction or nerve paresis. It may occur in association with brainstem and cerebellar injury. Differentiation from other vertical deviation, such as superior oblique paresis, is often difficult, but the absence of torsional deviation is one diagnostic clue.

DISORDERS OF VERGENCE AND ACCOMMODATION[6,20,21]

Decompensated Phoria

Patients with pre-existent latent deviation may lose the ability to maintain fusion after head trauma. Before the development of a manifest deviation the patient may experience esthenopia.

Central Disruption of Fusional Amplitudes

Central control of fusion may be disrupted as a squeal to head trauma. Patients are usually esotropic and may also manifest hypertropia and excyclotorsion.

Paresis of Convergence

A transient or permanent paresis of convergence may occur after head trauma. In contrast to convergence insufficiency, paresis of convergence most often has a sudden onset. The patient experiences diplopia with near effort. Ductions of each eye are full, and deviation is comitant across all fields of gaze.

Paresis of Accommodation

Transient paresis of accommodation may also occur as squeal of head trauma. Blunt trauma to the globe may interrupt parasympathetic innervation by damaging the short posterior ciliary nerves as they enter the globe. Patients may experience blurring of near objects. Evaluation for accommodative paresis is challenging because tests of accommodative amplitude depend on the patients effort. Recovery of accommodative amplitude occurs in most cases within 1–2 months.

Paresis of Divergence

Trauma related injury to the pontomedullary junction may produce divergence paresis. The patient may experience a sudden onset of horizontal diplopia, especially with distant objects. The esotropia is greater in the distance. Patients may be able to achieve singular binocular vision with near targets.

REFERENCES

1. Baker RS, Epstein AD. 'Ocular Abnormalities from Head Trauma' Survey of Ophthalmology 1991;35:245–67.
2. Baker RS, Epstein AD. Ocular motor abnormalities from head trauma. Surv Ophthalmol 1994;35:245–67.
3. Van Stavern GP, Biousse V, Lynn MJ, Simon DJ, Newman NJ. Neuro-Ophthalmic manifestations of head trauma. J Neuro-Ophthalmol 2001;21(2):112–7.
4. Smith JL. Some neuro-ophthalmological aspects of head trauma. Clin Neurosurg 1966;13:181–196.
5. Sabates N, Gonce M, Farris B. Neuro-ophthalmological findings in closed head trauma. J Clin Neuroophthalmol 1991;11:273–277.
6. Kowal L. Ophthalmic manifestations of head injury. Austra New Zealand J Ophthalmol 1992;20:35–40.
7. Moster ML, Volpe NJ, Kresloff MS. Neuro-ophthalmic findings in head injury. Neurol 1999;52(Suppl 2):A23
8. Annegers JF, Grabow JD, Kurland LT, Laws ER. The incidence, causes, and secular trends of head trauma in Olmsted County, Minnesota, 1935–1974. Neurology 1980;30:912–919.
9. Suchoff IB, Kapoor N, Waxman R, et al. 'The occurrance of ocular and visual dysfunction in an acquired brain injured patient sample' Journal of the American Optometric Association 70:301–309,1999.
10. Keane JR. Neurologic eye signs following motor vehicle accidents. Arch Neurol 1989;46:761–762.
11. Clinical Guideline 4. Head Injury. Triage, Assessment, Investigation and Early Management of Head Injury in Infants, Children and Adults. National Institute for Clinical Excellence: London, June 2003.
12. Thurman DJ, Jeppson L, Burnett CL, Beaudoin DE, Rheinberger MM, Sniezek JE. Surveillance of traumatic brain injury in Utah. West J Med 1996;165:192–196.
13. Lepore F. Disorders of ocular motility following head trauma. Arch Neurol 1995;52:924–926.
14. Mariak Z, Mariak Z, Stankiewicz A. Cranial nerve II – VII injuries in fatal closed head trauma. Eur J Ophthalmol 1997;7:68–72.
15. Banks M, Lessell, Simmons MD. Neuro-ophthalmology and Trauma. Int Ophthalmol Clin Ocular Trauma 2002;42(3):1–12.
16. Leigh RJ, ZeeDS. The neurology of Eye Movements, 2nd edition. Philadelphia, DA,FA Davis 1991.
17. Lepore FE; Disorders of ocular motility following head trauma. Arch Neurology 1995;52:924–6.
18. Ciuffreda KJ,Ciuffreda YH,Kapoor N, et al. Oculomotor consequences of acquired brain injury, in visual and vestibular consequences of acquired brain injury. In: Suchoff IB, Ciuffreda KJ, Kapoor N, eds. Santa Ana, CA, Optometric Extension program Foundation, 2001a:77–88.
19. Griffin JR, Grishan JD; Binocular anomalies: Diagnosis and vision therapy, 3rd edition. Boston, MA, Butterworth Heinmann, 1995.
20. Cohen M, Gros Wasser Z, Barchadski R, et al. Convergence insufficiency in Brain injuried patients. Brain Injury 1989;3:187–191.
21. Cooper J. Accomodative dysfunction, in diagnosis and management in vision care. In: Amos J Boston, Butterworth, MA, 1998;431–59.

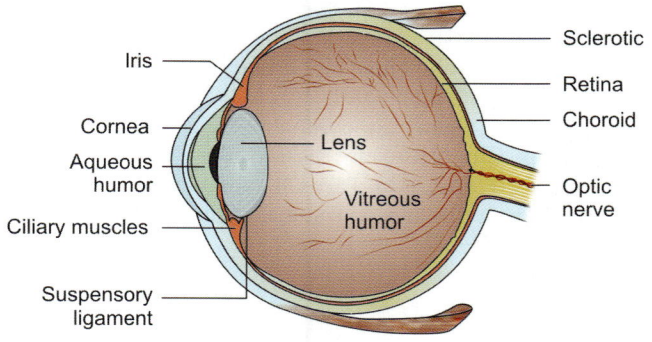

13 Prevention and Rehabilitation

13.1 PROTECTIVE GEARS AND STANDARDIZATION

• SM Bhatia

GENERAL

Eye sight is the most precious of all the senses gifted to the mankind. While we routinely tend to neglect this all important gift, we do not realise that its neglect can lead to many eye problems including loss of sight, loss of livelihood and can bring untold miseries in life. It is, therefore, extremely important that we guard this God gifted sense by taking essential precautions against accidental injuries to the eyes, which may lead to numerous problems later on. Be it at home, workplace, leisure or sports field, there is a need to follow the set norms for the protection of the eyes.

First of all we do not use the personal protective equipment or (PPE), and if we do at all, we do not even know what the appropriate PPE for use at our workplace or sports field is? Many a times, we use a product which is substandard and does not conform to the specifications. We tend to have a false sense of complacence that we are using a PPE. This can lead to adverse impact on the eyes in case of accident(s) and sometimes may be more dangerous than not using the PPE. However, using the right type of PPE can never be over-stressed (undermined).

Why Protection of Eyes is Required?

Eyes are one of the most vital and sensitive organs of the living beings. Located in the face they are prone to injuries which can result in the partial or total loss of sight. This will result in avoidable handicap to the human beings of all ages irrespective of the color or creed.

Anatomy of the Eye and Its Proneness to Injury

Anatomy of eye (Fig. 13.1.1) is such that it provides ready opportunity for injury. The eye consists of:
- The eyeball or globe
  - Five-sixth of the globe is well protected within the socket
  - Remaining one-sixth of the globe is exposed to the outside environment.

It is this one-sixth part of the globe consisting of front part of the ocular surface layer which provides opportunity for the foreign particles, chemicals and gases to get in and cause ocular trauma.

An eye represents an enormous emergency when exposed. Its structure provides tremendous opportunity for foreign particles/bodies for absorption into the human body causing bodily harm or the eye itself can be permanently damaged/injured.

Eyes being the part of the face, get can get greatly affected as most injuries to the face come from flying

Fig. 13.1.1: Structure of human eye

248

objects, usually very small particles or particulates. When a particulate hits the face, it might cause a cut or scratch on the skin and the skin will repair itself over time—given the proper medical attention. If by chance, the particulate hits the eye, it causes direct damage, and it is far more difficult for the eye to repair itself. It has been established that almost 70% of eye accidents result from flying or falling objects, or sparks striking the eye. The goal of face protection is mainly to shield the eyes from injury.

- Surveys of the injured workers have indicated that nearly three-fifths of the objects striking the eyes were smaller than the head of a pin. Most of the particles were said to be traveling faster than a hand-thrown object when the accidents occurred.
- Contact with chemicals is responsible for one-fifth of all occupational eye injuries.
- Other accidents are caused by objects swinging from a fixed or attached position, such as tree limbs, ropes, chains or tools, which were then pulled into the eye while the worker was using them.

Eye injuries occur at an estimated rate of 1,000 per day in the American workplace. The statistics for India would be far more alarming for three reasons: (1) there is practically no or negligible protection equipment provided at the work place and if provided at all, the workers shun the use of the protection equipment citing it as cumbersome and unnecessary, (2) many accidents go unreported both by the workers and the factory managements. The workers are not aware of their rights and factory managements do not want to pay compensation and want to avoid payment of fines and (3) there are little and largely unenforced legal requirement to report such accidents in a structured manner to assess the number of accidents and causes for formulating policy guidelines on mandating the use of appropriate eye protection equipment at workplace or for other occupational use.

Apart from the regularity with which these types of accidents occur, there are several other reasons why face and eye protection at the workplace are so important. One reason is compliance—mainly in the western world. Eye and face protection must be provided whenever necessary to protect against chemical, environmental, radiological or mechanical irritants and hazards. The Occupational Safety and Health Administration (OSHA) [of United States of America (USA)] can fine an employer for not providing an eyewash station or for not complying with the general duty clause to provide a safe and healthy work environment.

In India also, we have a legislation to regulate the safety of workers and safety at work place. This legislation, called **the Factories Act, 1948** is largely modelled on the erstwhile British legislation. Its provisions concerning the safety and protection of eyes have not been updated with need of the times; even though it has been amended several times, having been last amended in 1987.

- **The Factories Act, 1948**
- Last amended in 1987
- **Article 35 of the Act** covers the requirements relating to "protection of the eyes". The provisions of the Act relating to this vital aspect are reproduced below:
- **"35. Protection of Eyes:** In respect of any such manufacturing process carried on in any factory as may be prescribed, being a process which involves—risk of injury to the eyes from particles or fragments thrown off in the course of the process, or risk to the eyes by reason of exposure to excessive light, the State Government may by rules require that effective screens or suitable goggles shall be provided for the protection of persons employed on, or in the immediate vicinity of, the process.

It is important to note that the law does not make it mandatory for the workers to use the eye protection equipment. Further one of the most important area of exposure, i.e. exposure to chemicals is absent from the provisions of the Act concerning the protection of eyes.

TYPES OF EYE TRAUMA

Injury to eyes can be caused by the exposure to the following:
- Chemicals and fumes
- Particulates traveling at great speeds
- Radiation (X-rays and other harmful radiations)
- Light radiation, e.g. ultraviolet light
- Welding-related radiations
- Sports related injuries.

Chemicals and Fumes

Most chemicals get absorbed by the skin and eyes and can result in extreme emergencies at work-place. Property of the chemical determines how rapidly it will be absorbed by the skin. Chemicals which are soluble in the lipids will be absorbed more rapidly. It should be remembered that *moist skin is ten times more absorbent than the dry skin.* Thus, eyes being moist most of the times become extremely permeable when exposed to lipid soluble chemicals. Temperature of chemicals and the surrounding environment also aggravates the absorption. Condition of the tissue in direct contact/injury/inflammation and sensitivity increases the absorption. Eyes and skin act as the transport media for chemicals that can negatively impact other body organs/systems.

Some chemicals have only local impact but do not impact other systems. Hydrochloric acid is the example of this type of chemical. It burns locally but does not have any systemic effect. However, when it comes in contact with eyes, it can permanently damage the eyesight.

Some chemicals do no harm locally but greatly affect other systems. Example of this type is the nitroglycerine paste, which when placed on the skin does not have any affect on the site but moving through the skin and transported throughout the body affects a widespread systemic vascular tone change.

Some chemicals have dual impact, i.e. one type of impact at site of contact and a different effect somewhere in a dissociated body system. Chemical *methyl isocyanate* in gaseous form emitted during the Bhopal Gas Tragedy is the example of having local as well as systemic impact on many body systems. The initial effects of exposure were coughing, vomiting, severe eye irritation and a feeling of suffocation. The acute symptoms were burning in the respiratory tract and eyes, blepharospasm, breath-lessness, stomach pains and vomiting. The causes of deaths were choking, reflexogenic circulatory collapse and pulmonary edema. Long-term systemic impacts included blindness, other eye diseases, diseases of the reproductive system, diseases of the respiratory system and many more. Another example of this type of chemical is the *Hydrofluoric acid* which causes devastating chemical burns on the skin. The fluoride within the acid penetrates below the surface, where it binds with calcium and magnesium. This results injury to the nerves and bones and has the potential of causing hypocalcemia within the circulating bloodstream resulting in electrocardiography (ECG) abnormality and possibly cardiac arrest. Eye exposure to hydrogen fluoride (fumes or liquid) may cause prolonged or permanent visual defects, blindness, or total destruction of the eye.

Exposure to toxins—both chemicals and metals, may develop many diverse symptoms depending on the toxin exposure. These may include blurred vision, decrease in visual activity, photophobia, excessive tearing and blindness and altered odor. Eyeball may be completely destroyed by an overwhelming exposure to a toxic chemical material.

Some of the more common surface toxins to which the eyes may be exposed (and the first aid to tackle the emergency) include:

Acids

In case of exposure to acids, the epithelial tissue reacts with the acid forming a tough coagulum. Acids act with the proteins found within the tissue causing a process called *coagulation necrosis*. The tissue becomes thickened and rubbery either stopping or slowing the absorption of acids below the surface. The process actually acts as a naturally protective barrier against acid penetration. However, highly concentrated acids have the ability to overcome the protective barrier and cause deeper, more severe injury similar to alkalis.

Any injury to the eye must be treated aggressively by the first responder to arrive with the patient. Neutralization of an acid or alkali should never even be considered on the surface of the eye or inside the eye due to excessive heat generation during the neutralization reaction—resulting in further aggravation of the injury. The one and only treatment for this type of injury is rapid and immediate irrigation and transportation to a medical facility. Use a device like the Morgan Therapeutic Lens[1] or a similar device, if possible. At the work place, the eyes should be washed at the eyewash stations before moving the victim to the nearest medical facility. When the exposure to acids occurs at other places (outside work place) where there is no eyewash station, immediate action shall be to wash the eyes in abundant quantity of water (preferably under running water at low pressure) till the victim can be moved to the nearest medical facility. Irrigation may be stopped with medical advice if pH of the waste fluid is at 7 (after irrigation for 30–60 minutes).

Alkalis

Exposure to alkalis may damage the tissues through liquefaction of the fatty substance within the tissue of the eyes. This allows alkali to penetrate deeper into the underlying structures, causing a much more devastating injury as compared to acidic chemicals.

Alkalis have 20 times greater dose response on the eyes than the acids. Chemicals of pH greater than 11.5 cause more devastating impacts.

More the penetration and damage by alkalis lesser the pain experienced by the victim. Similar to the third degree burns, deep alkali burns destroy the corneal nerves, desensitize the tissues. The extent of penetration also depends on the toxicity of the alkali involved, for example, ammonium hydroxide penetrates the fastest followed by sodium hydroxide, potassium hydroxide and calcium hydroxide in that order.

Damage to the underlying structure of the eye and the circulatory system may lead to necrosis of tissue and loss of the globe. Opacification of the cornea and related underlying structures may lead to blindness without loss of globe. In either case, alkalis have the ability to evoke serious injury to the eyes.

As in the case of acid burns, any injury to the eye due to alkali must be treated aggressively by the first responder. Neutralization of alkali like the acid should not even be considered whether on the surface of the eye or inside the eye due to excessive heat generation during the neutralization reaction—resulting in further aggravation of the injury. The one and only immediate treatment for injury due to exposure to alkali is rapid and immediate irrigation and transportation to a medical facility. Use a device like the Morgan Therapeutic Lens[1] or a similar device, if possible. At the work place the eyes should be washed at the eyewash stations before moving the victim to the nearest medical facility. When the exposure to alkali occurs at other places (outside work place) where there is no eyewash station, immediate action shall be to wash the eyes in abundant quantity of water (preferably under running water at low pressure) till the victim can be moved to the nearest medical facility. Irrigation may be stopped only with medical advice if pH of the waste fluid is at 7 (after irrigation for at least 60 minutes).

Solvents

Such solvents as petrol, alcohols, toluene, acetone, etc. are the most commonly used solvents in the industry thus posing hazards particular to the eyes. These chemicals are fat soluble—mixing and disrupting fats found in the tissues of the eyes—causing normally transparent tissues to become opaque and dehydrated. The effects are epithelial sloughing and pain. The symptoms generally persist several days and most heal without lasting damage.

As in the case of acids and alkalis, the immediate treatment in case of exposure to solvents like petrol, alcohols, toluene, acetone, etc. is to wash the eyes with excess of water and take the victim to the nearest medical centre for treatment.

Surfactants and Detergents

These chemicals are used to promote wetting. They also disperse and dissolve fatty substances and decrease foaming. Short-term exposure to such chemicals can cause epithelial sloughing and pain in the eyes but do not cause long-term injury. These types of chemicals are also used in the household as shampoos and soaps and practically everyone is exposed to them.

In case of sustained exposure to surfactants and detergents, the immediate treatment remains the same as in case of acids and alkalis, i.e. to wash the eyes with excess of water and take the victim to the nearest medical center for treatment. The eyes should be continuously irrigated till they can be medically treated.

Lacrimatory Agents

These chemicals stimulate corneal nerve endings, causing reflex lacrimations and stinging pain. In low doses, they usually have self-limiting impact. In higher doses, conjunctival inflammation may result, but this injury is also mostly self-limiting not requiring medical follow-up care. Teargas is the most common lacrimator containing capsicum and does not harm permanently.

Effects of the lacrimatory agents can usually be dealt with short-term irrigation followed by use of topical anesthetic like pontocaine topical (generic name: tetracaine topical) which will take care of burning in the eyes and lacrimation.

Specks in the Eye

- Do not rub the eye.
- Flush the eye with large amounts of water.
- See a doctor if the speck does not wash out or if pain or redness continues.

Cuts, Punctures, and Foreign Objects in the Eye

- Do not wash out the eye.
- Do not try to remove a foreign object stuck in the eye.
- Seek immediate medical attention.

Metals and Metal Powders

Metal powders and salts can cause severe damage to the eyes, if the ocular surface is exposed. Many metals bind with proteins and form metallic complexes which may further result in the formation of permanent granular deposits within the ocular tissues. Solubility within the cornea determines the toxicity of the metallic salt. Mercury has the highest solubility followed by tin, silver, copper, zinc and lead in that order. Iron may cause only little damage to the ocular tissues but as a foreign body causes a staining of the surrounding tissue termed as "rust ring".

Most metals and salts are stable solids with minimal potential for exposure unless ingested or unless the material is present in the air as dust, vapor (at normal temperatures), or fumes (if heated). Sodium and potassium metals and sodium hydroxide are extremely corrosive in the presence of moisture. Lithium aluminium hydride is extremely reactive (fire and explosion hazard).

> In case of exposure to metallic powders and metallic salts, the first aid treatment remains the same as for acids, alkalis, and other chemical toxins, i.e. immediate washing of the eye with plenty of water. *Do not rub the eye.* In addition the victim should try to keep the eyelids open so that any lodged particles can be washed out. Medical help should sought at the earliest. Irrigation with such devices as Morgan's therapeutic lens will be of great help in reducing irritation in the eyes.

Exposure to Hydrogen Fluoride

Hydrogen fluoride (HF) is the most lethal of the exposures next to cyanides and cyanide derivatives one can get at work place. Therefore, one must be extremely careful while working in the environments which have HF as the intermediate, or by-product or the intended product itself.

- If you think you may have been exposed to HF, you should remove your clothing, rapidly wash your entire body with water under the emergency shower, and get medical care as quickly as possible.
- Removing your clothing:
  - Quickly take off clothing that may have hydrogen fluoride on it. Any clothing that has to be pulled over the head should be cut off the body as pulling it over the head may *expose the eyes* to HF which may be very harmful.
  - If you are helping other people remove their clothing, try to avoid touching any contaminated areas, and remove the clothing as quickly as possible.
- Washing yourself:
  - As quickly as possible, wash any HF from your skin with large amounts of water.
  - If your eyes are burning or your vision is blurred, rinse your eyes with plenty of plain water for considerable length of time.
  - If you wear contact lenses, remove them after washing your hands thoroughly with soap and put them with the contaminated clothing. Do not put the contacts back in your eyes (even if they are not disposable contacts). If you wear eyeglasses, wash them thoroughly with soap and plenty of water. You can put your eyeglasses back on after you have washed them.
- Disposing of your clothes:
  - After you have washed yourself, place your clothing inside a plastic bag. Avoid touching contaminated areas of the clothing. If you cannot avoid touching contaminated areas, or you are not sure which areas are contaminated, put the clothing in the bag using tongs, tool handles, sticks, or similar objects. Anything that touches contaminated clothing should also be placed in the bag.
  - Seal the bag, and then seal that bag inside another plastic bag. Disposing of your clothing in this way will help to protect you and other people from any chemicals that might be on your clothes.
  - When emergency personnel arrive, tell them what you did with your clothes. The health department or emergency personnel will arrange for further disposal. Do not handle the plastic bags yourself.

EYE PROTECTION EQUIPMENT

Following types of eye protective equipment is available for use:
- Safety spectacles
- Safety goggles
- Shields
- Protective visors
- Dust masks
- Light polarisers.

Safety Spectacles and Glasses

Safety spectacles provide protection to the eyes from flying particles which can cause severe eye trauma. These should made from toughened glass lenses or plastic lenses and can have plastic or metallic frame. Lenses should not be removable as they could fall out and cause eye injury in the wake of flying particles. In certain dusty environments, spectacles with side shields should be used.

Standards for Safety Glasses

Following Indian Standard (IS) and organization for International (ISO) standards are available for safety glasses:
1. IS/ISO 8980 (Part 1):2004 Ophthalmic Optics-Uncut finished Spectacle lenses-Part 1-Specification for single vision and multifocal lenses.
2. IS/ISO 18369-1: 2006 Ophthalmic Optics-Contact lenses- Part 1 Vocabulary. Classification system and recommendation for labelling specification.
3. IS/ISO 18369-2:2006 Ophthalmic Optics-Contact Lenses-Part 2:Tolerances.
4. IS/ISO 18369-3:2006 Ophthalmic Optics-Contact Lenses-Part 3 Measurement methods.
5. IS/ISO 18369-4:2006 Ophthalmic Optics-Contact Lenses-Part 4 Physico-chemical properties of contact lens materials.

These IS have been prepared by adopting the ISO on the subject of spectacle lenses and contact lenses.

Prevention against Ultraviolet (UV) Exposure

- Bright outdoor light can cause eyes to instinctively squint or tear, a natural defence against the sun's harmful UV-rays. Sun protection for your skin is prevalent as the dangers of skin exposure to UV rays is well-known. But, the effects of the sun on the eyes can be just as overwhelming if they are not protected.
- UV damage to the eye can result in multiple diseases, such as: cataracts, skin cancer on the eyelids, and macular degeneration. The two unique types of UV rays affect different parts of the eye. ultraviolet A (UVA) rays penetrate all the way to the back of the eye, while ultraviolet B (UVB) rays tend to cause damage to the cornea and lens.
- Using prevention:
  - In order to prevent damage to the eyes, it is necessary to wear proper glasses. Different sunglasses have different UV classifications, and it is preferable to obtain sunglasses with 100% UVA and UVB protection. At a minimum, the sunglasses should be at least UV400.
  - Tints in colors yellow, pink, or blue should be avoided. These colors do not fully protect the eyes from the sun. Darker tints are better, but some dark tints could be illegal to use while driving in some countries.
- UV protection for children.
  It is estimated that in united states (US) and the European Union (EU) three out of every four parents do not protect their child's eyes from the bright sun. In Britain, particularly, nearly a third of parents do not buy sunglasses for their children and those that do put price into more consideration than protection. In India, this aspect of eye protection of children is not given any importance at all. When choosing sunglasses for the children, it is important to choose dark sunglasses with the standard mark of quality and safety, such as Indian Standards Institute (ISI) Mark in India, consumer electronics (CE) Mark of safety in the European Community, Kitemark in UK, American National Standards Institute (ANSI) mark in USA, etc.
- People with light-colored eyes are at more risk from sun damage than people with dark-colored eyes.
- Wearing cheap sunglasses with no UV protection may be a greater danger as it causes pupils to dilate and allow more harmful rays into the eyes. Not all quality sunglasses are expensive. Buying sunglasses that filter both UVA and UVB rays, in addition to having the standard quality marks like ISI Mark, CE mark, ANSI Mark, Kitemark etc. are crucial to knowing that the sunglasses are of good quality and safe to use.

Safety Goggles

Safety goggles have features which make them versatile for using as eye protectors (Fig. 13.1.2). Some of the features of the safety goggles are:
- Cheaper and more versatile than spectacles
- Can lead to discomfort if worn for long durations. This discourages their regular usage by workers
- Some designs can be worn over the prescription lenses
- Cup-type goggles protect against flying particles, welding glares or radiation

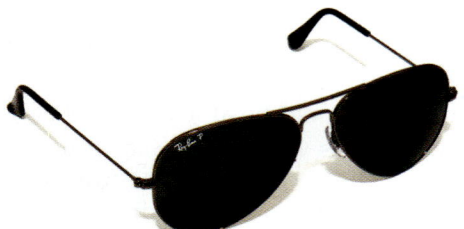

Fig. 13.1.2: Safety goggle

• Wide vision goggles (specific to a process or purpose) give protection against flying particles, welding glare, radiation, dust, fumes and splashes.

Face Shields and Eye Protectors

Face shields are of various types. These can be hand held, fixed to the helmet or strapped to the head. They protect the face and the eyes from splashes, flying particles and welding glare and radiations. These shields can also be fixed between the operator's head/face and the work station (job) to prevent splashes.

Standards for Eye Protectors and Shields

1. IS 5983: Specification for eye protectors—this standard covers the optical and non-optical requirements for eye protectors, which include the following:

   Optical requirements (IS 7524 – Part 1):
   – Refractive, astigmatic and prismatic powers
   – Diffusion of light
   – Quality of material and optical surface
   – Light transmittance
   – Color chromaticity.

   Non-optical requirements (IS 7524 – Part 1):
   – Stability at elevated temperature
   – Robustness
   – Resistance to corrosion
   – Suitability for disinfection
   – Flammability
   – Resistance to high speed particles
   – No-adherence of molten metals
   – Resistance to penetration of hot solids
   – Proof against chemical splashes
   – Protection against gas and dust.

2. IS 8519: Guide for selection of Industrial Safety Equipment for body protection—this standard codifies various types of industrial hazards, typical industrial applications where such hazards occur and type of body and eye protection equipment which should be used for such hazards.

3. IS 8521: Part 1—specification for Industrial Safety Face shields, Part 1—with plastic visors—this standard covers the requirements of three types of industrial safety face shields (which also shield eyes from splashes) with plastic visors namely: (1) type 1, (2) type 2 and (3) type 3. Type 3 face shields are further classified into class 1 and class 2 for attachment to a full brim or brimless helmet.

   These types include face shields with or without crown protectors and cover physical requirements which include:
   – Impact resistance
   – Penetration resistance
   – Visible transmittance
   – Flammability
   – Suitability for disinfection

4. IS 8521: Part 2 covers specification for face shields with wire-mesh visor. Although this type of face shield does not protect against liquids and fumes, it protects the eyes against larger solid particles. This standard covers the materials of construction, design, headgear, visor and visor support and disinfection requirements.

5. IS 15321: Molten metal splash protective hoods— the standard covers the materials of construction, which include fabric, fasteners, threads, etc. Requirements for design, sizes, seam strength, packing, marking and sampling for testing are also covered.

6. IS 8940: Code of practice for maintenance and care of industrial safety equipment for eye and face protection—this standard lays down recommended practices in selection, maintenance and care of safety equipment for protection eyes and face in order to obtain optimum effective use from these devices.

   The goggles should have light weight frame, and should be strong enough to hold their shapes. Frames shall not be made of nitrocellulose or other flammable materials. Materials of construction should not corrode easily and should be amenable to sterilization. In case of environments having risk of exposed electrical wiring or contacts, goggles with metallic frames shall not be used. Where there is danger of moderate or heavy impact, hardened lenses should be used. Plastic lenses should be used for processes where sparks or pitting is expected. The standard also covers the requirements for fitting and adjustment and advises that this should only be undertaken by trained technicians. Goggles should be kept in a suitable protective case if they are not required to be used continuously. The users should be trained to clean their goggles. Company issued goggles should be thoroughly cleaned and sterilized before reissue. Convenient dispensing stations with commercial cleaning solutions should be provided for quick removal of grease and oil. Carbon tetrachloride, gasoline (petrol), naphtha or other petroleum solvents should not be used for cleaning the goggles and other equipment. Drying of goggles and shields with excessive heat should be avoided.

The standard also suggests five types of sterilization processes for the safety equipment. Standard also specifies the inspection methodology and repairs in case the safety equipment requires any repairs to make it useable.

Other Related Standards

1. IS 1179: Indian Standard for equipment for eye and face protection during welding.
2. ANSI Z – 87.1: American Standard for practice for occupational and educational eye and face protection.
3. ISO 4854: International Standard on personal eye protestors—optical test methods.
4. ISO 4855: International Standard on personal eye protestors—nonoptical test methods

Emergency Showers and Eyewash Stations and Systems (Fig. 13.1.3)

Face and Eye Washing Stations

Face and eye washing stations are used for face washing and emergency eye and body washing in laboratory, industrial, or factory environments. Body and eye washing systems and stations are required when there is a potential danger for the body or eyes to be exposed to corrosives, strong irritants, or toxic chemicals in the form of solids, liquids, gases and fumes. In such cases, washing systems and stations must be available and accessible to workers. The proper selection of such systems and stations is based on the properties of the chemicals being used and the

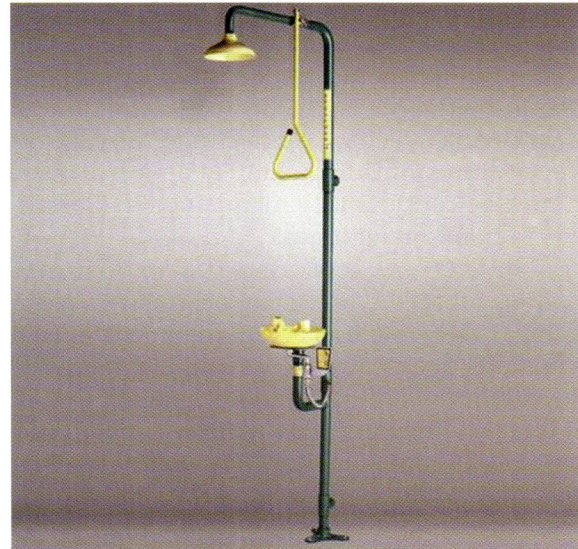

Fig. 13.1.3: Typical emergency shower and eyewash station

tasks being undertaken. The type of equipment should match the expected hazards.

Emergency eyewash station is designed to flush only the eye and face area. There are three major types of emergency wash stations:
1. Eye wash bowls
2. Drench hoses at sinks
3. Plastic eyewash bottles.

Boric acid eyewash, an antiseptic commonly used in commercial "artificial tears" and eyewash products, should be essentially stocked in an emergency eye-wash station.

Emergency shower, also called a drench or deluge shower, is used to flush the worker's entire head and body in case of exposure. Emergency shower should never be used to flush a worker's eyes as the higher rates of pressure can cause damage to the eye.

Automatic shower system are designed to flush eyes for the appropriate period of time in case of exposure to the dangerous chemicals. These systems use a solenoid valve to control the water flow in tandem with a timer so that the flushing occurs for the desired time period.

Hand wash stations are critical for hand cleansing to prevent the spread of bacterial infections or to remove contaminants after gloves and protective equipment are removed and accidently transferring the contaminants to the eyes.

Hand sanitizing system can range from a one station to a four-station sink and often includes hands-free foot pump operations, a heater to keep water temperature warm, or built-in lifting handles. A portable hand washing station may also be used; however, these units have limited amounts of water and must be continuously maintained to be sure the unit is available at all times.

The first 10–15 seconds after exposure to a hazardous substance, especially a corrosive substance, are critical. Delaying immediate treatment, even for a few seconds, may cause serious injury, particularly to the eyes.

Emergency showers and eyewash stations provide on-the-spot decontamination. They allow workers to flush away hazardous substances that can cause injury.

Accidental chemical exposures can occur even with good engineering controls and safety precautions. It is, therefore, essential to look beyond the use of goggles, face shields, and procedures for using personal protective equipment. Emergency showers and eyewash stations are a necessary backup to minimize the effects of accident exposure to chemicals. Emergency showers can also be used effectively in extinguishing clothing fires or for flushing contaminants off clothing.

"Flushing Fluid" Used in the Emergency Showers and Eyewash Stations

All emergency showers and eyewash stations use a "flushing fluid"—normally water.

The ANSI standard defines "flushing fluid" as any of potable (drinking) water, preserved water, preserved buffered saline solution or other medically acceptable solutions. Local laws pertaining to the flushing fluid may apply in some cases. The Indian standard (IS 10592) indirectly implies the use of clean potable water as the flushing fluid as it specifies the pressure and flow for *"water"* to be used in showers and flushing systems for these to be effective.

Duration for the Contact Area to be Rinsed/Flushed

For emergency showers and eyewash stations to be effective, the ANSI Standard for Emergency Eyewash and Shower Equipment (ANSI Z358.1-2004) recommends that the affected body part must be flushed immediately and thoroughly for at least 15 minutes using abundant supply of clean fluid under low pressure. Water does not neutralize contaminants—it only dilutes and washes them away. This is the reason why large amounts of water are needed for emergency showers.

However, other references recommend a minimum 20 minute flushing period if the nature of the contaminant is not known. The flushing or rinsing time can be modified if the identity and properties of the chemical are known. For example:

- A minimum 5 minute flushing time is recommended for mildly irritating chemicals
- At least, 20 minutes for moderate-to-severe irritants,
- Twenty minutes for non-penetrating corrosives
- At least, 60 minutes for penetrating corrosives.

Non-penetrating corrosives are chemicals which react with human tissue to form a protective layer which limits the extent of damage. Most acids are non-penetrating corrosives. Penetrating corrosives, such as most alkalis, hydrofluoric acid and phenol, enter the skin or eyes. Deeply-penetrating corrosives require longer water flushing (a minimum of 60 minutes) than non-penetrating corrosives (a minimum of 20 minutes).

In all cases, if irritation persists, repeat the flushing procedure. It is important to get medical attention as soon as possible after first aid has been given. A physician (preferably an ophthalmologist) familiar with procedures for treating chemical contamination of the eyes and body should be consulted.

Note: The total amount of water in self-contained systems should exceed the volume required to deliver water at the recommended flow rates and flushing times.

Selection of the Type of Equipment

Emergency showers, also known as *drench or deluge showers,* are designed to flush the user's head and body. ***They should not be used to flush the user's eyes because the high rate or pressure of water flow could damage the eyes in some instances. Eyewash stations*** are designed to flush the eye and face area only. There are *combination units* available that contain both features: a shower and eyewash.

The need for emergency showers or eyewash stations is based on the properties of the chemicals that workers use and the tasks that they do at the workplace. The selection of protection—emergency shower, eyewash or both—should match the expected hazard.

In some jobs or work areas, the effect of a hazard may be limited to the worker's face and eyes. Therefore, an eyewash station may be the appropriate device for worker protection. In other situations, the worker may risk part or full body contact with dangerous substances. In these areas, an emergency shower would be more appropriate.

A combination unit has the ability to flush any part of the body or all of the body. It is the most effective protective device and should be used wherever possible. This unit is also appropriate in work areas where detailed information about the hazards is lacking, or where complex, hazardous operations involve many chemicals with different properties. A combination unit is useful in situations where there are difficulties handling a worker who may not be able to follow directions because of intense pain or shock from an injury.

Specifications for the Equipment

Emergency eyewash and shower equipment should conform to the following specifications (every country has a specification for this type of equipment; some of the widely recognized standards including Indian Standard are listed below):

1. IS 10592: Specification for Industrial Emergency Showers, eye and face fountains and combination units, published by Bureau of Indian Standards, India.
2. ANSI Z358.1: Emergency Eyewash and Shower Equipment, published by the ANSI, USA
3. The AS4775 Australian standard for emergency eye wash and emergency shower equipment.

The above standards are similar in nature and cover minimum performance requirements expected from emergency showers, eye and face fountains and the combination units (containing a shower and eyewash, or eye/face wash, and/or drench hose into one common assembly). As per the standards, these units should preferably be located as near to the workplace as possible, and in any case not more than 15 meters from the workplace. The water used in these showers should be of potable quality and delivered at the comfortable temperature between 15°C and 35°C. The standards require the showers to be designed to deliver water at the minimum rate of 110 liters per minute.

The objective of Australian Standard AS4775 is to provide uniform minimum requirements for equipment performance, installation, use, maintenance and training of users, along with relevant test procedures.

AS4775 specifies minimum performance for eye wash and shower equipment for the emergency treatment of the eyes or body of a person who has been exposed to materials which may cause injuries. It covers the following types of equipment:

- Emergency shower equipment
- Eyewash equipment
- Eye/face wash equipment
- Combination shower and eyewash equipment
- Facilities for disabled persons.

It also includes performance and user requirements for the following supplemental equipment:

- Drench hoses
- Self-contained (portable) equipment.

There are some 3,000 dangerous goods scheduled in the Australian Code. Whether they be acids, alkalis, solvents, waxes, peroxides, poisons or hot materials, they represent a risk, not only in fire situations, but in everyday handling, packing, transporting and using. Emergency showers are an essential adjunct to any handling or storing situation and they are called up in a number of Australian Standards. Showers are needed for decontamination, corrosive splash and burn victims. The examples are many.

Although portable models are available, it is always a good practice to select a plumbed model whenever possible. Portable models should be able to deliver the same volumes of water, as well as meet the dimensions for plumbed models, as specified in the standards. However, portable stations are necessary for mobile crews, temporary locations, or when the plumbed model is under repair. In order to prevent any secondary eye infections, the water in self-contained models should be treated to prevent bacterial growth in the water itself. Changing the water supply weekly is another good preventative measure.

Emergency Showers

The emergency shower should deliver a pattern of water with a diameter of at least 50 cm (20 inches) at

150 cm (60 inches). This diameter ensures that the water will come into contact with the entire body—not just the top of the person's head. ANSI standard (ANSI Z358.1) also recommends that the shower head should be between 200 cm and 240 cm (82–96 inches) from the floor. The minimum volume of spray should be 75 liters/minute (20 gallons/minute) for a minimum time of 15 minutes.

The shower should also be so designed that it can be activated in less than 1 second, and it remains operational without the operator's hand on the valve (or lever, handle, etc.). This valve should not be more than 170 cm (69 inches) in height. If enclosures are used, ensure that there is an unobstructed area of 85 cm (34 inches) in diameter.

Eyewash and Eye/Face Wash Stations

As per ANSI Standard eyewash stations should be designed to deliver fluid to both eyes simultaneously at a volume of not less than 1.5 liters/minute (0.4 gallons/minute) for 15 minutes. However, the volume should not be at a velocity which may injure the eyes. The unit should be between 85 cm and 115 cm (33 to 45 inches) from the floor, and a minimum of 15 cm (6 inches) from the wall or nearest obstruction.

The user should be able to open their eyelids with their hands and still have their eyes in the liquid. As with the shower, the unit should also be so designed that it can be activated in less than 1 second, and it remains operational without the operator's hand on the valve (or lever, handle, etc.) with the valve being located in an easily accessible and operable place. Since the nozzles in eyewash stations need to be protected from airborne contaminants, the units should be so designed that the removal of these covers may not require a separate motion by the user when the unit is activated.

Personal Wash Stations

Designed to deliver flushing fluid immediately, personal wash stations can be used while transporting the victim to the permanent eyewash station or medical facility. These stations do not replace the requirement to have a 15 minute-supply eyewash station. The expiry date of the fluid should be printed permanently on the unit.

Drench Hoses

This type of equipment is usually considered to be secondary to proper emergency showers and eyewash stations (e.g. having a drench hose does not mean that it replaces the need for showers/stations). Drench hoses may be used to "spot" rinse an area when a full shower is not required, to assist a victim when the victim is unable to stand or is unconscious, or to wash under a piece of clothing before the clothing is removed.

Combination Units

This name refers to equipment that shares a common plumbing fixture. Any of the fixtures such as shower, eyewash, eye/face wash or drench hose may be in this combination, but most commonly it refers to a shower and an eyewash station. It is important that pressure and volume requirements for each piece of the unit (as described above) are in compliance with the code.

Location of Emergency Equipment

To be effective, the equipment has to be accessible. ANSI recommends that a person be able to reach the equipment in no more than 10 seconds. In practical terms, considering that the persons who need the equipment will be injured, and may not have normal use of their vision. Recommendations for this distance in linear terms range from 15 meters to 30 metres.

However, the "10 second" rule may be modified depending on the potential effect of the chemical. Where a highly corrosive chemical has been the cause of the injury, an emergency shower and eyewash station may be required within 3–6 meters (10–20 ft) from the hazard. These units should be installed in such a way that they do not become contaminated from corrosive chemicals used nearby.

The location of each emergency shower or eyewash station should be identified with a highly visible sign. The sign should be in the form of a symbol that does not require workers to have language skills to understand it. The location should be well lit.

Other recommendations include that the emergency shower or eyewash station should:
- Be located as close to the hazard as possible
- Not be separated by a partition from the hazardous work area.

- Be on an unobstructed path between the workstation and the hazard (workers should not have to pass through doorways or weave through machinery or other obstacles to reach them).
- Be located where workers can easily see them—preferably in a normal traffic pattern.
- Be on the same floor as the hazard (no stairs to travel between the workstation and the emergency equipment).
- Be located near an emergency exit where possible so that any responding emergency response personnel can reach the victim easily.
- Be located in an area where further contamination will not occur.
- Provide a drainage system for the excess water (remember that the water may be considered a hazardous waste and special regulations may apply).
- Not come into contact with any electrical equipment that may become a hazard when wet
- Be protected from freezing when installing emergency equipment outdoors.

Temperature of Water/Flushing Fluid

The 2004 version of the ANSI standard, which is the currently valid version, recommends that the water should be "tepid" but does not give a specific temperature, while the IS specifies a comfortable temperature range of 15 to 35°C. Other standards will use the term "lukewarm water". ANSI does provide a guideline that the water temperature should be under 38°C and above 15.5°C. Temperatures higher than 38°C are harmful to the eyes and can enhance chemical interaction with the skin and eyes. Long flushing times with cold water (less than 15.5°C can cause hypothermia and may result in not rinsing or showering for the full recommended time (ANSI 2004). With thermal burns (burn injuries to the skin), the American Heart Association noted that optimal healing and lowest mortality rates are with water temperatures of 20–25°C.

It must be remembered that any chemical splash should be rinsed for a minimum of 15 minutes but rinsing time can be up to 60 minutes to flush out the entire chemical. The temperature of the water should be one that can be tolerated for the required length of time. Too cold or too hot water will inhibit workers from rinsing or showering as long as they should.

Anti-scalding devices (temperature control valve or thermostatic tempering valve) should be installed. Constant flow meters and other devices that will help maintain a constant temperature and flow rate should also form part of the installation.

For cold or outdoor locations, emergency showers with heated plumbing are available. In hot climates, outdoor emergency showers should also have a tempering valve so that workers are not exposed to water that is too hot.

Examples of Areas that may Require This Equipment

Work areas and operations that may require these devices include:

- Battery charging areas
- Laboratories
- Spraying operations
- High dust areas
- Dipping operations
- Hazardous substances dispensing areas.

Other Factors to be Considered while Selecting and Using This Type of Emergency Equipment

The following factors should also be considered as part of a hazard analysis when decisions are being made about the selection and use of emergency showers, eyewash stations or combination units:

Potentially Hazardous Substances in the Immediate Work Area

All hazardous substances need to be properly identified. A review of Material Safety Data Sheets (MSDSs) and labels can help to evaluate the hazard. To select the appropriate eyewash and shower equipment, one must know about the chemicals being used and their potential risks.

Number of Workers in an Area with a Hazardous Substance

More than one emergency shower or eyewash station may be required in an area where many workers use hazardous substances. Evaluate how many workers are using the hazardous chemicals, and provide more equipment where necessary to ensure each worker's protection.

Isolated Workers

The installation of an audible or visual alarm can alert other workers when the emergency shower or eyewash station is being used. An alarm is especially important if only one worker happens to be working in that area. A victim may need help in getting to the eyewash if temporarily blinded. Valves can also be connected electrically to warning lights or buzzers in central areas to alert other workers/safety of people.

Comfort and Warmth

Extra-overalls and foot covers should be stored near emergency showers. Clothes contaminated with corrosive or toxic chemicals need to be removed from the injured person. Consider installing a privacy curtain (but remember to maintain the "obstacle free" diameter dimension as stated in the ANSI and IS).

Quality of the Flushing Fluid

Changing the fluid in self-contained systems frequently and cleaning the units regularly can prevent inadvertent use of contaminated fluid. Manufacturer's instructions should also be referred for details of any precautions required in this aspect. Even in plumbed eyewash stations, the water may contain contaminants such as rust, scale and chemicals. Systems should be flushed and cleaned regularly and filters should preferably be installed to clean out these contaminants. IS requires installation of filters in the system to filter out particles which may injure the eyes.

Neutralized Solutions

Eyewash bottles and some portable units cannot supply enough fluid to adequately dilute and wash away contaminants. The use of buffered solutions can improve the efficiency of the portable eyewashes because these solutions can increase the first aid potential of the small amount of fluid, and can partially neutralize the contaminant.

Limitations for Different Types of Emergency Wash Systems

Plumbed Emergency Showers and Eyewash Stations

Studies have shown that despite the 15-minute flushing requirement, users usually flush exposed body parts (and eyes) for much less time (5 minutes or less). The reasons were always related to the extreme discomfort users experienced using cold water. In cold climates the water temperature in indoor plumbed systems can be as low as 2–7°C and forcing the use of cold water in case of accidents could compromise the eyesight of the victim(s).

Drinkable tap water may not provide the best flushing solution. Tap water may contain many contaminants and could aggravate the injured body part. Some municipal water supplies also contain chlorine which can irritate and leach salt from the eye tissue. The tap water may contain rust, scale and chemicals. Running the water continually keeps the water line fresh. Plumbed emergency eyewash stations should use water that is periodically tested and treated to remove chemical contaminants.

Portable, Self-contained Eyewash Stations

Portable, self-contained eyewash stations have a limited amount of fluid. As a result, maintenance is critical to ensure that units are fully charged at all times. These eyewash stations also require ongoing maintenance of the buffered saline solution. The agents used to control bacterial growth are effective only for limited periods of time. Also, small amebae capable of causing serious eye infections have been found in portable and stationary eyewash stations. Consequently, it is important to monitor the shelf life of the solution and replace the solution when it has expired.

Eyewash Bottles

Eyewash bottles or personal eyewash units supplement plumbed and self-contained stations, but in no way can replace them. They are portable and permit immediate flushing of contaminants or small particles. However, eyewash bottles are very difficult for the user to handle, especially when alone and when both eyes have been exposed (e.g. holding the eyelids open while handling the unit is unpractical). Also, one bottle cannot flush both eyes simultaneously. Since the fluid supply lasts for only a short period of time, the bottle may not able to wash the eyes sufficiently.

The main purpose of such a unit is to supply immediate flushing. Once accomplished, the user should proceed to a self-contained or plumbed eyewash and flush for the required flushing/rinsing period.

Inspection and Maintenance of the Safety Equipment

It is recommended that one worker in the work area should be made responsible for inspecting and operating (activating) the emergency shower, eyewash station, combination units, and drench hoses at least on weekly basis. Such a periodical check will make sure that the flushing fluid is available in the system as well as clear the supply line of any sediments and minimize microbial contamination caused by 'still' or sitting water. This worker should keep a signed, dated record. The ANSI standard also recommends a complete inspection on an annual basis. The IS 10592 requires that systems shall be activated daily to flush out deposits and contaminants and to verify that the unit is operational.

A specific Indian Standard Code of Practice for maintenance and care of safety equipment (IS 8940) has been published by Bureau of Indian Standards.

Preventive maintenance inspections should be done every 6 months to check for such problems as valve leakages, clogged openings and lines, and adequacy of the fluid volume. A work record of these inspections should be kept. Replacement parts should be kept on hand to prevent the system from becoming non-functional. If the system breaks down for any reason, the workers in the area should be properly warned and protected by deploying another mobile unit. Personal eyewash equipment should be inspected and maintained according to the manufacturer's instructions and at least annually for overall operation.

> Caring for your protective eyewear
> - Care for your protective eyewear in a manner that will extend the life of your equipment and help to ensure that it provides the maximum protection when you need it the most!
> - Use polycarbonate lenses with antiscratch coating.
> - Wear an eyewear retainer strap that will let the glasses hang around your neck when not in use.
> - Store protective eyewear in a case or an old sock before tossing them into a tool chest or the seat of a car or pickup.
> - Clean your protective eyewear with eyeglass cleaning solutions, or wash and wipe them with a soft, clean cloth.
> - Use antifog solutions to keep your lenses from fogging when in use.

Training of Workers

All workers require instructions in the proper use and location of emergency showers or eyewash stations before any emergencies occur. It should never be assumed that workers are already aware of the proper procedures. While written instructions should be made available to all workers and posted by the side of the emergency shower and eyewash station, the workers should be given training in the use of equipment as many of them may not be literate. Part of the instructional process should include a "hands-on" drill on how to find equipment.

The wearing of contact lenses can be dangerous because chemicals can become trapped under a contact lens. Any delays caused by removing contact lenses in order to rinse eyes could result in injury. Training should include instructions in contact lens removal.

Selection of Eye Protection Equipment

> Choose the best protection, make sure it fits, keep it clean and wear it!

The first step in the selection of appropriate eye protection equipment is to conduct the hazard assessment of the work place.

Hazard Assessment

Because workers who wear protective eyewear still suffer injuries, how much protection is enough? To answer that question, begin with a hazard assessment to determine which of several eye hazards exist for each job:

- Dust, concrete, metal and other particles
- Chemicals such as acids, bases, fuels, solvents, lime and wet or dry cement powder
- Falling or shifting debris, building materials and glass
- Smoke and noxious or poisonous gases
- Welding light and electrical arcs
- Thermal hazards and fires
- Blood borne pathogens (hepatitis or HIV) from blood, body fluids and human remains.

The Proper Type of Eye Protection must be Selected to Match the Type of Hazard

As indicated above, the most common types of eye protection include the following:
- Safety glasses with side protection/shields
- Goggles
- Face shields

- Welding helmets
- Full-face respirators.

Safety glasses are designed to withstand impact from common workplace hazards and to provide the minimum level of protection required in the workplace.

- Safety glasses with side protection are required any time there are hazards from flying particles or objects such as minor dust or chips.
- Safety glasses are commonly used as protection against impact and low-intensity optical radiation from soldering and the sun.
- Goggles are stronger than safety glasses and are used for protection from high impacts, particles, chemical splashes and welding light.
- Faceshields are used for even higher impact tasks and protect the wearer's face and eyes from dangers such as critical chemicals and blood borne hazards.
- Welding helmets protect the user from the intensity of welding light, which can cause severe burns to the eye and surrounding tissue.

Selecting Appropriate Protective Eyewear

- As per the regulations of OSHA of USA, all protective eyewear must meet the ANSI Z87.1 Eye and Face Protection Standards.
- Safety eyewear must have "Z87" or "Z87+" marked on the frame and, in some cases, the lenses too.
- Safety eyewear with polycarbonate lenses affords the highest impact resistance and greater eye safety (marked Z87+).
- Protective eyewear should be properly fitted and comfortable to wear.
- When other PPE such as a half-face respirator is required, protective eyewear must be selected to fit so that both types of PPE work properly.
- Glasses that are not snug against the face create gaps in protection. The biggest gaps are usually near the corners of the glasses and allow more exposure to hazards coming at an angle from above or below.
- Adjustable-temple glasses, eyewear retainers, and straps help hold the glasses in the proper position, close to the face.
- Safety glasses may have hard or soft nose pieces, padded temples, and a variety of other features can be added to improve comfort at incremental cost.

Types of Protection

To ensure that workers wear the proper type of protective eyewear, the following list from the National Institute for Occupational Safety and Health (NIOSH) of the USA provides guidance:

- Nonprescription and prescription safety glasses
- Goggles
- Face shields
- Welding helmets
- Full-face respirators.

Safety Glasses

Safety glasses with side protection provide minimum protection and are for general working conditions where there may be minor dust, chips or flying particles. Side protection includes side shields and wraparound-style safety glasses.

Safety glasses should have an antifog treatment. Polycarbonate lenses are lightweight and provide the best impact protection, but generally are not as scratch-resistant as glass unless treated with a hard coating.

Occupational Safety and Health Administration eye and face protection standard, 29 CFR 1910.133, requires that eye and face protection be certified by the ANSI as per ANSI Z87.1 standard. Look for the ANSI Z87.1 mark on the lens or frame.

Goggles

Goggles provide higher impact, dust and chemical splash protection than safety glasses. Goggles for splash or fine dust protection should have indirect venting. Use direct-vented goggles for less fogging when working with large particles. Safety goggles designed after ski-type goggles with high air flow minimize fogging while providing better particle and splash protection than glasses.

Safety glass users should graduate to goggles when there is more than occasional particle hazards, such as when cutting wood. The assessment, in many cases, comes down to the severity of the hazard.

In some activities, safety glasses are not enough protection for workers who clean mixers and hoppers. The goggles and even anti-fog products occasionally fog up. With face shields, chips can still get under the shield. The solution in such cases is to use chipper's goggles, which look like large swimmer's goggles and cup around the eye to seal out particles and dust.

Hybrid Safety Glasses or Goggles

Safety glasses with foam or rubber around the lenses provide better protection from dust and flying particles than conventional safety glasses. Wraparound safety glasses that convert to goggles with a soft plastic or rubber face seal may offer better peripheral vision than conventional goggles. Johnson cautions, however, to avoid hybrids or wraparounds when more impact protection is needed than safety glasses provide. In those cases, use goggles.

Prescription Safety Glasses

Workers who wear nonsafety prescription glasses should wear tight-fitting goggles over the glasses. Because contact lenses may present a significant corneal abrasion risk when working in dusty areas, contact lens wearers should wear unvented goggles.

Wear goggles over prescription safety glasses in high-dust environments. If worn alone, prescription safety glasses should have side protection.

Prescription safety lenses with tempered glass or acrylic plastic lenses are not suitable for high impact. Do not use these types of safety glasses when working in debris areas unless covered by goggles or a face shield. Use polycarbonate lenses when working in high-impact areas.

Face Shields

When protecting the eyes, do not forget to guard against injuries to the face. For highest impact protection, face shields protect the full face from spraying, chipping, grinding and critical chemicals or blood borne hazards.

Never wear face shields, which provide secondary protection, without primary eye protection (safety glasses or goggles). Wear safety glasses or goggles under face shields to provide protection when the shield is lifted, Johnson says. Primary protection helps to prevent particles that get under the shield from lodging in the eyes.

Specialty Protection

Use other types of protection, such as filtered helmets or goggles, for tasks such as welding or working with lasers. Lenses for welding light protection must be marked with an appropriate "shade number" for the task. Remember to protect the eyes even when the helmet is lifted. Welder's helpers, other workers and bystanders should have welding light protection when near torch cutting or welding. Use ANSI Z136-certified eye protection for laser light hazards.

While full-face respirators provide the best general dust, chemical and smoke protection, they may not necessarily be Z87.1-compliant for impact protection, or seal properly over glasses. Use prescription inserts compatible with a respirator. Respirators should be professionally fitted.

What is the Difference between Glass, Plastic, and Polycarbonate Safety Lenses?

All three types of safety lenses meet or exceed the requirements for protecting your eyes.

Glass Lenses

- Are not easily scratched
- Can be used around harsh chemicals
- Can be made in your corrective prescription
- Are sometimes heavy and uncomfortable.

Plastic Lenses

- Are lighter weight
- Protect against welding splatter
- Are not likely to fog
- Are not as scratch-resistant as glass.

Polycarbonate Lenses

- Are lightweight
- Protect against welding splatter
- Are not likely to fog
- Are stronger than glass and plastic
- Are more impact resistant than glass or plastic
- Are not as scratch resistant as glass.

Ensure a Proper Fit

One way to make sure that safety glasses provide adequate protection is for them to fit properly, according to Winston Wolfe, president of Olympic Optical.

Safety glasses should rest firmly on top of the nose and close to, but not against, the face. The nose piece should not slide down the face due to sweat or moisture. "If the glass slides down even a small amount, the user will lose some protection".

Safety glasses should have a three-point fit, meaning the frame should touch the face in three places—at the nose bridge and behind each ear. Temples should wrap around the head, with slight pressure behind the ear, not above the ear.

Protective eyewear works best when employees know how to use it properly. Employers should ensure proper training for employees. Combined with machine guards, screened or divided work stations, and other engineering controls, using the correct protective eyewear can help keep workers safe from any type of eye hazard.

SPORTS-RELATED EYE INJURIES AND PROTECTION

Eye Injury and Sports

Eye injuries are the leading cause of blindness in children in the US and other developed nations. Most of these occur in school going children and are sports-related. Ninety percent of these injuries can be avoided with protective eyewear.

Following facts bring out the enormity of the problem:

- More than 100,000 eye injuries in the US each year are estimated to be sports-related. In india too the problem is equally serious, if not worse.
- Sports-related eye injury is treated every 13 minutes in emergency rooms in the health facilities in the US.
- An estimated 27% of all eye injuries in children aged 11–14 years are sports-related.
- Children under age 15 years account for 43% of sports and recreational eye injuries.
- The sports responsible for the greatest number of injuries in the US are baseball, ice hockey, and racquet sports.

In 2002, 15% of children and 33% of adults reported wearing eye protection always or most of the time when participating in sports, hobbies, or other activities that can cause eye injuries. This figure has slightly improved due to increased awareness, campaign of the Blindness Associations and enforcement by the authorities. Polycarbonate lenses provide the best eye protection for many sports because they are lightweight, scratch resistant, thin, and can be designed to meet most eyewear designs or prescriptions.

Risk ratings for individual sports

- *High risk of eye injury:* Air rifle, baseball, basketball, boxing, cricket, fencing, hockey, lacrosse, full-contact martial arts, paintball, racquetball, softball, squash.
- *Moderate risk of eye injury:* Badminton, fishing, football, golf, soccer, tennis, volleyball.
- *Low risk of eye injury:* Bicycling, diving, non-contact martial arts, skiing (snow and water), swimming, wrestling.
- *Eye safe:* Track and field, gymnastics.

Baseball

Baseball is the leading cause of sports-related eye injury among children aged 14 years and under in the US and other countries where baseball is popular.

Basketball

Basketball is a leading cause of sports-related eye injury in athletes aged 15–24 years. The odds of an eye injury for basketball players are one in 10. Of 1,092 injuries sustained by National Basketball Association players during a 17 months period in 1992 and 1993, 5.4% involved the eye.

Football and Soccer

Soccer ball-related ocular injuries disproportionately affect young players. Females are affected more frequently than previously reported, and have more severe visual consequences than previously recognized.

Golf

Golf-related ocular injuries account for 1.5% to 5.6% of all sports injuries. The incidence of ocular injuries caused by golf-related trauma is low compared with that for other sports-related injuries.

Ice Hockey and Field Hockey

As of July 2007, National Collegiate Athletic Association (NCAA) field hockey players are permitted to wear a face mask, soft protective head covering, or eye protection in the form of plastic goggles.

Lacrosse (Women)

The 2007 NCAA Women's Lacrosse Rules and Interpretations mandates: "All field players must properly wear eye protection." Eye protection must meet the most current **American Society for Testing and Materials (ASTM) Specification Standard F803 for women's lacrosse**. Eye injuries were a frequent occurrence in women's lacrosse before the rule was added. Before protective eyewear was mandated, eye injuries occurred 15 times more often in women's lacrosse than in men's.

Racquet Sports (Badminton, Table Tennis, Tennis, Racquetball, Squash)

Tennis, badminton, and squash form the highest percentage of eye injuries to a casualty clinic. In the case of squash and tennis injuries, follow-up treatment and/or admission to hospital was required in 100% of cases.

Thirty-seven cases of ocular injury incurred while persons were playing racquetball were found in reviewing records of 1,071 emergency room patients in a three-month period. Ocular safety devices are strongly recommended to help to prevent racquetball injuries. Tennis is a leading source of eye injury in female adults.

Standards for Protection at Play

The eye protection needed for the sport is determined by various standards set by ASTM which are:

- *ASTM F803:* Eye protectors for selected sports (racket sports, women's lacrosse, field hockey, baseball, basketball)
- *ASTM F513:* Eye and face protective equipment for hockey players
- *ASTM F1776:* Eye protectors for use by players of paintball sports
- *ASTM F1587:* Head and face protective equipment for ice hockey goal fenders

- *ASTM F910:* Face guards for youth baseball
- *ASTM F659:* High-impact resistant eye protective devices for Alpine skiing.

Annexure

Morgan therapeutic lens is the ideal equipment to meet the requirement for constant irrigation of the eyes till the affected person can reach the medical facilities.

The ideal treatment for eye injury or disease is to have someone constantly dropping medicine into the eye. The old fashioned eye cup provided some relief, it was filled with a solution and tipped over the eye. The trouble with that is that there is one good washing and from then on there is rewashing in the same old dirty fluid.

The Morgan therapeutic lens was developed to meet a need Dr Morgan recognized during his duty in Vietnam as part of the American Medical Association's Volunteer Physicians for Vietnam Program.

Conditions in Vietnam produced a wide range of serious illnesses among the civilian population. Dr Morgan discovered the less-than-sterile conditions under which he was having to work often resulted in postoperative infections. Taking the ideas of two "commonly accepted methods" of irrigating the eye he moulded a lens to completely cover each eye, punctured a hole (chimney he calls it) in the lens, inserted a tube leading to a bottle of fluid. At first he moulded the lens for each sick eye but soon he realized that a standard mould would fit because the lens floats on a cushion of fluid, never touching the eye itself.

The Morgan therapeutic lens is a continuous bath, running all the time with clean, sterile fluid, usually Lactated Ringer's Solution. It does not have to be used by a doctor although it usually is. Some industries stock Dr Morgan's lens to have on hand for accidents involving chemicals or debris in workers' eyes. The fluid keeps the eye cool and moist and continually washes out bacteria, dead cells, or whatever foreign matter may have caused injury to the eye.

13.2 COMPENSATION IN OCULAR INJURIES

• Mukesh Yadav

INTRODUCTION

As we rely so much on our eyes in everyday life, an eye injury can be very distressing. Eye injuries can vary from minor discomfort to more serious injuries such as loss of sight (blindness) or even removal of the eye. As the eye is very sensitive, even a minor injury can cause impairment of vision. Therefore, it is important to get medical treatment and care immediately for any type of eye injury.

Eye injuries are most often caused by road traffic accidents or accidents at work place. In a car accident the small pieces of glass from a shattered windscreen can cause damage to the inner or outer parts of the eye. The severe impact against the airbag could cause damage to the eye socket. Eye injuries from accidents at work can happen due to non-availability of safety equipment or inadequate training, especially if the work is hazardous.

WHAT ARE THE TYPES OF EYE INJURY?

One may experience pain or symptoms immediately after the accident or it could take several days. Some of the most common eye injuries include:

- Foreign body entering the eye
- Scratches or irritation on the outer part of the eye
- Chemical burns
- Blurred vision
- Light sensitivity
- Swollen eyelids
- Double vision
- Eye socket fractures.

An eye injury should be treated carefully to enable a full recovery. This could mean one have to take time off work, lose earnings and have to pay for recovery treatment. To help ease the financial burden, it is important that one who suffers should take advice on making a claim for eye injury compensation.

WHAT ARE THE LAWS (STATUTES) AND PROVISIONS FOR COMPENSATION IN INDIA?

- *Constitutional provisions:* For violation of Fundamental Rights (Compensation for Custodial Deaths, Rape Victims, Death or injury due to criminal Act).
- Under Criminal Procedure Code: Section 357 CrPC
- Under Workmen Compensation Act (WCA), 1923
- Under Motor Vehicle Act (MVA), 1898
- Under Common Law (Law of Tort) for negligence.

WHO IS LIABLE FOR COMPENSATION UNDER WCA?

If personal injury is caused to a workman by accident arising out of and in the course of his employment, his employer shall be liable to pay compensation in accordance with the provisions of WCA [this Chapter]: [Section 3 (1)].

When Employer is not Liable for Compensation under WCA?

The employer shall not be so liable:

- In respect of any injury which does not result in the total or partial disablement of the workman for a period exceeding 3*[three] days; [Section 3 (1)(a)].
- In respect of any injury, not resulting in death, caused by an accident which is directly attributable to [Section 3 (1)(b)].
  i. The workman having been at the time thereof under the influence of drink or drugs or
  ii. The willful disobedience of the workman to an order expressly given, or to a rule expressly framed, for the purpose of securing the safety of workmen or
  iii. The willful removal or disregard by the workman of any safety guard or other device which he knew to have been provided for the purpose of securing the safety of workmen.

If a workman employed in any employment specified in Part A of Schedule III contracts any disease specified therein as an occupational disease peculiar to that employment, or if a workman, whilst in the service of an employer in whose service he has been employed for a continuous period of not less than 6 months (which period shall not include a period of service under any other employer in the same kind of employment) in any employment specified in Part B of Schedule III, contracts any disease specified therein as an occupational disease peculiar to that employment, or if a workman whilst in the service of one or more employers in any employment specified in *Part C of Schedule III* for such continuous period as the Central Government may specify in respect of each such employment, contracts any disease specified therein as an occupational disease peculiar to that employment, the contracting of the disease shall be deemed to be an injury by accident within the meaning of this section and, unless the contrary is proved, the accident shall be deemed to have arisen out of, and in the course of, the employment.[3]

Provided that if it is proved: (a) that a workman whilst in the service of one or more employers in any employment specified in Part C of Schedule III has contracted a disease specified therein as an occupational disease peculiar to that employment during a continuous period which is less than the period specified under this subsection for that employment and (b) that the disease has arisen out of and in the course of the employment; the contracting of such disease shall be deemed to be an injury by accident within the meaning of this section.

Provided further that if it is proved that a workman who having served under any employer in any employment specified in Part B of Schedule III or who having served under one or more employers in any employment specified in Part C of that Schedule, for a continuous period specified under this sub-section for that employment and he has after the cessation of such service contracted any disease specified in the said Part B or the said Part C, as the case may be, as an occupational disease peculiar to the employment and that such disease arose out of the employment, the contracting of the disease shall be deemed to be an injury by accident within the meaning of this section. If a workman employed in any employment specified in Part C of Schedule III contracts any occupational disease peculiar to that employment, the contracting whereof is deemed to be an injury by accident within the meaning of this section, and such employment was under more than one employer, all such employers shall be liable for the payment of the compensation in such proportion as the Commissioner may, in the circumstances, deem just.

The State Government in the case of employments specified in Part A and Part B of Schedule III, and the Central Government in the case of employments specified in Part C of that Schedule, after giving, by notification in the Official Gazette, not less than 3 months' notice of its intention so to do, may, by a like notification, add any description of employment to the employments specified in Schedule III, and shall specify in the case of employments so added the diseases which shall be deemed for the purposes of this section to be occupational diseases peculiar to those employments, respectively, and thereupon the provisions of subsection (2) shall apply as if such diseases had been declared by this Act to be occupational diseases peculiar to those employments [Section 3(3)].

Amount of Compensation

Subject to the provisions of WM Act, the amount of compensation shall be as follows, namely:

- Where death results, an amount equal to 40% from the date of injury of the monthly wages of the deceased workman multiplied by the relevant factor; or an amount of ₹ 20,000 whichever is more [Section 4(1)(a)].
- Where permanent total disablement from the injury, an amount equal to 50% from the monthly wages of the injured workman multiplied by the relevant factor; or an amount of ₹ 24,000, whichever is more [Section 4(1)(b)].

Explanation I: For the purposes of clause (a) and clause (b), "relevant factor", in relation to a workman means the factor specified in the second column of Schedule IV against the entry in the first column of that Schedule specifying the number of years which are the same as the completed years of the age of the workman on his last birthday immediately preceding the date on which the compensation fell due.

Explanation II: Where the monthly wages of a workman exceed ₹ 1,000, his monthly wages for the purposes of clause (a) and clause (b) shall be deemed to be ₹ 1,000 only,

- Where permanent partial disablement
  - In the case of an injury disablement results from such injury as specified in Part II of Schedule I, such percentage of the compensation which would have been payable in the case of permanent total disablement as is specified therein as being the percentage of the loss of earning capacity caused by that injury
  - In the case of an injury not specified in Schedule I, such percentage of the compensation payable

in the case of permanent total disablement as is proportionate to the loss of earning capacity (as assessed by the qualified medical practitioner) permanently caused by the injury [Section 4(1)(c)].

- *Explanation I:* Where more injuries than one are caused by the same accident, the amount of compensation payable under this head shall be aggregated but not so in any case as to exceed the amount which would have been payable if permanent total disablement had resulted from the injuries.

Explanation II: In assessing the loss of earning capacity for the purposes of subclause (ii), the qualified medical practitioner shall have due regard to the percentages of loss of earning capacity in relation to different injuries specified in Schedule I

- Where temporary disablement a half-monthly payment, whether total or partial injury result from the sum equivalent to 25% of monthly wages of the workman, to be paid in accordance with the provisions of sub-section 2 [Section 4(1)(d)].
- The half-monthly payment referred to in clause (d) of subsection (1) shall be payable on the 16th day: (i) from the date of disablement where such disablement lasts for a period of 28 days or more, or (ii) after the expiry of a waiting period of 3 days from the date of disablement where such disablement lasts for a period of less than 28 days; and thereafter half-monthly during the disablement or during a period of 5 years, whichever period is shorter [Section 4(2)].

WHAT IS THE AMOUNT OF DEDUCTION ALLOWED?

A sum proportionate to the duration of the disablement in that half-month.

Provided that:

a. There shall be deducted from any lump sum or half-monthly payments to which the workman is entitled the amount of any payment or allowance which the workman has received from the employer by way of compensation during the period of disablement prior to the receipt of such lump sum or of the first half-monthly payment, as the case may be

b. No half-monthly payment shall in any case exceed the amount, if any, by which half the amount of the monthly wages of the workman before the

accident exceeds half the amount of such wages which he is earning after the accident [Section 4(2)(a((b)].

WHAT IS MEANT BY MEDICAL TREATMENT ALLOWANCE/ PAYMENT?

- *Explanation:* Any payment or allowance which the workman has received from the employer toward his medical treatment shall not be deemed to be a payment or allowance received by him by way of compensation within the meaning of clause (a) of the proviso [Section 4(2)].
- On the ceasing of the disablement before the date on which any half-monthly payment falls due, there shall be payable in respect of that half-month a sum proportionate to the duration of the disablement in that half-month [Section 4(3)].

WHEN COMPENSATION NOT GIVEN/PAYABLE?

- Save as provided by 2*[subsections (2), (2A)] and (3), no compensation shall be payable to a workman in respect of any disease unless the disease is directly attributable to a specific injury by accident arising out of and in the course of his employment [Section 3(4)].
- Nothing herein contained shall be deemed to confer any right to compensation on a workman in respect of any injury if he has instituted in a Civil Court a suit for damages in respect of the injury against the employer or any other person; and no suit for damages shall be maintainable by a workman in any Court of law in respect of any injury [Section 3(5)].

a. If he has instituted a claim to compensation in respect of the injury before a Commissioner [Section 3(5)(a)].

b. If an agreement has been come to between the workman and his employer providing for the payment of compensation in respect of the injury in accordance with the provisions of this Act [Section 3(5)(b)] [Section 3(5)] .

COMPENSATION TO BE PAID WHEN DUE AND PENALTY FOR DEFAULT

Compensation under section 4 shall be paid as soon as it falls due [Section 4A(1)] In cases where the employer does not accept the liability for compensation to the extent claimed, he shall be bound to make provisional payment based on the extent of liability which he accepts, and, such payment shall be deposited with the Commissioner or made to the workman, as the case may be, without prejudice to the right of the workman to make any further claim. [Section 4A (2)].

Where any employer is in default in paying the compensation due under this Act within 1 month from the date it fell due, the Commissioner may direct that, in addition to the amount of the arrears, simple interest at the rate of 6% per annum on the amount due together with, if in the opinion of the Commissioner there is no justification for the delay, a further sum not exceeding 50% of such amount, shall be recovered from the employer by way of penalty [Section 4A (3)].

EXAMPLES OF COMPENSATION AMOUNTS AWARDED FOR EYE INJURIES

Please note these figures are estimates of what is commonly awarded for similar eye injuries. It is advisable to seek medical advice from his/her doctor or local hospital as soon as possible following an eye injury as they will be able to recommend the best treatment for you. The doctor/hospital records of your eye injury are used when making your compensation claim.

If one has suffered an eye injury and it was someone else's fault, then one could be entitled to make a claim for compensation under various provisions of law in India, like under the Motor Vehicle Act and Workmen's Compensation Act and Law of Tort.

CLAIM OF COMPENSATION UNDER MOTOR VEHICLE ACT

1. The amount of compensation so arrived at in the case of fatal accident claims shall be reduced by one-third in consideration of the expenses which the victim would have incurred toward maintaining himself had he been alive.
2. Amount of compensation shall not be less than ₹ 50,000.
3. General damages (in case of death): The following general damages shall be payable in addition to compensation outlined above:
   i. *Funeral expenses:* ₹ 2,000
   ii. *Loss of consortium, if beneficiary is the spouse:* ₹ 5,000
   iii. *Loss of estate:* ₹ 2,500

iv. *Medical expenses:* Actual expenses incurred before death supported by bills/vouchers but not exceeding as onetime payment: ₹ 15,000.
4. General damages in case of injuries and disabilities:
   i. *Pain and sufferings:*
      a. Grievous injuries: ₹ 5,000
      b. Non-grievous injuries: ₹ 1,000
   ii. *Medical expenses:* Actual expenses incurred supported by bills/vouchers but not exceeding as onetime payment ₹ 15,000
5. *Disability in nonfatal accidents:* The following compensation shall be payable in case of disability to the victim arising out of nonfatal accidents:
   Loss of income, if any, for actual period of disablement not exceeding 52 weeks. Plus either of following:
   a. In case of permanent total disablement the amount payable shall be arrived at by multiplying the annual loss of income by the multiplier applicable to the age on the date of determining the compensation or
   b. In case of permanent partial disablement such percentage of compensation which would have been payable in the case of permanent total disablement as specified under item (a) above.
      Injuries deemed to result in permanent total disablement/permanent partial disablement and percentage of loss or earning capacity shall be as per Schedule I under Workmen's Compensation Act, 1923.
6. National income for compensation to those who had no income prior to accident.
   Fatal and disability in nonfatal accidents:
   a. *Non-earning persons:* ₹ 15,000
   b. *Spouse:* One-third of income of the earning surviving spouse.

In case of other injuries only "general damage" as applicable.

Note: Calculation of compensation and amount worked out in Schedule suffer from several defects:
The calculation of compensation and the amount worked out in the Schedule suffer from several defects. For example, in item 1 for a victim-aged 15 years, the multiplier is shown to be 15 years and the multiplicand is shown to be ₹ 3,000. The total should be ₹ 3,000 × 15 = ₹ 45,000 but the same is worked out at ₹ 60,000. Similarly, in the second item the multiplier is 16 and

the annual income is ₹ 9,000; the total should have been ₹ 144,000 but is shown to be ₹ 171,000.

To put it briefly, the table abounds in such mistakes. Neither the Tribunals nor the Courts can go by the ready recknoer. It can only be used as a guide. Besides, the selection of multiplier cannot in all cases be solely dependent on the age of the deceased. For example, if the deceased, a bachelor, dies at the age of 45 years and his dependants are his parents, age of the parents would also be relevant in the choice of the multiplier.

But these mistakes are limited to actual calculations only and not in respect of other items.

Illustrations of eye injury claims under various provisions of Law in India: What is proposed to be emphasised is that the multiplier cannot exceed 18 years' purchase factor. This is the improvement over the earlier position that ordinarily it should not exceed 16.

CONVENTIONAL AMOUNT TO BE AWARDED IN CASE OF NON-EARNING MEMBERS

In the case of Hazi Zainullah Khan (dead) by L.Rs. vs. Nagar Mahapalika, Allahabad 1994 the Supreme Court, while dealing with the question of compensation payable in respect of a student of 14 years, has held that ₹ 150,000 will be a just compensation. Thus, it can be taken to be the conventional amount for awarding compensation for non-earning members of the family like the young children and students. This view finds support from the Schedule II to the Motor Vehicles Act, 1988 which provides that notional income for the purpose of compensation to those who had no income can be taken to be ₹ 15,000 per annum out of which one-third has to be deducted for notional personal expenses and thereafter, on application of appropriate multiplier, the compensation can be ascertained. The multiplier for the children aged up to 15 years has been set out as "15". On applying the same, the compensation payable in case of the children up to 15 years will come to ₹ 150,000.

COMPENSATION FOR LOSS OF VISION

The appellant lost his left eye and made a claim as having lost his complete vision in that eye but medically it was assessed that loss of vision was only 80%. The Commissioner on an application being made to it by the appellant assessed the compensation payable to him as 100% under Schedule I, Part I at item No. 4. The assessment of compensation at ₹197,000 was reduced to ₹ 100,000.

METHOD OF CALCULATION OF WAGES

In this Act and for the purposes thereof the expression "monthly wages" means the amount of wages deemed to be payable for a month's service (whether the wages are payable by the month or by whatever other period or at piece rates), and calculated as follows, namely:

a. Where the workman has, during a continuous period of not less than 12 months immediately preceding the accident, been in the service of the employer who is liable to pay compensation, the monthly wages of the workman shall be one-twelfth of the total wages which have fallen due for payment to him by the employer in the last 12 months of that period [Section 5(a)].

b. Where the whole of the continuous period of service immediately preceding the accident during which the workman was in the service of the employer who is liable to pay the compensation was less than one month, the monthly wages of the workman shall be 5*** the average monthly amount which, during the 12 months immediately preceding the accident, was being earned by a workman employed on the same work by the same employer, or, if there was no workman so employed, by a workman employed on similar work in the same locality] [Section 5(b)].

- In other cases including cases in which it is not possible for want of necessary information to calculate the monthly wages under clause (b), the monthly wages shall be thirty times the total wages earned in respect of the last continuous period of service immediately preceding the accident from the employer who is liable to pay compensation, divided by the number of days comprising such period [Section 5(c)].

- *Explanation:* A period of service shall, for the purposes of 4*, 5*[section] be deemed to be continuous which has not been interrupted by a period of absence from work exceeding 14 days.

- Any half-monthly payment payable under this Act, either under an agreement between the parties or under the order of a Commissioner, may be reviewed by the Commissioner, on the application either of the employer or of the workman accompanied by the certificate of a qualified medical practitioner that there has been a change in the condition of the workman or, subject to rules made under this Act, on application made without such certificate [Section 6(1)].

- Any half-monthly payment may, on review under this section, subject to the provisions of this Act, be continued, increased, decreased or ended, or if the accident is found to have resulted in permanent disablement, be converted to the lump sum to which the workman is entitled less any amount which he has already received by way of half-monthly payments [Section 6(2)].

COMMUTATION OF HALF-MONTHLY PAYMENTS

Any right to receive half-monthly payments may, by agreement between the parties or, if the parties cannot agree and the payments have been continued for not less than 6 months, on the application of either party to the Commissioner be redeemed by the payment of a lump sum of such amount as may be agreed to by the parties or determined by the Commissioner, as the case may be.

NOTICE AND CLAIM

No claim for compensation shall be entertained by a Commissioner unless notice of the accident has been given in the manner hereinafter provided as soon as practicable after the happening thereof and unless the claim is preferred before him within 2 years of the occurrence of the accident or, in case of death, within 2 years from the date of death: [Section 10(1)].

HOW APPLICATION CAN BE MADE?

- Every such notice shall give the name and address of the person injured and shall state in ordinary language the cause of the injury and the date on which the accident happened, and shall be served on the employer or upon [any one of] several employers, or upon any person responsible to the employer for the management of any branch of the trade or business in which the injured workman was employed [Section 10(2)].
- The State Government may require that any prescribed class of employers shall maintain at their premises at which workmen are employed a notice-book, in the prescribed form, which shall be readily accessible at all reasonable times to any injured workman employed on the premises and to any person acting bona fide on his behalf [Section 10(3)].

POWER TO REQUIRE FROM EMPLOYERS STATEMENTS REGARDING FATAL ACCIDENTS

Where a Commissioner receives information from any source that a workman has died as a result of an accident arising out of and in the course of his employment, he may send by registered post a notice to the workman's employer requiring him to submit, within 30 days of the service of the notice, a statement, in the prescribed form, giving the circumstances attending the death of the workman, and indicating whether, in the opinion of the employer, he is or is not liable to deposit compensation on account of the death [Section 10A(1)].

If the employer is of opinion that he is liable to deposit compensation, he shall make the deposit within 30 days of the service of the notice [Section 10A (2)].

If the employer is of opinion that he is not liable to deposit compensation, he shall in his statement indicate the grounds on which he disclaims liability [Section 10A (3)].

Where the employer has so disclaimed liability, the Commissioner, after such enquiry as he may think fit, may inform any of the dependants of the deceased workman, that it is open to the dependants to prefer a claim for compensation, and may give them such other further information as he may think fit [Section 10A (4)].

REPORTS OF FATAL ACCIDENTS AND SERIOUS BODILY INJURIES

Where, by any law for the time being in force, notice is required to be given to any authority, by or on behalf of an employer, of any accident occurring on his premises which results in death [or serious bodily injury], the person required to give the notice shall, within 7 days of the death [or serious bodily injury], send a report to the Commissioner giving the circumstances attending the death [or serious bodily injury] [Section 10B (1)].

Provided that where the State Government has so prescribed the person required to give the notice may instead of sending such report to the Commissioner send it to the authority to whom he is required to give the notice [Section 10B (1)].

The State Government may, by notification in the Official Gazette, extend the provisions of subsection (1) to any class of premises other than those coming within the scope of that subsection, and may, by such notification, specify the persons who shall send the report to the Commissioner [Section 10B (2)].

Nothing in this section shall apply to factories to which the Employees' State Insurance Act, 1948, (34 of 1948.) applies.

What are the Rules for Medical Examination?

Where a workman has given notice of an accident, he shall, if the employer, before the expiry of 3 days from the time at which service of the notice has been effected, offers to have him examined free of charge by a qualified medical practitioner, submit himself for such examination, and any workman who is in receipt of a half-monthly payment under this Act shall, if so required, submit himself for such examination from time to time [Section 11(1)].

Provided that a workman shall not be required to submit himself for examination by a medical practitioner otherwise than in accordance with rules made under this Act or at more frequent intervals than may be prescribed [Section 11(1)].

If a workman, on being required to do so by the employer under subsection (1) or by the Commissioner at any time, refuses to submit himself for examination by a qualified medical practitioner or in any way obstructs the same, his right to compensation shall be suspended during the continuance of such refusal or obstruction unless, in the case of refusal, he was prevented by any sufficient cause from so submitting himself [Section 11(2)].

If a workman, before the expiry of the period within which he is liable under subsection (1) to be required to submit himself for medical examination, voluntarily leaves without having been so examined the vicinity of the place in which he was employed, his right to compensation shall be suspended until he returns and offers himself for such examination [Section 11(3)].

Where a workman, whose right to compensation has been suspended under subsection (2) or subsection (3), dies without having submitted himself for medical examination as required by either of those subsections, the Commissioner may, if he thinks fit, direct the payment of compensation to the dependants of the deceased workman [Section 11(4)].

Where under subsection (2) or subsection (3) a right to compensation is suspended, no compensation shall be payable in respect of the period of suspension, and, if the period of suspension commences before the expiry of the waiting period referred to in clause (d) of subsection (1) of section 4, the waiting period shall be increased by the period during which the suspension continues [Section 11(5)].

WHAT ARE THE DUTIES OF WORKMAN FOR MEDICAL EXAMINATION AND INSTRUCTIONS OF QUALIFIED MEDICAL PERSONNEL (QMP)?

Where an injured workman has refused to be attended by a QMP whose services have been offered to him by the employer free of charge or having accepted such offer has deliberately disregarded the instructions of such medical practitioner, then, if it is proved that the workman has not thereafter been regularly attended by a qualified medical practitioner or having been so attended has deliberately failed to follow his instructions and that such refusal, disregard or failure was unreasonable in the circumstances of the case and that the injury has been aggravated thereby, the injury and resulting disablement shall be deemed to be of the same nature and duration as they might reasonably have been expected to be if the workman had been regularly attended by a QMP [whose instructions he had followed], and compensation, if any, shall be payable accordingly [Section 11(6)].

PENALTIES

Whoever:

a. Fails to maintain a notice-book which he is required to maintain under subsection (3) of section 10 or [Section 18A (a)].

b. Fails to send to the Commissioner a statement which he is required to send under subsection (1) of section 10A or [Section 18A (b)].

c. Fails to send a report which he is required to send under section 10B or [Section 18A (c)].

d. Fails to make a return which he is required to make under section 16, shall be punishable with fine which may extend to 3*[five hundred] rupees [Section 18A (d)].

No prosecution under this section shall be instituted except by or with the previous sanction of a Commissioner, and no Court shall take cognizance of any offence under this section, unless complaint thereof is made 4*[within 6 months of the date on which the alleged commission of the offence came to the knowledge of the Commissioner] [Section 18A].

Schedule I
[See Secs. 2 (1) and 4]
[Part-I List of Injuries Deemed to Result in Permanent Total Disablement]

S. No.	Description of injury	Percentage of loss of earning capacity
1.	Loss of both hands or amputation at higher sites	100
2.	Loss of a hand and a foot	100
3.	Double amputation through leg or thigh or amputation through leg or thigh on one side and loss of other foot	100
4.	Loss of sight to such an extent as to render the claimant unable to perform any work for which eyesight is essential	100
5.	Very severe facial disfigurement	100
6.	Absolute deafness	100

Schedule I
List of Injuries Deemed to Result in Permanent Total Disablement

S. No.	Description of injury	Percentage of loss of earning capacity
[1][25	Loss of one eye, without complication, the other being normal	40
[1][26	Loss of vision of one eye, without complications of disfigurement of eyeball, the other being normal	30
[6][26-A	Loss of partial vision of one eye	10

APPLICATION FOR CLAIM

No application for the settlement of any matter by a Commissioner, [other than an application by a dependant or dependants for compensation] shall be made unless and until some question has arisen between the parties in connection therewith which they have been unable to settle by agreement. [Section 22(1)].

An application to a Commissioner may be made in such form and shall be accompanied by such fee, if any, as may be prescribed, and shall contain, in addition to any particulars which may be prescribed, the following particulars, namely:

a. A concise statement of the circumstances in which the application is made and the relief or order which the applicant claims.

b. In the case of a claim for compensation against an employer, the date of service of notice of the accident on the employer and, if such notice has not been served or has not been served in due time, the reason for such omission.

c. The names and addresses of the parties.

Except in the case of an application by dependants for compensation a concise statement of the matters on which agreement has and [of] those on which agreement has not been come to [Section 22(2)].

If the applicant is illiterate or for any other reason is unable to furnish the required information in writing, the application shall, if the applicant so desires, be prepared under the direction of the Commissioner [Section 22(3)].

GLOSSARY OF TERMS

- "Commissioner" means a Commissioner for Workmen's Compensation appointed under section 20 [Section 2 (b)].
- (c) "Compensation" means compensation as provided for by this Act [Section 2 (c)].
- "Dependant" means any of the following relatives of a deceased workman, namely:
  i. A widow, a minor legitimate son, and unmarried legitimate daughter, or a widowed mother.
  ii. If wholly dependent on the earnings of the workman at the time of his death, a son or a daughter who has attained the age of 18 years and who is infirm.
  iii. If wholly or in part dependent on the earnings of the workman at the time of his death
    a. A widower
    b. A parent other than a widowed mother

c. A minor illegitimate son, an unmarried illegitimate daughter or a daughter legitimate or illegitimate if married and a minor or if widowed and a minor.

d. A minor brother or a unmarried sister or a widowed sister if, a minor.

e. A widowed daughter-in-law.

f. A minor child of a pre-deceased son.

g. A minor child of a pre-deceased daughter where no parent of the child is alive.

h. A paternal grandparent if no parent of the workman is alive [Section 2 (d)].

- "Employer" includes anybody of persons whether incorporated or not and any managing agent of an employer and the legal representative of a deceased employer, and, when the services of workman are temporarily lent or let on hire to another person by the person with whom the workman has entered into a contract of service or apprenticeship means such other person while the workman is working for him [Section 2 (e)].

- "Managing agent" means any person appointed or acting as the representative of another person for the purpose of carrying on such other person's trade or business, but does not include an individual manager subordinate to an employer 1* [Section 2 (f)].

- "Minor" means a person who has not attained the age of 18 years [Section 2 (ff)].

- "Partial disablement" (temporary and permanent) means, where the disablement is of a temporary nature, such disablement as reduces the earning capacity of a workman in any employment in which he was engaged at the time of the accident resulting in the disablement, and, where the disablement is of a permanent nature, such disablement as reduces his earning capacity in every employment which he was capable of undertaking at that time: provided that every injury specified [in Part II of Schedule I] shall be deemed to result in permanent partial disablement [Section 2 (g)].

- "Total disablement" means such disablement, whether of a temporary or permanent nature, as incapacitates a workman for all work which he was capable of performing at the time of the accident resulting in such disablement: 8*[Provided that permanent total disablement shall be deemed to result from every injury specified in Part I of Schedule I or from any combination of injuries specified in Part II thereof where the aggregate percentage of the loss of earning capacity, as specified in the said Part II against those injuries, amounts to one hundred percent or more [Section 2 (l)].

- "Serious bodily injury" means an injury which involves, or in all probability will involve the permanent loss of the use of, or permanent injury to, any limb, or the permanent loss of or injury to the sight or hearing, or the fracture of any limb, or the enforced absence of the injured person from work for a period exceeding twenty days [Section 10B, Explanation]

- "Qualified medical practitioner" means any person registered under any [Central Act, Provincial Act or an Act of the Legislature of a [State] providing for the maintenance of a register of medical practitioners, or, in any area where no such last-mentioned Act is in force, any person declared by the State Government, by notification in the Official Gazette, to be a qualified medical practitioner for the purposes of this Act [Section 2 (i)].

- "Seaman" means any person forming part of the crew of any 6*** ship, but does not include the master of 7*[the] ship [Section 2 (k)].

- "Wages" includes any privilege or benefit which is capable of being estimated in money, other than a travelling allowance or the value of any travelling concession or a contribution paid by the employer of a workman toward any pension or provident fund or a sum paid to a workman to cover any special expenses entailed on him by the nature of his employment [Section 2 (m)].

- "Workman" means any person (other than a person whose employment is of a casual nature and who is employed otherwise than for the purposes of the employer's trade or business) who is:

i. A railway servant as defined in section 3 of the Indian Railways Act, 1890 (9 of 1890), not permanently employed in any administrative, district or subdivisional office of a railway and not employed in any such capacity as is specified in Schedule II

ii. Employed in any such capacity as is specified in Schedule II. whether the contract of employment was made before or after the passing of this Act and whether such contract is expressed or implied, oral or in writing; but does not include any person working in the capacity of a member of the Armed Forces of the Union; and any reference to a workman who has been injured shall, where the workman is dead, include a reference to his dependants or any of them.

- The exercise and performance of the powers and duties of a local authority or of any department [acting on behalf of the Government] shall, for the purposes of this Act, unless a contrary intention appears, be deemed to be the trade or business of such authority or department. The [State Government], after giving, by notification in the Official Gazette, not less than 3 months' notice of its intention so to do, may, by a like notification, add to Schedule II any class of persons employed in any occupation which it is satisfied is a hazardous occupation, and the provisions of this Act shall thereupon apply [within the State] to such classes of persons: provided that in making such addition the [State Government] may direct that the provisions of this Act shall apply to such classes of persons in respect of specified injuries only [Section 2 (n)].

BIBLIOGRAPHY

1. The Motor Vehicle Act, 1988
2. The Workmen's Compensation Act, 1923, [5th March, 1923]
3. U.P. State Road Transport Corpn. vs. Trilok Chandra (1996) 4 S. C.C. 362: 1996 Acc. C. J. 831.
4. Hazi Zainullah Khan (dead) by L.Rs. vs. Nagar Mahapalika, Allahabad 1994 [1] S.C.C. (Cr.) 1568: (1994) 2 Acc. C.C. 426
5. Puttamma vs. D.V. Krishnappa (1999) 2 Acc. C.C. 491 (Karn.) (D.B).
6. Amar Nath Singh vs. Continental Constructions Ltd., New Delhi, (2001) 1 Lab. L.J. 184 at p. 185 (S.C).

Index